Living with Arthritis

I dedicate this book to my parents

JOAN AND GORDON POWELL

who never lost hope

Living with Arthritis

Julie Barlow

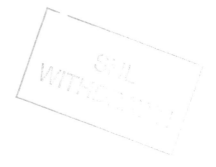

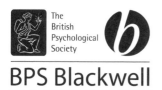

BPS Blackwell

This edition first published 2009 by the British Psychological Society and Blackwell Publishing Ltd
© 2009 Julie Barlow

BPS Blackwell is an imprint of Blackwell Publishing, which was acquired by John Wiley & Sons in February 2007. Blackwell's publishing program has been merged with Wiley's global Scientific, Technical, and Medical business to form Wiley-Blackwell.

Registered Office
John Wiley & Sons Ltd, The Atrium, Southern Gate, Chichester, West Sussex, PO19 8SQ, UK

Editorial Offices
350 Main Street, Malden, MA 02148-5020, USA
9600 Garsington Road, Oxford, OX4 2DQ, UK
The Atrium, Southern Gate, Chichester, West Sussex, PO19 8SQ, UK

For details of our global editorial offices, for customer services, and for information about how to apply for permission to reuse the copyright material in this book please see our website at www.wiley.com/wiley-blackwell.

The right of Julie Barlow to be identified as the author of this work has been asserted in accordance with the Copyright, Designs and Patents Act 1988.

Library of Congress Cataloging-in-Publication Data

Barlow, Julie (Julie Helen)
   Living with arthritis / Julie Barlow.
      p. cm.
   Includes bibliographical references and index.
   ISBN 978-1-4051-0809-6 (hardcover : alk. paper) – ISBN 978-1-4051-0810-2 (pbk. : alk. paper)
1. Arthritis–popular works. 2. Arthritis–Psychological aspects. I. Title.

   RC933.B342 2009
   616.7'22–dc22

                                                        2008044723

A catalogue record for this book is available from the British Library.

Set in 10/13pt Palatino
by SPi Publisher Services, Pondicherry, India
Printed and bound in Malaysia by Vivar Printing Sdn Bhd

The British Psychological Society's free Research Digest e-mail service rounds up the latest research and relates it to your syllabus in a user-friendly way. To subscribe go to www.research-digest.org.uk or send a blank e-mail to subscribe-rd@lists.bps.org.uk.

1   2009

Contents

List of Abbreviations   vii
Acknowledgements   ix

1. **Introduction**   **1**

2. **Arthritis and Disease Management**   **7**
Osteoarthritis   8
Rheumatoid Arthritis   10
Ankylosing Spondylitis   14
Juvenile Idiopathic Arthritis   16
Metaphysical Explanations for Arthritis   18
Complementary and Alternative Medicine   22
Chapter Summary   27

3. **Onset, Diagnosis and Duration of Disease**   **28**
Onset, Personality and Stress   28
Diagnosis   37
Duration   38
Chapter Summary   41

4. **Life with Arthritis**   **43**
Disease Symptomatology and Impact   44
Emotional Reactions and Activity Restrictions   46
Social Issues   50
Resistance to Disruption   52
Children with JIA and their Parents   56
Chapter Summary   64

5. **The Psychological Impact on Person and Family**   **66**
Psychological Impact on the Person   66
Mediators and Moderators of Psychological Wellbeing   72

Positive Aspects of Psychological Wellbeing 86
Children with JIA 88
Chapter Summary 99

6. The Social Impact on Person and Family **101**
Parenting with Arthritis 101
Social Support 105
Children and Parents 111
Social Impact: Society 113
Working with Arthritis 116
Chapter Summary 126

7. Health Care and Patient Education **128**
The Experience of Health Care 128
Patient Education 146
Chapter Summary 158

8. Psycho-Educational Interventions **160**
Cognitive Behavioural Interventions 161
Interventions Based on Emotional Disclosure 163
Social Support Interventions 165
Multi-Component Interventions Focused
    Primarily on Exercise 168
Multi-Component Self-Management Interventions 174
Personal Development Interventions 188
Interventions for Enhancing Employment Potential 190
Interventions in JIA 194
Effectiveness of Psycho-Educational Interventions 197
Chapter Summary 206

9. Agenda for the Future **209**
Under-Researched Groups 209
Under-Researched Psychosocial Domains 211
Expand Research on Positive Dimensions 213
Health Care and Interventions 215
Longitudinal Studies 219
Chapter Summary 219

Appendix: Malcolm Macdonald's Arthritis Journey 220
References 226
Index of Citations 275
General Index 291

Abbreviations

AAR	adolescent arthritis and rheumatism
ACR	American College of Rheumatology
ANS	autonomic nervous system
anti-TNF	anti-tumour necrosis factor
AS	ankylosing spondylitis
ASE: Function	Arthritis Self-Efficacy Function
ASMP	Arthritis Self-Management Programme
CAM	complementary and alternative medicine
CBCL	Child Behaviour Check List
CBT	cognitive behavioural therapy
CDC	Centers for Diseases Control and Prevention
CDSMC	Chronic Disease Self-Management Course
DMARD	disease-modifying anti-rheumatic drug
ESR	erythrocyte sedimentation rate
FMS	fibromyalgia syndrome
GP	general practitioner
HADS	Hospital Anxiety and Depression Scale
HPA	hypothalamic-pituitary-adrenal
HRQOL	health-related quality of life
IWPD	INTO Work Personal Development Programme
JIA	juvenile idiopathic arthritis
LBP	low back pain
MHLC	Multi-Dimensional Health Locus of Control Scale
MMPI	Minnesota Multiphasic Personality Inventory
NAAB	National Arthritis Advisory Board (USA)
NAAP	*National Arthritis Action Plan: A Public Health Strategy*
NSAID	non-steroidal anti-inflammatory drug
OA	osteoarthritis

PASE   Parent's Arthritis Self-Efficacy Scale
PIL   purpose in life
RA   rheumatoid arthritis
RNP   rheumatology nurse practitioner
SMART   Self-Management Arthritis Relief Therapy
SMC-AS   Self-Management Course for People with Ankylosing
            Spondylitis
WHO   World Health Organization

Acknowledgements

I extend my grateful thanks to the many research and practitioner colleagues I have worked with on arthritis-related studies that feature in this book, including Mary Grant, Jenny Hainsworth, Karen Harrison, Roy Jones, Thilo Kroll, Steve Macey, Lesley Powell, Ian Rowe, Karen Shaw, Janice Sheasby, George Struthers, Laura Swaby, Andy Turner, Bethan Williams, Chris Wright and Suzanne Wright. Thanks are extended to people living with arthritis who have taken part in my research studies, giving freely of their time and perspectives.

1

Introduction

Arthritis is a topic worthy of attention and one in which psychology and psychologists have crucial roles to play. For example, psychological theories may enable greater understanding of this painful, long-term condition and can be used to inform development of psychological interventions aiming to aid adaptation. Such interventions may be delivered by psychologists or psychologists may design and provide tutor training for interventions that can be delivered by others, including health and social care professionals, voluntary organisations or lay people living with arthritis who take on the role of peer educators.

Arthritis is a generic label used for over 100 different types of musculoskeletal, connective tissue and non-articular conditions, the most prevalent forms being osteoarthritis (OA), rheumatoid arthritis (RA) and ankylosing spondylitis (AS) in adults (Taal, Seydel *et al.*, 1993) and juvenile idiopathic arthritis (JIA) in children. Other forms of arthritis (e.g. systemic lupus erythematosus, Scleroderma, Sjogren's syndrome, psoriatic arthritis, and gout) are less common. Most forms of arthritis follow an unpredictable course of exacerbations and remissions, resulting in varying degrees of physical disability. Prognosis is uncertain, and, since there is no cure, treatment is ameliorative, aiming to alleviate inflammation, reduce pain and preserve or improve function. Medication remains the mainstay of medical management and can improve disease outcomes for many. However, medication can be associated with adverse side effects (Kean *et al.*, 1997; Thompson *et al.*, 1985), which are often a cause of concern for patients and their carers (J. Barlow, Harrison & Shaw, 1998). Other treatments that may be offered include physiotherapy, occupational therapy and podiatry. People with arthritis often require long-term monitoring and care by general practitioners (GPs) and/or hospital-based rheumatology clinics for more severe cases and conditions (e.g. RA). Despite regular treatment, many patients experience severe functional disability after 20 years of living with the disease (Fries *et al.*, 1996). Indeed, a recent community-based, UK study reports the rates of work disability among people with RA at 1, 2, 5 and 10 years after symptom onset as 14 per cent, 26 per cent, 33 per cent and 39 per cent respectively (Barrett *et al.*, 2000). The authors conclude that the move to earlier, more aggressive medical treatment has failed to influence the rates of work disability among this patient group. Thus, it is not surprising to find that many people with arthritis turn to complementary medicine (Resch *et al.*, 1997), express a strong desire to learn 'something I can do myself' (J. Barlow, Pennington & Bishop, 1997) and participate in psycho-educational interventions.

Arthritis is one of the most common, long-term conditions affecting millions of people worldwide. In the US, prevalence rates of self-reported arthritis are projected to increase from 15 per cent (37.9 million) in 1990 to 18.2 per cent (59.4 million) by 2020 (Helmick *et al.*, 1995) with older people, women, and those with less education or lower incomes being at greater risk. In the UK, diseases of the musculoskeletal system account for 46 per cent of all disability reported by adults living in private households (Martin *et al.*, 1988). The burden of rheumatic diseases is related to treatment and outcomes, described by Fries and Spitz (1980) as death, discomfort, disability, drug toxicity, dollars and dissatisfaction, mainly associated with current treatment. To this can be added quality of life for individuals living with arthritis, and their families. The burden of disease from a societal perspective is measured in monetary terms. Data from the US, Canada, the UK, France and Australia suggests that the cost of rheumatic diseases accounts for 1 to 2.5 per cent of the gross national product (March & Bachmeier, 1997). Until 1999 arthritis was not considered a major public health problem anywhere in the world, despite being the largest single cause of physical disability (Badley & Tenant, 1993) and being associated with increased rates of mortality (Pincus & Callahan, 1993). The US is the only country to have recognised that arthritis demands a public health approach. Following publication of the *National Arthritis Action Plan: A Public Health Strategy* (NAAP), the Centers for Diseases Control and Prevention (CDC) initiated a major programme in 1999 to both measure and reduce the impact of arthritis. The programme involves three core strategies:

1. fostering development of state arthritis programmes;
2. strengthening public health science;
3. developing health communication, health education, and health system quality improvement activities to reduce the burden of arthritis.

The last of these involves the development of tools and strategies to be used by state health departments and other partners. One strategy under development is a health communication campaign to increase physical activity among people with arthritis. In addition, the CDC has developed an online training programme for state health departments and others interested in a public health approach to arthritis. The CDC is also attempting to improve the clinical care received by people with arthritis by piloting system changes such as routine monitoring of functional status, ongoing self-management support and easy access to physical and occupational therapy in primary care.

At an international level and with the support of the World Health Organization, the period 2000–2010 has been designated the Bone and Joint Decade by health professionals from different specialities, scientific and patient organisations and governments. The overall purpose is to mobilise an offensive against diseases affecting the musculoskeletal system, particularly in terms of the development and promotion of improved therapeutic options.

This book aims to provide an overview of arthritis that is grounded in the realities of living with a long-term condition often characterised by pain, fatigue, physical limitations and psychological sequela such as anxiety and depression. Life with arthritis involves a continual process of adjustment, which is a useful illustration of how the human spirit can survive, maintain a sense of hope and even flourish in the face of adversity.

As well as the growing body of literature in psychosocial rheumatology, the book draws on my own research and research conducted with colleagues based in the Self-Management Programme, Applied Research Centre in Health & Lifestyle Interventions, Coventry University and in healthcare provision. I view the person with the condition as central to my research and have learned a great deal by simply listening to the stories of people with different types of arthritis covering the full age span – from young children to 90-year-olds. The lessons learned and the rich depth of understanding offered by qualitative approaches is used to complement quantitative investigations of pertinent issues. Thus, qualitative studies and associated quotes from such studies are used extensively in many sections of the text. A substantial section of the book is devoted to interventions with a psychological basis. Anything that promotes a positive change is of vital importance in the search to assist people with arthritis make the adjustments needed to attain a satisfactory quality of life. Indeed, psycho-educational interventions, especially those involving lay people as tutors, are well established in psychosocial rheumatology. One could speculate that this development has occurred in the face of the inability of medicine to offer a cure or successful alleviation of symptoms with no associated adverse side effects.

In Chapter 2, the disease characteristics of the main types of arthritis are described, along with epidemiological data, risk factors and disease management strategies that are typically employed. The book will focus on four main types of arthritis (i.e. RA, OA, AS in adults and JIA in children), allowing perspectives from across the age span (e.g. childhood to the older elderly) to be considered and, in the case of JIA, the perspectives of close family members. The chapter concludes by considering metaphysical explanations for arthritis and the use of complementary medicine.

Chapter 3 adopts a historical approach by reviewing early attempts to link personality characteristics with the onset of arthritis, particularly RA and AS. The difficulties of identifying causal links between personality and arthritis and links between stressful events and disease onset are discussed. The problems that can arise in obtaining a diagnostic label for the specific type of arthritis and the overlap between physiological and psychological symptomatology are reviewed. Finally, the relationship between disease duration and wellbeing, particularly depressed mood, is examined.

Chapter 4 describes the experience of living with arthritis from the perspectives of children through to older adults, and includes insight into the perspectives of carers (partners or parents). The chapter draws on the growing body of qualitative studies that aim to provide a picture of arthritis grounded in lived experiences and to generate rather than to test theory. An increasing number of such studies are appearing in the literature, a trend that reflects the increasing emphasis on patient-centred approaches to health care, and the need to listen to the voices of consumers (users) of services. This focus is in keeping with a number of

White Papers published in the UK (e.g. *Saving Lives: Our Healthier Nation*). Key areas perceived as problematic by people with arthritis and their carers are developed. For example, the essential task of managing persistent pain, chronic fatigue and feelings of loss of control are presented. This chapter sets the scene for later discussions of coping and self-management.

The psychological and social aspects of life with arthritis are intertwined. However, for the purpose of presentation, they are dealt with in Chapters 5 and 6 under the broad headings of psychological impact and social impact. The theme of considering both the people with arthritis and their carers is continued. In contrast to Chapter 4, most studies of psychological impact are based on quantitative methods, with many aiming to test psychological models. Reflecting the focus of the majority of psychological studies, the increased vulnerability to depression will be discussed in depth, including the relationship between pain, disability and depression. Other issues covered include the concept of control that emerges as a salient issue for people living with the disease.

Chapter 6 focuses on the way that arthritis can interfere with social relationships, and gives particular emphasis to studies of social support, spouses and other family members. The social model of disability is explored and issues connected with working life, resultant economic impact and the visibility of arthritis are discussed. The notion of visibility is examined in relation to children, adolescents and the myths about arthritis that are present in society (e.g. that arthritis is a disease of old age).

Chapter 7 discusses healthcare issues in arthritis, such as understanding more about the relationship between patient and healthcare professional, particularly in terms of encouraging individuals to play a role in their disease management. The issue of disease duration in relation to the amount of knowledge and coping skills attained by people with arthritis is reviewed. This leads to consideration of arthritis patient education focusing on the use of informational strategies and written materials as simple interventions that can be widely distributed at relatively low cost.

Chapter 8 covers the use of more complex psychological interventions in arthritis, many of which draw on social cognitive theory in their guiding principles. The most common interventions are based around cognitive-behavioural techniques and lifestyle management (e.g. exercise, diet). Self-management is well established in the field of arthritis, and encompasses lay-led interventions delivered in community settings. Given that people with arthritis spend the majority of the time managing their condition in the home environment, becoming a successful self-manager is of paramount importance. Interventions for children with JIA are included, although there are few studies published in this area.

Key issues covered are summarised in Chapter 10 and the way forward for psychosocial rheumatology is identified in the form of a research agenda.

2

Arthritis and Disease Management

Rheumatic diseases are among the oldest diseases known to man. They were recognised by Hippocrates in the fourth century BC, and the discovery of skeletal remains in North America suggest that rheumatoid arthritis may have existed 3000 years ago (Goemaere *et al.*, 1990). Similarly, the remains of ancient Egyptian mummies indicate the presence of ankylosing spondylitis. The term 'rheuma' was used in the first century AD, to indicate a flow of pain through the joints. The term 'rheumatology' first appeared in a textbook edited by Hollander and Comroe and published in 1949.

Classification of rheumatic conditions is hindered by the lack of aetiological evidence for many diseases. Nonetheless, classification systems have been developed, primarily by the American College of Rheumatology (ACR) 1987. At present, classification is determined by clinical and laboratory findings, including observation of abnormal anatomical structures and organ systems, the presence of suspected aetiological mechanisms, genetic factors and, occasionally, infectious agents, and the general manifestations of disease (Sangha, 2000). Thus, individual manifestation may suggest a broad category of disease or a syndrome rather than a firm diagnostic label. This situation is confounded even more by the potential overlap, clinically and pathologically, of many rheumatic conditions. The role of psychological factors in masking or overlapping physical disease has been acknowledged in the literature (J. Barlow, Macey & Struthers, 1993; Creed & Ash, 1992). However, is not clear how often psychological factors are considered in practice.

Rheumatic disease, or the more commonly used term 'arthritis', has no clear boundaries. Rather the term arthritis is used to refer to over 100 different conditions. This book focuses on RA, OA, AS and JIA.

These types of arthritis have been selected for the following reasons. Firstly, OA is the most prevalent type of arthritis worldwide; secondly, RA tends to be the most common condition seen in many rheumatology clinics. Together, OA and RA account for a large percentage of disability worldwide (Sangha, 2000). The condition of AS has a similar prevalence to RA but differs in terms of the sex ratio (i.e. it is one of the few types of arthritis to have a male predominance). Finally, JIA is one of the most common diseases of childhood and can have long-lasting impact on both the child's and family's wellbeing. Each of these conditions is described in more detail below.

Osteoarthritis

Osteoarthritis (OA) is generally acknowledged to be the most prevalent form of arthritis and is a significant cause of disability, particularly among older people. For example, it is estimated that OA accounts for 12.3 per cent of all activity limitations in the USA (La Plante, 1988). Since there is no discrete onset, laboratory abnormality or pathognomic features, the condition is classified according to the joint affected (e.g. hip, knee, hand, spine, or other). Estimates of the prevalence of OA are imprecise due to the difficulties of diagnosis. Thus, prevalence rates vary according to the reporting methods used, the age and gender of study participants and the number of joints studied. Early epidemiological studies in the UK, using radiographic change as the detection criterion, found that almost everyone aged 65 and over had OA in at least one joint (Lawrence *et al.*, 1966). The incidence of moderate or severe OA in one or more joints increases with age; therefore, as the proportion of older people in the population increases, a growing number of older adults are likely to develop OA. Indeed, age is the principal predictor of OA regardless of joint site.

Risk factors for OA vary according to the joint affected and include age, female gender, obesity, genetic predisposition, occupation, trauma, repetitive use and excessive mechanical loading of joints (Croft *et al.*, 1992; Schneider *et al.*, 2005; Vingard, 1994). The last of these risk factors leads to a higher prevalence of OA among certain occupations, including mining (Felson *et al.*, 1994), ballet dancers (Andersson *et al.*, 1989) and athletes such as runners, weight lifters and footballers (Kujala *et al.*, 1995, Turner *et al.*, 2000). It should be noted that age, intensity and duration of the physical activity causing strain on joints and the risk of injury associated with certain physical pursuits (e.g. football) are likely to be influential factors determining disease onset. (See the Appendix for an account of arthritis from an ex-professional footballer's perspective.) Both hand and knee OA appear to be more common among women (i.e. 1.5:1 to >4:1), suggesting that female sex hormones may represent a predisposition to disease onset and/or severity (Rosener *et al.*, 1986). However, there is an absence of clearly supportive data to confirm this notion. Obesity has been associated with OA of the knee but is less associated with OA of the hand or hip (Oliveria *et al.*, 1999). The importance of avoiding obesity was demonstrated in a prospective study showing that a weight loss of 5 kg was associated with a 50 per cent risk reduction of developing symptomatic OA of the knee (Felson *et al.*, 1992). A particular pattern of high fat distribution in the abdominal cavity has been linked to possible metabolic abnormalities or fertility problems (Zaadstra *et al.*, 1993). Basically, a high waist-to-hip ratio (an apple body shape) has been linked to risk of OA whereas a pear-shaped body has not.

In contrast to most other long-term conditions, smoking may have a protective effect in OA (Felson *et al.*, 1989). One possible biological mechanism through which smoking may play a protective role concerns the stabilisation of cartilage by tar and/or nicotine. This issue is likely to attract a great deal of attention, although it is unlikely that smoking would be recommended as a prophylactic due to its many adverse effects on health. Other factors that have been implicated in the development of OA include bone density and diet. However, further studies are needed to affirm these proposed linkages. An early study of 2389 older people with three or more symptoms of arthritis (Elder, 1973) found that people attributed their symptoms to ageing, the weather (e.g. cold, damp), injuries and heredity. Although there is no scientific evidence to support such claims, changes in temperature and humidity are consistently reported to influence perceptions of pain and stiffness by people living with the disease.

Osteoarthritis is characterised by progressive loss of articular cartilage and secondary reactions in the bone causing joint pain and stiffness, particularly at the start of movement. Bony enlargement of affected joints (osteophytes) can occur and mobility can become progressively restricted. The symptoms of OA are unpredictable and can follow a fluctuating course. Hutton (1995) suggests that since there is no treatment that can influence disease progression, clinical management should be based on principles of logic and not doing harm. Control of pain is through low-toxicity analgesia (e.g. acetaminophen or paracetamol), and although considered a non-inflammatory condition, non-steroidal anti-inflammatory drugs (NSAIDs) are often prescribed. Two surveys conducted in the US found that a significantly higher proportion of patients preferred NSAIDs to acetaminophen (Pincus *et al.*, 2000; Wolfe *et al.*, 2000). Exercise, use of splints, use of aids (e.g. walking stick) can assist mobility. Interestingly, physical therapy is viewed as a cornerstone of treatment in Europe whereas rehabilitation and physical therapy do not form key features of treatment in the US, despite being recommended in the ACR guidelines (Sangha, 2000). A systematic review of exercise therapy in patients with OA of the hip or knee found that the positive effects on pain and physical function were not sustained over time unless patients attended booster sessions after the treatment period (Pisters *et al.*, 2007). However, exercise therapy did have longer-term positive effects on patient global assessment of effectiveness. Outcome for people with severe hip or knee OA can be improved with joint replacement, which tends to last between 10 and 20 years. Use of specific measures for assessing hip function (e.g. Oxford hip score) reveals that hip replacement results in less pain and functional difficulty for the majority of patients (McMurray *et al.*, 1999). However, Orbell *et al.* (1998) suggest that the extent of functional improvement following joint replacement surgery varies considerably. Measurement of physical functioning in OA can be difficult due to the use of adaptive aids, which make movements easier to accomplish. Measures that do not specify 'movement without the use of aids' may tend to underestimate the true degree of physical impairment. Most people with OA remain under the care of a general practitioner, and are only referred to hospital-based clinics when problems become severe. For example, people with severe OA of the hip may be referred to an orthopaedic surgeon if ability to walk becomes seriously impaired and a hip replacement is thought to be the best option. As may be expected, co-morbidity is common among older people with OA.

Rheumatoid Arthritis

Rheumatoid arthritis (RA) is a chronic, multisystemic, autoimmune disorder of unknown cause. It affects the majority of races with a prevalence of approximately 1 per cent (Schumaker, 1988), although prevalence is lower among rural Sub-Saharan Africans and Caribbean Blacks and is higher among Pima Indians in the USA (Silman & Hochberg, 2001). Onset typically occurs between the ages of 20 and 50, and is more prevalent amongst women, with a gender ratio of 2.5:1 (Sangha, 2000).

The precise aetiology of RA remains largely unknown, although several interactive, risk factors are believed to be implicated. Family studies suggest there is a genetic predisposition to RA. For example, severe RA appears at four times the expected rate among first-degree relatives of people with RA who test positive for rheumatoid factor. Furthermore, approximately 10 per cent of people with RA have an affected first-degree relative (Silman & Hochberg, 1993). The hereditary predisposition has been linked to the human leukocyte antigen, HLA-DR4, although the precise mechanism is poorly understood (Hazes & Silman, 1990). The predominance of RA among women has led to investigation of sex hormones, menstrual and reproductive factors as possible risk factors. For example, it is widely known that pregnancy can be associated with disease remission, followed by exacerbations during the postpartum period (Spector *et al.*, 1990). Although evidence is inconclusive, there are indications that oral contraceptives protect or postpone development of severe RA (Spector & Hochberg, 1990). Several studies report an increased prevalence of RA among smokers (e.g. Silman *et al.*, 1996). Furthermore, smoking has been associated with greater disease severity independent of age, disease duration or treatment (Masdottir *et al.*, 2000). Other factors thought to predispose individuals to the development of RA include low socioeconomic status (Berkanovic *et al.*, 1996), low levels of education (Callahan & Pincus, 1988), stress (Persson *et al.*, 1999) and trauma (Al-Allaf *et al.*, 2001). Regarding the last of these, a case-control study compared 262 RA outpatients with age- and sex-matched controls (262) attending non-rheumatology outpatient clinics. Fifty-five (21 per cent) of the RA patients reported significant physical trauma (e.g. injury) during the previous six months before disease onset, compared with 17 (6.5 per cent) of the controls. Interestingly, history of trauma was more common among patients who were seronegative for rheumatoid factor. The authors suggest that those with seronegative RA might have a different form of inflammatory arthritis that is precipitated by physical trauma.

There is evidence of an increased mortality rate among people with RA (Spector & Scott, 1988) that is attributed to the disease itself, infection, renal, respiratory, gastrointestinal and cardiovascular disease. Regarding the last of these, a large study of 2262 deaths of patients with RA found that approximately 40 per cent were attributed to cardiovascular causes (Pincus & Callahan, 1986). There is evidence that stress, age, male gender, high functional impairment and low education are predictors of mortality (Wolfe *et al.*, 1994). Chehata *et al.* (2001) found that although individual measures of disease activity at a single point in time were not predictive of mortality, the mean level of disease activity over time did have a significant relationship. High levels of sustained inflammation appeared to be important predictors of premature death. A study in The Netherlands maintains that life expectancy is reduced by approximately seven years in men and approximately three years in women (Vandenbrouke *et al.*, 1984). A population-based study conducted in Minnesota found evidence of a widening mortality gap between patients with RA and the general population (Gonzalez *et al.*, 2007). The widening gap was due to the lack of improvement in survival among patients with RA compared to improvements in overall mortality rates in the general US population.

In RA, the synovial membrane becomes thickened and inflamed, eventually resulting in degeneration of the cartilage and ultimately the joint. Primary symptoms are persistent pain, stiffness, swollen joints and fatigue. Anaemia is a common. Rheumatoid arthritis is a systemic condition, and therefore people can feel generally unwell in addition to experiencing problems with specific joints. Typically, joints in the hands and feet are affected, with mild to severe structural damage resulting in varying degrees of physical dysfunction (Meenan *et al.*, 1991) that can pose problems for activities of daily living. Individual prognosis is uncertain (Parker *et al.*, 1990), with some people experiencing only mild disease of brief duration whilst others have a relentless progressive polyarthritis with marked functional impairment and disability. The condition can follow an unpredictable course of exacerbation and remission. The economic impact of RA in England for the year 1992 has been estimated at £1.256 billion (McIntosh, 1996), with 48 per cent of costs attributed to medical expenses and over 52 per cent of costs (£0.65 billion) due to lost productivity. Figures such as these make inability to work (i.e. work disability) a key issue in the management of RA and other types of arthritis that affect people during their working years.

Many people with inflammatory arthritis, including those with RA, are prescribed NSAIDs as the first-line drug treatment that is designed to reduce pain and swelling. Unfortunately, NSAIDs can have side effects on the digestive system (e.g. indigestion) and thus are often prescribed alongside proton-pump inhibitors which reduce indigestion and protect the stomach. Developments in the field include the use of NSAIDs called COX-2 inhibitors which are easier on the stomach but have been linked to increased risk of heart attacks and stroke. A second-line treatment comprises disease-modifying anti-rheumatic drugs (DMARDs) that aim to slow down the effects of the disease rather than relieve symptoms. It is important that patients are monitored for side effects if taking DMARDs (e.g. gold injections, methotrexate). Corticosteroids or 'steroids' are useful for reducing inflammation but can have a number of side effects if given at a high dosage for a long period of time. A recent development concerns biological therapies, such as anti-tumour necrosis factor (anti-TNF) that is given as an infusion or regular subcutaneous injections. The long-term side effects of anti-TNF are not known. Analgesics, such as paracetamol, may be used to assist with the pain-relieving effects of other drugs. Useful websites for finding out more about the drugs used to treat RA and other forms of arthritis are www.arc.org.uk or www.arthritis.org.

People with RA are advised to carry out regular, gentle exercise and to learn how to protect affected joints thus avoiding unnecessary strain. Splints may be used to help prevent permanent joint deformity. Finally, where joints become damaged beyond repair, joint replacement may be necessary to relieve pain and to improve function. Hip or knee replacements can be successful in reducing pain and increasing physical functioning among many people with arthritis. However, for some patients with RA, replacement surgery is less successful and they continue to experience pain and functional limitations after a period of 12 months (Keefe *et al.*, 1991). Gender differences have been identified among patients with RA referred for orthopaedic surgery in Finland (Hakkinen *et al.*, 2006) in that women had greater disability than men. Pain, muscle strength and disease activity had a major impact on disability, especially among the female patients.

People with RA often require long-term monitoring and care by specialised rheumatology clinics. The per-case cost of treatment for RA is 1.5 times greater than for OA (Yelin, 1998). However, the lower cost of treating OA has to be offset against its greater prevalence, and thus the overall economic impact is highest in OA. The situation is further complicated by the toxicity of NSAIDs used to treat RA, OA and AS where gastrointestinal complications can result from NSAID usage (e.g. bleeds, perforations). Disease-related resource utilisation tends to be higher for RA, whereas for OA a large proportion of medical costs relate to the side effects of NSAIDs that may necessitate additional physician visits, diagnostic procedures and hospitalisation (Sangha, 2000). In recent years, the psychosocial burden of disease has received more recognition, although conversion of psychosocial burden and quality of life into reliable and valid economic parameters remains to be achieved.

Ankylosing Spondylitis

Ankylosing spondylitis (AS) is one of a group of diseases referred to as seronegative spondylarthropathies. This group of diseases include psoriatic arthritis, Reiter's syndrome, reactive arthritis, and arthritis associated with inflammatory bowel disease, ulcerative colitis and Crohn's disease. Ankylosing spondylitis is characterised by an early age of onset (under 40) and is one of the few rheumatic diseases to exhibit a male predominance, with reported sex ratios in the region of 3:1 male to female (Kahn & van der Linden, 1990). However, it has been suggested that the true ratio may be nearer 1:1 (Russell, 1985). Whilst the debate about male:female ratio remains unresolved, it is acknowledged that the diagnosis of AS is often missed in women, and more women are now being diagnosed with the disease (Arnett, 1989). Consensus regarding methodologies and diagnostic criteria is necessary before the issues of gender-differentiated clinical profiles and prevalence rates of AS can be explained. Prevalence estimates range between 0.1 per cent and 2 per cent (Gran & Husby, 2003), although there may be many subclinical cases that do not receive a diagnosis.

Disease aetiology remains unknown, although an association with the human leukocyte antigen HLA-B27 was identified over 20 years ago (Brewerton *et al.*, 1973), suggesting that a genetic mechanism may be involved. Approximately 95 per cent of patients with AS have the HLA-B27 antigen compared with only 7 per cent in the population as a whole (Ebringer *et al.*, 1978). Possession of this antigen does not necessarily mean that AS is inevitable. A trigger factor, possibly an intestinal infection, is believed to be responsible for the onset of symptoms. Some patients assert that onset occurred following trauma (Jacoby *et al.*, 1985). However, the disease may have been present in a subclinical form and become more active due to the treatment received for the trauma (e.g. immobilisation). For many people, disease onset is gradual and insidious, affecting mainly the spine and sacroiliac joints, although other parts of the body (e.g. hips, shoulders, knees and eyes) can become involved. Onset may typically, but not always, manifest as sacroiliitis together with inflammation of entheses (points of union between tendon, ligament or capsule and bone) (McVeigh & Cairns, 2006). Gradual fusion of affected joints in the spine is known as 'ankylosis' and results in progressive functional impairment and the development of a typical hunched posture. Many people with AS will also develop osteoporosis. The disease is believed to follow a milder course among women, although consistent evidence to support this notion is lacking (Gran & Husby, 1990).

An international group, the Assessment in Ankylosing Spondylitis Society, is producing evidence-based recommendations for the management of AS (Zochling *et al.*, 2006). Traditionally, treatment has comprised medication and therapeutic exercise. The aim of medication, usually NSAIDs, is to reduce pain and inflammation thus enabling the patient to carry out regular strengthening and stretching exercises. The aim of the latter is to maintain mobility of affected joints, to improve or maintain posture and to achieve general fitness. The short-term effectiveness of a regular exercise programme has been demonstrated among hospital inpatients (Bulstrode *et al.*, 1987; Tomlinson *et al.*, 1986). However, the majority of people with AS are not admitted for inpatient care. Exercise has to be conducted in the home environment or in classes organised by physiotherapy departments and voluntary organisations, such as the National Ankylosing Spondylitis Society in the UK. One of the few studies among AS outpatients found positive effects of group exercise on thoracolumbar mobility, general fitness and self-reported estimates of global health (Hidding *et al.*, 1993). Van Tubergen and Hidding (2002) maintain that conventional treatment with NSAIDs and exercise is palliative and often does not control symptoms in the longer term.

A relatively new development in the treatment of AS is the use of anti-TNF drugs. These drugs have been used in the treatment of RA and are now licensed for use in the treatment of AS in some countries but are very expensive. McVeigh and Cairns (2006) argue that the high financial costs may be outweighed by the immense improvements in pain and function that can help some patients to remain in work and out of hospital. However, although anti-TNF can result in marked clinical improvements in trials, this treatment is not always effective and is not suitable for all AS patients (Claudpierre, 2005).

After diagnosis, some patients continue to be monitored in hospital-based clinics, whilst others may be referred back to community-based medical practitioners for long-term health care. People with AS can be referred to a physiotherapy department for advice on home exercise activities and may also receive a short course of hydrotherapy, although such treatment is dependent upon the availability of local facilities. Interestingly, there is evidence that people with AS tend to underestimate their functional difficulties (Hidding *et al.*, 1992) and use unusual movements or gadgets to assist in problem areas (Abbott *et al.*, 1994). Underestimation of functional difficulties and coping with daily activities through novel adaptations can mask true functional impairment in both clinical assessments and research studies.

Juvenile Idiopathic Arthritis

Contrary to the general belief that arthritis is a condition of 'old age', some forms of arthritis begin in childhood. Arthritis in children has been known as juvenile chronic arthritis (JCA), juvenile rheumatoid arthritis (JRA) or juvenile idiopathic arthritis (JIA). All of these terms appear in the published literature but refer to the same condition. The most recent term, JIA, will be used throughout this text. Juvenile idiopathic arthritis is one of the most common chronic diseases of childhood, with prevalence estimates ranging from 0.16 to 1.13 per 1000 children (Benjamin, 1990), suggesting that there are over 15,000 children with JIA in the UK, for example. Peak ages of onset are between 1 and 3 years, with incidence being twice as high among girls compared to boys (Cassidy & Petty, 1990). The disease is a significant cause of physical disability and blindness. Mortality has been estimated at between 2 per cent and 4 per cent (Cassidy & Petty, 1990), although the possibility of mortality remains a largely taboo area.

Classified as a heterogeneous group of disorders, JIA is characterised by persistent inflammation of the joints that presents before 16 years of age (Munthe, 1990). The condition is categorised into three subgroups:

1. systemic onset disease, characterised by fever and a rash;
2. pauciarticular disease (four or fewer joints affected in the absence of systemic features);
3. polyarticular disease where five or more joints are involved in the absence of systemic features.

Systemic onset disease affects between 10 per cent and 25 per cent of children with JIA, has a peak age at onset of 2 years and is equally prevalent among boys and girls. Onset is acute, with remittent fever, a rash, fatigue and possible inflammation of glands and vital organs (e.g. heart). Joint inflammation typically follows systemic onset. Complete recovery occurs in 50 per cent of cases, whilst a third will develop poly-articular JIA. The latter occurs in 30 per cent to 40 per cent of children with JIA, and predominates in younger girls. Arms, legs, hands and feet are affected, and prognosis tends to be poor. Children with poly-articular onset are those most likely to have active disease in adulthood and are at risk of permanent joint damage. Pauciarticular onset is the most common form of JIA, accounting for between 40 per cent and 50 per cent of cases. Onset typically occurs before the age of 5 years and, again, predominates among girls, usually affecting wrists, knees and ankles. Prognosis is generally good with the disease lasting for a few years only. Nonetheless, following a summary of outcomes from both retrospective and prospective studies, Duffy (2005) concluded that a significant number of patients continue to have active disease during adulthood and live with significant damage and disability. For example, a UK study of 231 adults with long-standing JIA found that 43.3 per cent had active arthritis as indicated by clinical parameters and 54.4 per cent had active disease using laboratory measures (e.g. C-reactive protein). The proportion with severe disability using a score of >1.5 on the Heath Assessment Questionnaire was 42.9 per cent (Packham & Hall, 2002).

The disease follows an unpredictable course, and thus for many children life with JIA fluctuates between periods of active disease and remission. Typical symptoms include pain, stiffness, swollen joints, fatigue, lack of appetite and general irritability. Prognosis is uncertain and in the absence of curative treatment, primary therapeutic goals are to reduce pain and inflammation, maintain joint function, promote muscle strength, prevent disability and control extra-articular manifestations such as iritis. Disease management is complex, involving a combination of diverse therapies (e.g. medication, wearing splints and exercise) and regular visits to various outpatient clinics such as rheumatology, ophthalmology and physiotherapy. In addition, JIA requires constant monitoring and performance of self-care activities. The responsibility for day-to-day disease management quickly shifts from health professionals to parents and children. Adolescents are expected to play a greater role in the management of their disease in accordance with their growing independence and autonomy.

The impact of JIA and its management upon the family is considerable. Up to one-third of the child's free time may be lost due to arthritis (Southwood & Malleson, 1993), and the family's involvement in health regimens can severely restrict personal time, holidays and leisure pursuits. Concordance involves the negotiated agreement between patients, or their representatives, and the medical team (Marinker *et al.*, 1997). Since the term *concordance* conveys equal respect for the health beliefs of both patients and medical practitioners, it is less value-laden than terms such as compliance and adherence. This issue is discussed further in Chapter 7. Concordance in relation to JIA is believed to be less than optimal and forms a major area of concern (Kroll *et al.*, 1999). Not only may poor concordance reduce the potential benefits of treatment for individual children and their families, but on a wider scale it may lead to increased healthcare costs (Rapoff & Christophersen, 1982; Varni & Wallander, 1984).

Metaphysical Explanations for Arthritis

Psychologists have long been aware of the interaction between perceptions of stress and the physical body. The immune system can be influenced by stress, with negative emotions (e.g. anger, fear and resentment) causing the formation of chemicals in the body. For example, it is accepted that stressful life events and daily hassles can aggravate many long-term diseases, including arthritis. Metaphysical explanations build on this understanding by using the body parts and functions as a map of the individual's wellbeing whereby the physical expression of illness is believed to reflect emotional imbalance, maladaptive patterns of learned behaviours or non-serving thought patterns. With the growth of interest in complementary medicine, it is worth considering metaphysical explanations for arthritis and whether the insights gained are of value for individuals with the disease. A detailed examination of metaphysics is complex and beyond the scope of this text; interested readers are referred to the burgeoning literature on this topic (e.g. Hay, 1984).

One of the basic premises of metaphysics is that we create our own reality. Since it is extremely unlikely that people deliberately and consciously chose to have pain and disease, it is important that individuals are not held to blame for their conditions. Rather, they are in need of assistance and support in attempts to find, understand and address the causes of their conditions and how they may promote healing (i.e. bring the whole system into balance). The insight provided by metaphysics is just that and should be used accordingly. Although typical patterns and associations have been noted and published, each person is unique and may not fit with established norms and views. The same holds for medical care; one person may react totally differently to the next when given NSAIDs for example.

The way the joints function determines the degree of freedom and grace expressed in our movements and the direction we are taking at a given point in time or in our lives in general (Shapiro, 1990). Any restriction in joint functioning is believed to indicate a problem in that area. Characteristic symptoms experienced by many people with arthritis include pain, stiffness, inflammation and fatigue. The metaphysical explanation views pain as a warning sign that the area corresponding to the pain needs attention and that the pain can be an indication of suppressed anger or bitterness. Stiffness of joints can indicate rigid thinking, self-criticism, or lack of self-worth. There can be fear around the notion of allowing new and different ideas to enter the mind and one's life. Metaphysically, inflammation is associated with unexpressed anger that manifests physically as hot, red, swollen joints that in turn cause restrictions of movement. Thus, there can be sensations of being restricted in one's life, restrained, confined or tied down. We may wish to be doing something different or even to be somewhere different. There may be a growing inability to be flexible in our thoughts and behaviours; an inability to 'go with the flow'. This state can reflect a lack of self-trust and a hardened attitude towards life. Rather than acknowledge these feelings about ourselves, we tend to project them outwardly towards others, placing ourselves in the role of victim rather than of co-creator of our world and the way we live (Shapiro, 1990). Fatigue can indicate weariness with life and a need for both mental and physical rest. We can experience an inner tiredness because we are trying to keep going or to cope with our life. Fatigue can suggest a loss of purpose and direction, and a need to increase the joy and love we experience.

The main sites of arthritis in the body are feet, knees, hips, spine, shoulders and neck. Feet, legs and spine are all concerned with support of the self, thus problems in these areas may be associated with feelings of lack of support. The feet are our foundation and control the direction we move in. Hence, as well as lack of support and insecurity, foot problems can indicate conflict with direction and movement. Similarly, the knees are connected to movement, direction, and flexibility; they are the body's shock absorbers (Shapiro, 1990). Fluid is associated with emotions, therefore swollen knees can indicate emotional defence or resistance against the way that life is unfolding. Resentment and anger can be 'stuffed' behind the knees with the resultant inflexibility and rigid thinking typified by comments such as 'Why should I change?' The hips are associated with moving forward in life, reflecting one's hopes, dreams, goals and also fears. As well as lack of support, the spine represents how well supported we feel in our lives and how we carry our own issue or burdens and the burdens of others. Hence, we can feel overburdened with cares, weighed down or sense that we have 'someone on our back'. The shoulders represent our ability to reach out and enjoy life, with pain indicating a fear of moving in the wrong direction or a failure to grasp life with both hands. Finally, the neck represents our support of ourselves, our ideas and our flexibility of outlook. A stiff neck can suggest an inability to look around and see all sides of the picture. In sum, problems with the main sites of arthritis represent notions of lack support, insecurity, inflexibility, and failure to reach out and enjoy life to the full.

In the metaphysical literature, arthritis is believed to indicate a lack of self-love (e.g. Belot, 1999). Furthermore, since the individual lacks love for the self, it is difficult for them to accept love from others. This situation can result in conflict within the body and conflict in relationships. Rheumatoid arthritis, where the immune system starts to attack itself, indicates a deep dislike of the self, arising from shame, guilt, a deep sense of worthlessness and self-criticism, or long-held anger, bitterness and stiff attitudes (Shapiro, 1990). The 'attack' on the self manifests as painful and limited movement, lack of fluidity, and difficulty in freely expressing feelings and beliefs. Thus, the person with RA can become unassertive, inhibited and self-sacrificing, unable to express strong emotions. It is interesting to note that this picture of RA is similar to the propositions regarding a stereotypical, RA personality (see Chapter 3).

The situation can be complicated by the fact that some fears or mistakes from past lives can be sources of dis-ease in this life (Stein, 1996), a concept known as non-serving karma. Put simply, karma involves the lessons we need to learn in this lifetime that bring opportunities for growth and healing. Thus, fears that do not appear to be related to any experiences in the present life may be linked to non-serving events in past lives. For example, a woman with a fear of giving birth may have died during childbirth in a previous incarnation, and may feel confused that she desires children but at the same time is terrified of becoming pregnant or of actually giving birth. A further complication is that some individuals offer to take on other people's karma (i.e. they take on the pain and dis-ease of other people as if it were their own). Despite the complexity of metaphysics, it may provide a useful alternative insight in terms of understanding and facilitating enhanced management of arthritis and the wellbeing of people living with the condition.

Healing occurs when the underlying emotions, non-serving behaviour patterns and thoughts are acknowledged and accepted, and the integrated wholeness of the body, mind, emotions and spirit is recognised (Shapiro, 1990). Stein (1996) describes the progression to physical dis-ease and its reversal as follows: negative life function → stress → resistance to change → emotional discomfort → mental discomfort → spiritual pain → physical dis-ease. Reversal is described: physical dis-ease → change and letting go → emotional release → mental (often karmic) release → spiritual reconnection → healing of the body.

Since physical manifestations are believed to be the result of non-serving thoughts and emotional reactions, it is logical to assume that the power of the mind can be harnessed to aid resolution. There is a range of healing modalities available to assist the individual in achieving this goal; these include meditation, visualisation, relaxation, prayer, counselling or energy medicines such as reiki or energy field healing. Such modalities can be used alongside traditional medicine and other complementary and alternative therapies such as reflexology, homeopathy or acupuncture. Thus, painkillers can be used to alleviate pain, freeing the individual to concentrate on working within, or self-healing, in order to achieve personal resolution, self-discovery and a sense of wholeness. Psychologists could have an important role to play in helping people to understand the messages of the physical body and how they are linked to cognitions, emotions and persistent behaviour patterns. Furthermore, psychologists are often conversant with strategies, such as reinterpretation of negative thoughts into positive statements, that could be of immense help to people trying to change their patterns of behaviour and cognitions. Some of the interventions detailed in Chapter 8 can be useful in giving people a different perspective on life with arthritis, one that is not dominated by the condition and its treatment; rather, they empower the individual to take steps towards self-fulfilment.

Complementary and Alternative Medicine

The terms 'complementary medicine', 'unconventional medicine' and 'alternative medicine' tend to be used interchangeably. The content and use of such therapies suggests that the majority are not intended to be used as an alternative to standard medical care but rather as an adjunct (i.e. in a complementary way). Moreover, the current and growing usage of such therapies suggests that they can no longer be considered 'unconventional'. Thus, the term complementary medicine is preferred and has been defined as 'A broad set of healthcare practices (i.e. already available to the public) that are not readily integrated into the dominant healthcare model, because they pose challenges to diverse societal beliefs and practices (cultural, economic, scientific, medical and educational)' (Eskanazi, 1998, p. 1622).

Many of the strategies employed by psychologists (e.g. cognitive-behavioural interventions, self-management training) can be considered complementary in that they are intended to be used alongside standard medical care and are designed to enhance the quality of patients' lives. The practice of relaxation is a useful example of a technique that already forms part of many psychologically based interventions, but can also be considered a complementary therapy in its own right. The value of relaxation for people with arthritis may lie in its stress-relieving effects, which in turn can help to reduce the experience of pain, combat fatigue and promote restful sleep. A controlled study of chronic, rheumatic back pain patients compared EMG biofeedback relaxation training with two control conditions (i.e. pseudotherapy and conventional medical care; Flor *et al.*, 1986). The biofeedback group improved on cognitive and behavioural measures but not on global pain, and viewed their treatment as more effective than the controls. Moreover, patients who improved reported continued use of relaxation as a means of controlling pain and tension, and increasing their sense of control. In contrast, patients who did not improve reported more help-lessness, more hopelessness and felt more dependent on health profes-sionals for their care. Interestingly, Affleck *et al.* (1992) found that the two most frequently used coping strategies utilised by patients with RA were taking direct action to reduce pain (e.g. applying warmth or cold to the painful areas) and relaxation. Moreover, patients using relaxation had lower levels of daily pain.

It is estimated that between 20 and 50 per cent of the general popula-tion have used complementary medicine (Fisher & Ward, 1994). Similar proportions of complementary and alternative medicine (CAM) users have been reported among people with arthritis attending rheumatol-ogy clinics (Breuer *et al.*, 2006; Osborn, 2001; Resch *et al.*, 1997; Vecchio, 1994), although higher rates of usage have been reported. In a Canadian survey of 103 rheumatology patients, 66 per cent had used complemen-tary medicine in addition to hospital-based therapies (Wainapel *et al.*, 1998). Similarly, a population-based telephone survey of 480 elderly patients with arthritis (aged >65) in the US found that 66 per cent had used complementary medicine and 28 per cent had consulted a CAM practitioner (Kaboli *et al.*, 2001). Respondents who consulted CAM practitioners were also those who made high use of healthcare services, suggesting the presence of a generally high service utilisation pattern among some people. Herman *et al.* (2004) report CAM usage among 69.2 per cent of a sample of Hispanic and non-Hispanic white men and women with OA, RA or fibromyalgia aged 18 to 84 years. Rates of usage did not differ by ethnicity. The use of CAM among children with JIA has received little research attention. However, a survey by Hagen *et al.* (2003) reports CAM usage among 64 per cent of child patients attend-ing a rheumatology clinic. Similarly, a survey of parents found CAM usage among their children with JIA to be 33.9 per cent (Feldman *et al.*, 2004). Not surprisingly, use of CAM was higher among children whose parents had themselves used CAM.

The cost of complementary medicine is usually borne by the recipi-ent rather than being provided as part of standard care services that are free at the point of delivery in healthcare systems such as that of the UK or maybe covered by medical insurance in countries such as the US.

Bearing this point in mind, it is surprising that there have been few studies of the relative costs of standard care versus complementary medicine. One exception is a survey of 120 older adults with OA (aged 55–75) recruited through community sources in the US (Ramsey *et al.*, 2001). Over 47 per cent of participants reported using at least one type of complementary medicine during a period of 20 weeks, most commonly massage (57 per cent), chiropractic services (20.7 per cent), and non-prescribed alternative medications (17.2 per cent). The mean cost per user for traditional therapies (ambulatory medical care services) was estimated at $1,148 per annum compared with $1,127 for complementary medicine services, with the highest costs being associated with massage and chiropractic services. Users made an average of 36 visits to complementary medicine practitioners compared with 21 visits to traditional medical practitioners. The only factor that was related to use of complementary medicine was that of lower health status.

Collectively, these studies suggest that the most popular types of CAM used by people with arthritis mirror those used in the general population, and include acupuncture, osteopathy, massage, homeopathy, herbal treatments, copper bracelets, aromatherapy, prayer and energy healing. In addition, many people try special diets, exercise, relaxation and self-management training, although these strategies are not always conceptualised as 'complementary'. Exercise was included in early surveys of CAM, but since exercise for arthritis has received greater recognition as a therapeutic modality in its own right it has been excluded from studies of complementary medicine. It remains to be seen whether modalities such as relaxation and massage move from being categorised as complementary to traditional as their popularity increases and they are offered by some hospital and primary care services.

The 21st century has witnessed a blurring of the boundaries between mainstream and complementary medicine, with some healthcare professionals beginning to practise CAM therapies themselves. For example, a survey of 157 rheumatology nurses in the UK found that 8.3 per cent (n = 13) practised CAM, with the most frequent therapies being aromatherapy, acupuncture, massage and reflexology (Osborn, 2001). Over 50 per cent of nurses had advised patients about CAM, particularly pain relief through acupuncture and aromatherapy. A similar survey among members of the Register of Qualified Aromatherapists showed that 74 per cent of aromatherapists (n = 269) had treated people with rheumatic disease, particularly OA (68 per cent) and RA (56 per cent)

(Osborn *et al.*, 2001). Lavender, rosemary and camomile were the most commonly used essential oils in the treatment of rheumatic disease symptoms (e.g. pain, stiffness) and consequences (e.g. mood disturbance).

Given the lack of knowledge regarding aetiology and cure for most types of arthritis, symptomatic relief is a major motivational factor influencing the decision to seek complementary medicine. Not surprisingly, relief from pain has been identified as a major factor in the decision to seek complementary care (e.g. Fautrel *et al.*, 2002; Wainapel *et al.*, 1998). Additional factors associated with CAM use are higher education, being female, aged under 55 years (Breuer *et al.*, 2006; Herman *et al.*, 2004; Zochling *et al.*, 2004), higher household income, and greater depression (Fautrel *et al.*, 2002). The link between use of CAM and analgesics appears variable, with some researchers finding greater use of analgesics (e.g. Fautrel *et al.*, 2002) whereas others report less use of analgesics among CAM users (e.g. Zochling *et al.*, 2004). Among children with JIA, CAM usage has been linked to longer disease duration (Hagen *et al.*, 2003) and greater use of CAM by parents (Feldman *et al.*, 2004).

Rao *et al.* (1998) used focus groups to understand arthritis patients' perceptions of CAM. Findings confirmed that, although patients are willing to look outside conventional medicine for relief, they do not stop using it; rather, they use both conventional and complementary medicine in combination. Similarly, Fautrel *et al.* (2002) found that CAM users continued to use traditional health resources. An investigation conducted in India focusing on patients with RA (n = 114) showed that the decision to use CAM was influenced by the belief that there is no cure for RA and that adverse reactions are rare in CAM (Chandrashekara *et al.*, 2002). The authors acknowledge that CAM use is a universal phenomenon, and conclude that it is important that healthcare practitioners are aware of patients' use of CAM in order to recognise and avoid interactions with medication. Not surprisingly, an exploration of participatory decision-making style conducted in the US found that patients were more likely to discuss their use of CAM with physicians who had a participatory style during consultations and involved patients in decision-making about treatment (Sleath *et al.*, 2005).

Given that CAM rarely forms an integral part of publicly funded healthcare systems, the majority of patients are forced to bear the costs themselves or to seek cover via medical insurance. Rao *et al.* (1998) found that the cost of CAM became an issue if the patient's symptoms failed to respond to the treatment received. A CAM consultation usually allows time for the recipient to discuss their condition, feelings and lifestyle in considerable depth and on a one-to-one basis with a complementary practitioner. This holistic stance may contrast with the patient's experiences in conventional healthcare systems, where time is a scarce resource and patients report that they are aware of other patients waiting and the pressures on doctors (J.H. Barlow, Bishop & Pennington, 1996).

Evidence for the effectiveness of CAM is beginning to accrue, particularly in relation to therapies such as acupuncture, homeopathy, chiropractic and herbal remedies. An interesting example of the last of these arises from the ancient folk practice of chewing on willow bark to relieve arthritis. It is now known that willow contains aspirin, which can alleviate the inflammatory effects of arthritis. Thus, there is now evidence for the basis of this folk medicine belief. Many patients attempt to influence their symptoms and the course of disease through the use of diet (e.g. McDougall *et al.*, 2002). A randomised, controlled trial of a vegan diet free of gluten showed that nine patients improved in terms of reduction in antibody levels compared to one patient in the control group who followed a well-balanced, non-vegan diet (Hafstrom *et al.*, 2001). However, it should be noted that an intent-to-treat analysis reduced the proportion of diet responders in the vegan group from 40.5 per cent to 34.3 per cent and there was also a high level of attrition, with only 22 out of 38 patients completing the trial in the vegan diet group. The authors do not provide any indication of why attrition was so high. Clearly it will be important to find out why patients find it difficult to maintain a strict diet and whether they perceive such diets to be of benefit in terms of how they feel rather than relying on laboratory indicators of disease activity. Breuer *et al.* (2005) examined the self-perceived efficacy of different CAM therapies among patients with rheumatological conditions. Acupuncture and homeopathy received the highest ratings of self-perceived efficacy among patients with spondylo-arthropathies and OA; satisfaction was lowest among patients with RA. Lack of perceived effectiveness and expense have been cited as the most frequent reasons for stopping CAM use (Rao *et al.*, 2003).

It is worth noting that the therapies (e.g. acupuncture, homeopathy) about which there is most scientific evidence are therapies that are amenable to research using similar methods to those used in drug and clinical trials (e.g. randomised controlled trials). Designing trials of other more diverse complementary approaches (e.g. reiki, Bowen technique, energy field healing) poses much more of a challenge. Making the results of such trials accessible to lay people is a further challenge that deserves to be more thoroughly addressed by researchers and complementary medicine practitioners alike. Training in the appraisal skills needed to understand the effectiveness of 'new treatments' and complementary medicine is sometimes included in self-management programmes (e.g. the Arthritis Self-Management Programme – Lorig & Holman, 1993). With the increased access to the internet, such training appears to be a vital component of patient management that cannot be ignored.

Chapter Summary

The four main types of arthritis that form the focus of this book have been introduced and the associated disease management strategies typically used have been described. In addition, the role of CAM has been considered, given that a relatively large proportion of people with arthritis use CAM modalities at some point during their disease journey. Subsequent chapters will focus more on psychosocial perspectives, commencing with issues around onset, diagnosis and disease duration.

3

Onset, Diagnosis and Duration of Disease

Onset, Personality and Stress

Personality

There are methodological problems associated with the nature of most studies examining the causal roles of personality and stress in the onset of arthritis. For example, studies are usually retrospective and identifying an appropriate comparison groups can be difficult. Nonetheless, early studies implicated personality and stress as predisposing factors leading to onset of RA (Booth, 1937; Jones, 1909). A review by Moos (1964) concluded that people with RA are conforming, conservative, compliant, subservient, depressed, sensitive, inhibited and anxious. It is interesting to note that this description of the RA personality coincides with metaphysical explanations of RA (see Chapter 2).

Later investigations have continued to focus on identifying an RA personality but have failed to find any differences between RA and other types of arthritis. A comparison of personality characteristics and stress at disease onset between patients with RA and OA failed to find evidence of a generalised, simple and distinct RA personality (Latman & Walls, 1996). However, there were indications that a subgroup of RA patients, characterised by high stress at disease onset, may experience a higher degree of disease severity. A cross-sectional comparison of healthy controls and women with RA, women with fibromyalgia syndrome (FMS), and women with chronic low back pain failed to find any differences between the three chronic pain groups (Amir *et al.*, 2000). Dimensions assessed included coping with a stressful situation, anger expression and suicide risk. Compared to the control group, all three chronic pain groups scored higher on avoidance coping and anger expression. Similarly, Zautra *et al.* (1999) found no differences between women with OA and women with FMS in terms of interpersonal stress, chronic pain or personality traits.

A few studies have examined the role of personality traits in relation to psychosocial adjustment and exercise. For example, Castenada *et al.* (1998) investigated the personality correlates of exercise behaviour in 70 men and 126 women with OA. The most frequently reported type of exercise was walking. Exercise was associated cross-sectionally with age, quality of well-being and extroversion. Thus, among this sample, people who were extroverts were more likely to use walking as a form of exercise. Lichtenberg *et al.* (1984) investigated associations between personality traits and pain among 40 people with knee OA. Pain severity was predicted by scores on hypochondriasis from the Minnesota Multiphasic Personality Inventory (MMPI). Hypochondriasis has been linked to neuroticism, which is associated with a wide range of symptom reporting. Similarly, self-rated symptoms and wellbeing among both inpatients and outpatients with RA has been linked with neuroticism (Persson & Sahlberg, 2002). In a comparison between early RA patients (< four years disease duration) and a reference group recruited from the community, neuroticism and socially desirable responses were significantly higher among the RA group (Krol *et al.*, 1998). Interestingly, the RA group had less emotional expression and avoided confrontational situations more than the reference group. A related analysis by Suurmeijer, van Sonderen, Krol *et al.* (2005) found that, among early RA patients with a more neurotic personality profile, there was evidence of more anxious and depressed feelings. Interestingly, extraversion had no direct effect on either depression or anxiety. A longitudinal investigation showed that higher neuroticism along with worse clinical status and lower educational level at the time of diagnosis were related to increased psychological distress at three- and five-year follow-up (Evers *et al.*, 2002). The personality trait of unmitigated communion (an extreme focus on relationships that has been associated with self-neglect) has been linked with psychological distress among women with RA (Danoff-Burg *et al.*, 2004). Similarly, Smith and Zautra (2002) found that, among women with RA and OA, those higher in interpersonal sensitivity (excessive sensitivity to the behaviour and feelings of others) reported more distress and disease activity during periods of interpersonal stress.

The role of optimism and pessimism has been investigated in relation to psychosocial adjustment and daily symptoms. Brenner *et al.* (1994)

examined the influence of optimism on psychosocial adjustment among 66 RA patients, and followed up a proportion of these 16 months from baseline. As may be expected, greater optimism was associated with better psychosocial adjustment both cross-sectionally and longitudinally. Moreover, optimism was found to precede increases in adjustment. Optimism has been associated with lower pain in early (< six months) and intermediate (1–7 years) RA patients (Treharne *et al.*, 2005). Drawing on their research programme investigating the effects of optimism on long-term conditions such as arthritis, asthma and fibromyalgia, Affleck, Tennen and Apter (2001) conclude that pessimism is mainly a predictor of daily sadness whilst optimism is a predictor of daily happiness. Optimism appeared to have a regulatory function on mood in patients' daily judgements of the efficacy of pain coping strategies. Interestingly, Affleck, Tennen and Apter suggest that neither optimists nor pessimists find pain-coping strategies to be successful in relieving pain; rather, they are helpful in improving mood. This suggestion is in accordance with the findings of many psycho-educational interventions that do not find any impact on absolute levels of pain but show evidence of improved mood (see Chapter 8).

Box 3.1 Methodological Note

The main methodological difficulty with studies of personality and stress among people with arthritis is that they are necessarily retrospective. People are identified after the onset of arthritis and then measures of personality are taken. Similarly, measures of stress in patients' lives (e.g. life events such as bereavement) are assessed retrospectively following diagnosis. Thus, it is not clear whether resultant associations are due to an underlying personality trait or prior life events, or are a reaction to developing painful, incurable conditions. Comparison of samples of people who are ill with samples of people who are well are interesting and can indicate the nature of differences in terms of personality or stress. However, they are usually plagued with similar methodological problems (i.e. based on retrospective data). The only sure method of determining issues of causality in the aetiology of arthritis would be to assess an extremely large sample of the general population and to follow them over many years in order to identify who develops arthritis.

Box 3.1 (cont'd)

One issue that is of equal interest and is, in essence, more easily resolved concerns the possible links between certain personality types and the ease with which people adapt to their condition or respond to psycho-educational interventions. However, data exploring these issues are sadly lacking.

Despite the lack of evidence to support linkages between certain personality traits and types of arthritis, beliefs deriving from clinical experience and anecdotal evidence can evolve into stereotypes of 'typical' patient groups. For example, compared with people with RA, people with AS are generally believed to be aggressive, active, less depressed, less emotional, more socially oriented, more highly motivated and to possess a high pain threshold (Williams, 1989). It is important to note that RA is more predominant in women with a typical age at onset of between 40 and 50, whereas AS is more predominant in men with a typical age at onset of between 20 and 30. In addition, the management of AS comprises regular performance of a relatively aggressive exercise regime whilst treatment for RA places greater emphasis on the importance of rest during periods of disease exacerbation and traditionally positions patients as passive recipients of care. Thus, stereotypic views of RA and AS patients appear to match the nature of the treatment demands for each condition combined with the male:female predominance.

One attempt to assess the validity of health professionals' beliefs compared patients with RA, AS and chronic low back pain (LBP) in terms of sthenia (non-complaining, active), ambition and education (Zant *et al.*, 1982). Results showed that, although AS patients had a significantly higher education level, they did not differ from the other patient groups or Dutch population norms on sthenia or ambition. Similarly, Stiles (1993) found no difference on personality traits between women with AS and either women receiving physical therapy for generalised aches and pains or healthy controls.

Overall, there remains little evidence of association between personality traits and various types of arthritis. However, there are indications that traits such as optimism may be advantageous in relation to attaining better psychosocial adjustment, whilst greater symptom reporting may be linked to neuroticism.

Stress

Although many of the characteristics associated with arthritis (e.g. depression) may be reactions to a painful, chronic and disabling disease rather than causal factors, there are indications that stress may trigger disease onset and may influence the course of established disease (Anderson *et al.*, 1985; Wegener, 1991). Disease onset has been shown to coincide with stressful life events (e.g. death of a close relative, divorce, conflict at work), as retrospectively reported by 40 per cent of RA patients and 7.5 per cent of OA patients (Nasser-Abdel, 1996). In contrast, Li *et al.* (2005) found no evidence of a link between a severe life event (death of a child) and RA. The study is somewhat unique in that it involves population-level data. The authors included all 21,062 parents whose child had died between 1980 and 1996 in Denmark (the exposed group) and matched 293,745 parents randomly selected from the general population on family structure (unexposed group). A total of 600 incident RA cases were identified (35 in the exposed group and 565 in the unexposed group) leading to the conclusion that there is no association between death of a child (a major life event) and onset of RA.

Traumatic experiences in childhood have been linked to the risk of arthritis (Kopec & Sayre 2004). Longitudinal data (n = 9159) from three cycles of a Canadian National Health Survey were analysed for new cases of arthritis using an interviewer-administered questionnaire. Childhood psychological trauma was measured using a seven-item questionnaire covering physical abuse, fearful experiences, hospitalisation, being sent away from home and parental disturbance. Results showed a 27 per cent increase in risk of developing arthritis among respondents reporting two or more traumatic events. A possible link between arthritis and childhood sexual abuse emerged from a phenomenological investigation (n = 21 women) that included measures of introversion and extroversion (Jahn, 1997). Arthritis was one of the most frequently reported somatic complaints along with migraines, sleep difficulty, nightmares and gastrointestinal problems. Clearly, this study has a small sample size and results are not generalisable. Also, arthritis may be part of an overall pattern of somatic symptoms following distressing and traumatic events. However, a similar finding emerged from a survey of 1359 white, middle-class, older (median age = 75 years) men and women recruited from a community setting (Stein & Barrett-Connor, 2000); 12.7 per cent of women and 5.4 per cent of men reported sexual assault. Among women, sexual assault was associated with an increased risk of arthritis and breast cancer. A dose-response effect was noted, whereby women reporting multiple episodes of sexual assault had a two- to threefold increased risk for arthritis or breast cancer. Whilst such findings may be a manifestation of the increase in somatic conditions following sexual abuse, it may be that, for a small proportion of people, a history of abuse is the trigger factor resulting in the pain, stiffness and inflammation that are characteristic of arthritis. It is interesting to note that survivors of abuse may be prone to feelings of anger and lack of love for the self and one's physical body, a scenario reminiscent of metaphysical explanations for arthritis. Equally, it is easy to understand how internalisation of anger and fear, irrespective of the cause, could manifest as pain, stiffness and restricted movement. Findings such as those reported above require further investigation in different populations and in terms of possible mechanisms of action. For example, the impact of a depressed and anxious mood following physical or sexual assault may in turn adversely affect immune functioning that may be involved in the onset of some types of arthritis.

The associations between stressful events, symptoms and daily mood have been examined among children with JIA (Schanberg *et al.*, 2000). Although based on a very small sample (n = 12), results show that diary methods of data collection are feasible among children aged between 7 and 15. Multilevel, fixed effects models showed that more negative daily mood and more stressful events were predictive of increased fatigue, stiffness and reduction in daily activities. Negative mood was associated with pain on a daily basis. A later study based on a larger sample (n = 51) showed that despite treatment with remittive agents and NSAIDs, children reported pain, stiffness and fatigue on over 70 per cent of days (Schanberg, Gil *et al.*, 2005). Moreover, increased pain, stiffness and fatigue were associated with daily fluctuations in stress and mood and resulted in a restriction of social activities but not educational attendance. The authors suggest that fatigue in children manifests later in the day and thus would not be expected to influence school attendance. The role played by arthritis-related stress has been examined among 75 children and young adults aged 8–18 year (LeBovidge *et al.*, 2005). After controlling for demographic and medical factors, greater levels of stress (both arthritis-related and non-arthritis-related) was associated with greater frequency of depressed and anxious moods and parent-reported adjustment problems. Youths' attitude towards illness moderated the relationship between arthritis-related stress and depression, and between episodic stress and depression. Manuel (2001) showed that maternal education moderated the relationship between daily hassles and psychological wellbeing among 92 mothers of children with JIA aged 5–16 years. Such information is useful when developing interventions. Overall, results support the notion of a relationship between stress, mood and arthritis symptoms among children and adolescents.

Similar findings have emerged from studies focused on adults. A detailed longitudinal investigation of the relationship between mood and pain linked to stress among people with joint pain was conducted by Affleck *et al.* (1994). More active inflammatory disease was associated with an undesirable daily event and greater pain on the day of the event and the following day. Patients with a history of negative events also reported more pain the following day. An unexpected finding was that patients with no recent history of major life events and with a high level of social support had lower levels of pain on the day after an undesirable event. This finding endorses the stress-buffering role that may be played by social support (see Chapter 6).

Links have been established between stress and immune system functioning in people with RA (Bradley, 1989; Wegener, 1991). A series of studies by Zautra and colleagues has examined the relationship between stress and disease activity. Using a combination of interviews and blood tests, an investigation of the relationship between life stress and immune parameters among 33 women with RA attending three routine monthly clinic checkups showed that stress resulted in negative immune system reactions (Zautra *et al.*, 1989). However, the precise mechanisms involved remain unclear. A later study (Zautra *et al.*, 1998) focused on interpersonal stress and disease activity among 20 married women (average age 55 years) who differed in the quality of their spousal relationships. Data were collected over a 12-week period and results showed that disease activity in RA increased following increased interpersonal stress. Interestingly, women with stronger marital relationships were less affected by interpersonal stress. Zautra *et al.* (1999) examined the role of stressful life events in disease flares among patients with RA (an autoimmune disease) and patients with OA (non-autoimmune disease). Although results supported the proposition that interpersonal stressors are predictive of disease activity, some individual differences emerged. Not all RA patients showed an association between stress and disease activity, and contrary to expectations, some OA patients who were depressed showed increased disease activity following interpersonal stress. Zautra, Yocum, Villanueva *et al.* (2004) examined immune activation markers during periods of stress and depressive symptoms among 45 female RA patients and compared these with 106 controls (no autoimmune disease). The pattern of autoimmune markers differed between the RA group and the controls. Moreover, greater immune activation was found among depressed RA patients in comparison with other groups. The authors concluded that results provide new evidence of the role played by psychosocial factors in the autoimmune processes in RA.

One interesting area that may offer further insight concerns ability to disclose emotional information. Emotional disclosure studies usually involve participants writing about traumatic experiences. In the context of RA, disclosure studies have reported reduction in disease activity (Smyth *et al.*, 1999), improved physical functioning, and reduced pain and affective disturbance (Kelley *et al.*, 1997). Along similar lines, Ishii *et al.* (2003) evaluated neuroendocrine and immune responses in peripheral blood following psychological stress induced by deep emotion in RA patients. Patients who were moved to tears were those whose condition was more easily controlled (by medication) than those who were emotionally affected but were not moved to tears. This could indicate that being less able to disclose emotion has an adverse effect on neuroendocrine and immune responses. Following earlier work showing that structured writing about stressful events can alleviate symptoms among people with RA, Stone *et al.* (2000) conducted a secondary data analysis to determine whether the process of writing mediated perceived stress, quality of sleep, affect, substance use and medication. There was no evidence of mediation; thus, the mechanism through which writing about stressful events can improve disease symptomatology remains unknown.

Dekkers *et al.* (2001) set out to investigate the potential mediating and moderating roles of social support, coping and physiological variables in the relationship between life events and health status. The sample comprised 54 RA patients with disease duration of < 12 months (38 women, 16 men, and mean age 56, SD 14.4). Although life events (major life events and daily hassles) correlated with psychological distress, there was no association between life events and disease activity (i.e. ESR – erythrocyte sedimentation rate – a blood test that indicates inflammation, or pain). The authors conclude that disease activity in this group of newly diagnosed patients may have been low and suggest that this fact may account for the absence of a relationship between life events and disease activity. Indeed, there was no evidence of mediation or moderation by any of the social support, coping or physiological variables included in the study. Clearly, there is further work to be done in clarifying the precise nature of the relationship between immune parameters and stressful events, particularly in relation to identifying protective mechanisms.

A meta-analysis of 56 publications by Geenen *et al.* (2006) aimed to better understand the potential impact of stressors on health status in RA, including the hypothalamic-pituitary-adrenal (HPA) axis and the autonomic nervous system (ANS). The HPA and ANS are both involved in inflammation and are activated by stress. One of the main findings was that major life events do not always affect disease status but may modify disease activity either positively or negatively depending upon the nature, duration and dose of the physiological stress response. Furthermore, following brief, naturalistic stressors, both self-perceived and clinicians' ratings of disease activity increased. Finally, enduring stressors (e.g. work-related or interpersonal) are associated with perceived health.

Overall, there appears to be consistent evidence of linkages between stressful events and more severe symptomatology, with variables such as social support acting as a buffer for adverse effects. In addition, personality studies suggest that being able to express emotions, such as anger, may assist wellbeing. Finding 'safe' ways to express powerful emotions can be difficult. How to deal with emotions and communicate one's feelings to family and friends is included in some multi-component interventions (see Chapter 8). Other strategies have included encouraging patients to release their feelings through the written word.

One issue likely to become more salient in the field of arthritis concerns the implications of genetic screening. Hereditary factors have been identified and associated with certain forms of arthritis (e.g. RA, AS), a fact reflected in anxiety about 'passing on' arthritis to children and grandchildren among adults with these conditions (Barlow & Cullen, 1996). Indeed, some families consider the hereditary risk 'too great', and decide not to have children at all (J.H. Barlow, Cullen, Foster, Harrison & Wade, 1999). Such issues have received little attention in the arthritis literature.

Diagnosis

One difficulty in diagnosing many forms of arthritis is the similarities between disease and psychological symptomatology. Intermittent pain, fatigue and sleep disturbance can be symptoms of both arthritis and depression. Thus acquiring a medical label for one's condition can be delayed, particularly where blood tests are not clear diagnostic indicators. Equally, the overlap of symptoms can work in the opposite direction, masking psychological distress. Hence, some people with arthritis may not receive appropriate physiological or psychological care when needed. Poor detection of major depressive disorder occurs when symptoms (e.g. fatigue) are attributed to RA and the possibility of concurrent psychological disorder is not considered (Creed & Ash, 1992). The authors of a study of depression in AS concluded that such oversights are not limited to RA, but can occur in other forms of arthritis (J. Barlow, Macey & Struthers, 1993).

A long delay between onset of symptoms and medical diagnosis is a characteristic of AS and is associated with greater disease severity and functional impairment (J.H. Barlow & Barefoot, 1996). Although issues of causality remain to be clarified, this set of variables (i.e. severity, functional impairment and diagnostic delay) is inversely related to performance of therapeutic exercise. It may be that waiting several years for a diagnosis leads to increased motivation to carry out treatment recommendations when finally being given a diagnostic label for one's condition. Alternatively, those with greater disease severity and worse functional outcomes may be more motivated to exercise compared with peers with a lesser degree of symptomatology. During the pre-diagnostic period people with AS are often considered 'neurotic' (Dekker-Saeys, 1976), and can be informed that pain, stiffness and fatigue are 'all in the mind', and do not have an organic cause. The impact of being given such opinions during the delay between symptom onset and diagnosis has not been fully examined. Contact with health professionals during this pre-diagnostic period appears to remain a source of unresolved anger and frustration for many decades after disease onset has occurred.

Delays in obtaining a diagnosis and subsequent medical care are not limited to adults, but have been reported by some parents of children with JIA (J. Barlow, Harrison & Shaw, 1998). Parents participating in focus groups recounted that the time between onset of symptoms and receiving a diagnosis was fraught with difficulties. Many parents reported that diagnoses had been 'slow' and in some cases their children's symptoms had been either 'missed' or 'dismissed'. Parents' experiences during this pre-diagnostic period had remained a source of anger and frustration, even where subsequent care was believed to be 'excellent'.

> Nicole was two and a half, her knees were swollen and bright red and she wasn't walking. There was something wrong with her. I didn't know what … I kept taking her to the doctor and in the end, the doctor told me I was a neurotic Mum. He said 'take your child home. There's nothing wrong with her.' (Mother)

> We nearly lost our son because the doctor said there was nothing wrong with him. He nearly died. (Father)

Delay in obtaining access to appropriate care for children presenting with musculoskeletal symptoms was investigated among 152 patients with JIA in a UK setting. (Foster *et al.*, 2007). The median time between onset of symptoms and first referral for a paediatric rheumatology multidisciplinary team assessment was 20 weeks, although the minimum was zero and the maximum was 416 weeks. In addition, 18 (11.8 per cent) of the children had been referred to multiple, secondary care specialities and had undergone multiple procedures, some of which were invasive (e.g. arthroscopy or synovial biopsy) and likely to be distressing for both child and family. However, none of these 18 children had been referred for ophthalmologic screening, physical therapy, or nursing input, and a diagnosis of JIA was rarely made. These children had untreated active disease at initial assessment by the paediatric rheumatology team.

Duration

The onset of arthritis can be a time of stress and uncertainty for the individual and their family. For many, obtaining a diagnosis can remove the uncertainty of unexplained symptoms, thereby reducing anxiety.

Nonetheless, patients have to come to terms with the fact that they have a painful, long-term condition characterised by a fluctuating disease course and an unpredictable prognosis. In this situation, one set of anxiety-provoking factors can be replaced by another. For example, Eberhardt *et al.* (1993), found that, two years after diagnosis, 33 per cent of RA patients had stopped working and 16 per cent had changed their pattern of work. The implications of such social and economic losses on lifestyle and psychological wellbeing are likely to be manifold. Sharpe *et al.* (2001) compared people with early RA (< 2 years' duration) with a chronic disease group of over two years' duration, and showed that the early RA group reported less disturbance on activity (70 versus 96 per cent), social life (49 versus 80 per cent), relationships (42 versus 61 per cent) and emotions (42 versus 61 per cent). However, the early group reported greater disturbance of appearance (34 versus 11 per cent), and finances (32 versus 20 per cent). Regarding the latter, it is likely that those recently diagnosed may need time off work whilst symptoms and disease are brought under control through treatment. This may explain percep-tions of greater impact on finance. Furthermore, the first experience of swollen joints may cause attention to be focused on the body and how others perceive it, hence the greater impact on appearance. Regardless, the proportions reporting disturbance suggest that, even at this early stage, the power of RA to interfere with various aspects of life is immense.

The influence of disease duration on psychosocial wellbeing, patient knowledge and coping ability has attracted attention from the research community and healthcare practitioners alike. Much of this attention has focused on people with RA. Healthcare practitioners can perceive newly diagnosed patients as more anxious and distressed than patients of more established disease duration and often attribute this difference to the increased coping ability of patients who have had many years to become accustomed to the dictates of arthritis and its treatment.

Understanding the relationship between disease duration and psychological wellbeing has centred largely on depression, with find-ings providing a somewhat mixed picture. Two studies report a rela-tionship between shorter disease duration and increased levels of depression in RA (Chaney *et al.*, 1996; Newman *et al.*, 1989). In contrast, Meenan *et al.* (1991) failed to find any differences in psychological distress between recently diagnosed RA patients and those with more established disease. Similarly, research in the US on people with recent onset RA suggests that the level of psychological distress equals that found in people with more established disease (Serbo & Jajic, 1991). Moreover, a study conducted in Sweden showed that psychological distress appears to remain fairly stable over a two-year period following diagnosis (Smedstad *et al.*, 1997). Similarly, Krol *et al.* (1998) showed that self-esteem among RA patients of < 4 years' duration remained stable over 12 months. One of the few studies to focus primarily on anxiety found no association between either state or trait anxiety and disease duration among people with RA living in the USA (van Dyke *et al.*, 2004). However, as may be expected, there was an association between depression and anxiety. A UK study of outpatients with RA (J.H. Barlow, Cullen & Rowe, 1999) adds further support to these findings: levels of depressed and anxious mood did not significantly differ between those with short (under one year) or longer (over one year) disease duration. In addition to depressed and anxious mood, the authors tested the hypothesis that beliefs about disease acceptance may differ between those whose disease was recently diagnosed versus those whose disease was of longer duration. A general measure of acceptance of illness (Felson *et al.*, 1984) was used to assess disease acceptance beliefs. Contrary to predictions, no significant differences were found in the degree of illness acceptance among those with short versus longer duration. Moreover, despite having considerably more experience of living with RA, patients with more established disease had similar levels of RA knowledge relative to patients of short disease duration. The desire for more education about RA and its wider impact was clearly expressed by all patients regardless of age or disease duration. (Patient education is discussed in more detail in Chapter 7).

Research on the relationship between disease duration and psychological distress conducted by Evers *et al.* (1997) offers some insight. A number of risk factors for psychological distress over a one-year period among newly diagnosed RA patients were identified. A decrease in distress was associated with being male, having less severe inflammatory activity at disease onset, and being part of a more extended social network at disease onset. A prospective study examined the relationship between psychological distress and traditional clinical variables over a two-year period. Smedstad *et al.* (1997) found that high levels of physical disability predicted an increase in depression during the following year, whilst other disease-related variables did not contribute to predictions of change in psychological distress. However, overall levels of psychological distress were relatively stable over time. A prospective, longitudinal study of early RA patients (< 4 years' duration) across three countries (The Netherlands, Norway and France) showed that their quality of life was at risk (Suurmeijer *et al.*, 2001). Interestingly, fatigue emerged as the aspect of RA that differentiated on disability, psychological wellbeing, social support and global health; the next most influential aspects were pain and swollen joints, with ESR showing least differentiating ability. This work is important, as it emphasises the salience of fatigue in the patient's experience of arthritis and its outcomes even among those whose disease is of relatively short duration. In general, much attention is paid to managing pain, whereas fatigue is relatively neglected and may not be resolved by taking prescribed medication. Clearly, more work is needed to identify patients with arthritis who are at most risk of psychological distress in order for appropriate interventions to be provided. Equally, patients need assistance in learning how to manage the critical symptom of fatigue not just in those with established disease but from the point of diagnosis onwards.

The issue of disease duration has rarely been examined in JIA. One exception is a study by Mullick *et al.* (2005) showing that longer duration of JIA was associated with a higher proportion of psychiatric disorders, including depression. It has been suggested that newly diagnosed adolescents are at increased risk of psychosocial distress (e.g. Daltroy *et al.*, 1992; Timko, Stovel, Moos & Miller, 1992). For example, Ennett *et al.* (1991) suggest that, compared to younger children, adolescents are more likely to have emotional problems and poor social competence. Furthermore, Billings *et al.* (1987) found adolescents to have more absences from school and less participation in family and peer activities. There may be gender differences, with behavioural problems being more prevalent among older boys (Daltroy *et al.*, 1992) and greater distress and fewer health-risk behaviours being found among girls (Timko, Stovel & Moos, 1992). Other authors have failed to find a gender effect.

Chapter Summary

Personality and stress have been proposed as possible causal factors involved in the onset of arthritis. Although there is little evidence of an association between personality traits and arthritis, there are indications that traits such as optimism may be linked to more positive psychosocial adjustment, whilst greater symptom reporting may be linked to neuroticism. In relation to stress, there appears to be consistent evidence of linkages between stressful events and more severe symptomatology, with variables such as social support acting as a buffer for adverse effects. In addition, personality studies suggest that being able to express emotions such as anger may assist wellbeing.

Delay between onset of symptoms and diagnosis may be more prevalent among types of arthritis with an early age of onset such as JIA and AS. The distress experienced by the individual and their family during this pre-diagnostic period has received little research attention, and psychological intervention may be needed to assist those affected in resolving any distress, anger and fear.

Much of the research on the influence of duration has focused on RA. In sum, the levels of psychological distress and arthritis knowledge among patients with RA do not appear to be greatly influenced by disease duration. As may be expected, those with more established disease tend to be older, have fewer educational qualifications, greater physical disability and higher co-morbidity. The findings of studies comparing patients with recent onset versus those with more established disease appear to suggest that a proportion of patients have psychological morbidity from the point of diagnosis onwards. Longitudinal studies following patients over 10, 20 or more years are needed in order to clarify the apparent persistence of psychological distress over the course of disease.

Regardless of the level of psychological distress, research has consistently shown that pain and physical functioning are important correlates of depression. This relationship is constant among RA patients with less than one-year disease duration (van der Heide *et al.*, 1994), among patients with up to three years' disease duration (Nicassio & Wallston, 1992) and among patients with established disease of more than 10 years' duration (Newman *et al.*, 1989). The robustness of this relationship suggests that pain management and perceptions of disability are important correlates of arthritis that demand attention from psychologists in the search to enhance the wellbeing of people with arthritis irrespective of disease duration.

4

Life with Arthritis

Understanding patients' experiences and perceptions about arthritis and its treatment is important for healthcare professionals, educators and researchers. Survey research has documented key life domains affected by arthritis, including psychological wellbeing (Anderson et al., 1985), social wellbeing (Fitzpatrick et al., 1991; Revenson et al., 1991), family relationships (J. Barlow, Macey & Struthers, 1993; J.H. Barlow, Cullen et al., 1999), employment (J. Barlow, Wright & Kroll, 2001; Lubeck, 1995), and restrictions in daily functioning and loss of independence (Taal, Johannes, et al., 1993). Survey research is of value in presenting evidence of the frequency and level of distress using standard measuring instruments that facilitate comparisons across studies and types of arthritis. However, greater insight into the range of experiences of arthritis is provided by qualitative studies that are grounded in the perceptions of people living with the condition. Indeed, Conrad (1990) asserts that the 'subtleties' and 'personal meanings' inherent in chronic illness are best investigated using qualitative methods. The aim is to increase understanding and to generate theoretical perspectives rather than to test theories. In the past, few researchers in the field of psychosocial rheumatology have adopted this approach, although recently there appears to have been a growing appreciation of the valuable insights provided by qualitative research and a greater willingness to accept its findings within the fields of both psychology and medicine. Studies combining quantitative and qualitative methods may have helped to pave the way in this regard. For example, interviews can provide useful insight regarding unexpected findings arising from a survey, or can inform development of an item pool when developing a new quantitative measure. In addition, there is increased pressure on healthcare professionals and providers to take account of 'consumer' views, including those of children. In keeping with this ethos, this chapter incorporates quotes from people with arthritis to exemplify key points and to enable readers to place their own interpretation on the ideas presented. One man's arthritis journey is presented in the Appendix. Many of the findings and insights presented in this chapter have arisen from studies that have set out to explore what it is like to live with arthritis. Thus, issues that emerge are those that are meaningful and memorable for respondents. Such issues tend to have a negative connotation revolving about the adverse impact of arthritis in respondents' lives. It can be hard for people with arthritis to recount any positive aspects of life, even in response to direct questions.

The onset of long-term conditions such as arthritis has been described as a 'biographical disruption', thus emphasising the adverse impact that such conditions can have on a person's life (Bury, 1991). People with arthritis have to deal with a continual flow of disruptions linked to the nature of the disease, its treatment and consequences that can have far-reaching implications for the quality of their lives. For example, arthritis is neither preventable nor curable by medical or behavioural interventions. It can follow an unpredictable disease course, with periods of spontaneous flare-up and remission, and often has an uncertain prognosis. Weiner (1975) suggests that RA patients are 'haunted' by uncertainty, hoping for extended periods of remission whilst concurrently aware of the likelihood of deterioration. The uncertainty of arthritis means that planning long-term activities is difficult since people are unable to predict how they will feel in the future. Even short-term planning can be fraught with worry and anxiety if symptomatology is highly variable from one day to the next, or even within the same day. Thus, uncertainty is a key aspect of arthritis that has to be resolved by people living with the condition.

Lay people tend to mix together descriptions of symptoms (e.g. pain, fatigue) with the impact of those symptoms on daily life (e.g. what they can or cannot do) and their resultant feelings about this disruption to their lives. Thus the following sections covering symptoms, emotional reactions, social issues and coping are not mutually exclusive.

Disease Symptomatology and Impact

Pain can dominate life for many people with arthritis. Toye (2003) interviewed 18 participants with osteoarthritis who were on a waiting-list for total knee replacement but scored low in terms of disease burden on a widely used, numerically based scoring system. Despite scoring low on disease burden, one man described being 'racked with pain' 24 hours a day such that he felt he could not do anything and the 'value' of his life had disappeared. He concluded by commenting that there's a 'lot to be said for this euthanasia'.

A study of 86 people with knee OA (mean age 61) in the UK confirmed the importance of pain as a major symptom (Tallon *et al.*, 2000), and showed that disability, instability of the knee joint and anxiety about knee OA were additional sources of distress for many patients. Pain emerged as a primary concern for participants in a longitudinal study by Turner *et al.* (2002) based on a sample of six people (four women, two men) with a median age of 53 (range 45–59) and a median disease duration of 22 years (range 5–24). Three respondents had OA, two had RA and one had AS. The sample was interviewed at three points in time over a six-month period, giving a total of 18 interviews, consistent with the prevailing trend among qualitative interview studies (i.e. 15 ± 10; Kavale, 1996). One woman described her battle with pain as a '24 hour long fight' and another expressed a preference for the pain of childbirth to the pain of arthritis:

> There is pain in childbirth and there is the pain of arthritis and given the two, I would have the childbirth pain any day. The pain in arthritis is such a weird pain to describe. The inflammation is all over you more or less and when it is in a joint, it is so severe it doesn't let up. Continual aggravation and pain! (Female respondent) (Turner *et al.*, 2002)

Although the salience of pain in the lives of people with arthritis cannot be denied, stiffness, fatigue and swollen joints add to the experience of daily life for many. Indeed, fatigue appears to be a major factor that interferes with daily living and can leave people 'too tired' to go out socially in the evenings, to interact with other family members or even to accomplish simple but necessary tasks such as eating and getting dressed.

> Even to go into the wardrobe and sort a few clothes is a mountainous task. Even light clothes because you have to put effort into getting things off the hanger and that is all exhausting. (Female respondent) (Turner *et al.*, 2002)

> Up until the end of May this year I was working full-time. I would come home and I was not fit to do anything else. In fact, sometimes, I was even too tired to eat. (Female respondent) (Turner *et al.*, 2002)

The fatigue of arthritis can form the major challenge in relation to working life. Several participants with AS interviewed by J.H. Barlow, Wright, Williams and Keat (2001) had difficulty 'making it to the end of the day', let alone the end of the week. In addition, fatigue was felt to threaten psychological wellbeing, home life, social life and leisure activities. Combating fatigue during working hours used up all reserves of energy. Consequently, participants were 'too tired to do anything' when they got home.

> I was finding it extremely difficult to cope with the fatigue, to the point where I would be fighting to stay awake during the afternoon. (Male respondent) (J.H. Barlow *et al.*, 2001)

> 'A busy day's work with AS, is like a busy week without AS. Evenings are only rest periods, with no energy left for amusements.' (Male respondent; J.H. Barlow *et al.*, 2001)

The above quote describes a situation that has consistently emerged in almost two decades of interviewing people with AS. Many are able to remain at work but bear the cost in terms of lack of energy to interact with family and friends outside of working life.

Emotional Reactions and Activity Restrictions

Interestingly, many people do not appear to view arthritis as an illness *per se*. Use of terms such as 'nuisance' and inconvenience' is in keeping with conceptualisations of arthritis as a biographical disruption (i.e. an uninvited interruption to the individual's life). The realities of living with arthritis are often described in terms of adverse emotional reactions, such as 'anger', 'frustration', 'nuisance' and feeling 'out of control' (e.g. Turner *et al.*, 2002). Toye (2003) reports a male participant who believes that his pain has turned him into a 'pain' and can be the cause of family breakdown. In a qualitative study of 32 patients attending a GP surgery with suspected RA they described their condition as an 'inconvenience' and, interestingly, few viewed themselves as 'ill'

(Donovan *et al.*, 1989). The distinction between arthritis-related symptoms and common illnesses (e.g. colds and flu) appears to be prevalent across many types of arthritis.

Feelings of anger are attributed to the restrictions that arthritis places on daily activities and leisure pursuits (i.e. loss of valued activities). For example, among people living with AS, activities that can be problematic include driving (due to difficulties turning one's head), carrying groceries, and having energy for leisure pursuits (Dagfinrud *et al.*, 2005). Lack of energy may have been connected with interrupted sleep, which was reported as one of the most frequent problem areas. Such difficulties can result in restriction of valued and routine activities, which in turn can result in a sense of loss and independence. The notion of having to rely on others, in particular partners, is keenly felt and leads to considerable frustration when people with arthritis are no longer able to carry out simple, routine tasks, such as housework, decorating, gardening and nurturing activities. A phenomenological explanation of living with RA refers to the difficulties of coping and the frustration at not being able to carry out daily activities (Ryan, 1996). This frustration leads to feelings of guilt, when other family members are forced to take over what are usually regarded as simple tasks (e.g. making a cup of tea).

The sense of loss associated with arthritis surfaces in many forms. For example, one woman felt that arthritis had 'robbed' her of her forthcoming retirement years (Turner *et al.*, 2002). She was angry that she would not be able to do the things that she had 'always longed to' when she retired and had been forced to reassess her retirement plans. Loss also emerges in relation to the gradual limitation on physical activities that can accompany progression of the disease. For example, people with arthritis cannot always continue valued leisure activities such as sports, dancing and swimming. Even the effort to get ready to go out can be too much, thus social interaction becomes less frequent and social network size reduces. Loss of valued activities due to arthritis reduces the sense of control that people have over their lives.

> I used to do a lot of sport and I had to give up all sports. I have had to give up work now and it is like life closing down, basically. You have fewer and fewer opportunities … (Turner *et al.*, 2002)

Ryan (1996) linked the physical limitations imposed by arthritis, the alteration in social roles and subsequent isolation to negative perceptions of self-esteem. A slightly different perspective is provided by Plach *et al.* (2004). They interviewed 20 women living with RA and conceptualised the physical limitations and changes to women's bodies as 'corporeality', which literally means 'being one's body'. Three themes were identified: a noncompliant body, a body out of synch and private body made public. The notion of having a body that does not conform, does not quite fit with the norm and suffering from a disease that has effects that are visible to all suggests that individuals may perceive a lack of control in their lives.

Given the number of losses involved in living with arthritis and lack of perceived control, it is not surprising to find that episodes of depression feature in the illness experience of many. Vulnerability to depressed mood has been reported in quantitative studies (see Chapter 5). Depressed mood can be temporary and follow on from initial diagnosis, a disease flare or loss of valued activity due to the physical restrictions imposed by progressive deterioration of affected joints. A few people appear to suffer extreme mood disturbance resulting in clinical depression and suicidal thoughts. The latter is illustrated in the following extract from an interview with an ex-professional footballer (aged 70), who has OA in both hips and was diagnosed at the age of 38. The importance of having a supportive partner is emphasised.

> I was very nearly suicidal and if it had not been for my wife, who knows what would have happened! I was very bitter about the way that football had treated me, or the way the football clubs I played for treated me. Lack of treatment, lack of information about pensions etc. and lack of interest in general about our futures and certainly lack of interest in our health. ...
> It is hard to describe the lack of mobility when you are young, not able to play games with your children, not to be able to dance with my wife. More mundane things – not being able to fasten shoelaces, can't put my socks on, can't lift feet to get trousers on, more embarrassing! Can't wash properly, can't reach your feet, can't sit on the toilet properly, believe me the list is endless. I still can't do a lot of these things even after the operations (hip replacements), but they have been life-saving. Unfortunately, I still was not able to work. So financially, it's been a struggle not having worked since I was 54. I had to leave my chosen trade through OA and work in a factory even though this was totally against my nature. I was unable to keep my quality of life money-wise. Simply because I could not earn the same amount I was able to earn at me trade and this meant I had to rely on a very understanding and helpful wife. (Turner, 2001)

This narrative exemplifies the links between gradual loss of simple everyday tasks that the majority of us take for granted (e.g. getting dressed, self-care) and the impact that such losses can have on psychological wellbeing, especially in an individual who is relatively young with a career in sport. The importance of a supportive, partner and family, who really understand the perspectives of the individual with arthritis, is emphasised. This short extract of one man's story of life with OA illustrates not only the wider impact of enforced changes to working life but also the impact of subsequent financial adjustments on the family as a whole. The difficulty of securing alternative employment featured consistently throughout the Turner study and is further exemplified in the following quote from a 50-year-old ex-professional footballer who developed OA in the right ankle following an injury.

> I eventually went to College (which I funded) and acquired an engineering qualification. I am now a draughtsman. Over the last two and a half years, I have had no rises due to my incapacity and have had to have extended periods of absence – 3 to 4 months – constant outpatient visits for many years. All in all, my general standard of living has been affected for many years. Since my first operation in 1989, it is not only myself but my family that have suffered greatly, having to care for me. My wife has to miss work at times. (Turner, 2001)

Loss of independence in relation to enforced changes in working lives can result in negative emotional reactions including depressed mood, frustration, bitterness, anger, mood swings, feelings of inadequacy, and loss of choice, self-esteem, self-confidence and job satisfaction. People can become anxious about their sickness record, their employability, and providing for themselves and their family in the future. A sense of being 'vulnerable' in relation to work can manifest as guilt or working harder in order to compensate for perceived shortcomings. Financial limitations through loss of earnings and the purchase of costly assistive devices (e.g. computer for communicating, automatic car for independence) are common concerns. This point is illustrated in the following quote.

> Working voluntarily and claiming benefits rather than being able to return to full-time employment has imprisoned me in a financial straitjacket. I know that I am set in a standard of living from which there is no escape and no hope of improvement. (J.H. Barlow, Wright, Williams & Keat, 2001)

Social Issues

Social comparisons

As in other long-term conditions, people with arthritis compare themselves to others in order to assess the degree of seriousness of their condition. Comparisons can be upwards or downwards. When first
attending an outpatient clinic, comparisons are typically downwards in
that fellow patients in the waiting room may be those with more established disease, greater disease progression and the likelihood of visible
changes to the physical body (e.g. swollen hands, hunched posture,
nodules on fingers). A minority of people with arthritis choose not to
attend meetings set up by voluntary organisations or group exercise
sessions for similar reasons (i.e. they anticipate that it will be difficult to
see people with the same condition who are worse than themselves).
Ryan (1996) raised the issue of seeing other inpatients with more
advanced disease during hospital admission and noted how patients
wondered whether they would have similar experiences, such as
becoming a wheelchair-user.

In other social settings, the individual may have a choice about
whether to compare upwards or downwards. Blalock, deVellis and
deVellis (1989) found that, of RA patients offered information about
other patients, 90 per cent chose to learn more about those with pain
greater than their own. However, when the topic of information was
coping ability, as may be expected, the majority chose to learn about
those who were coping well. Patients with RA compared themselves
not only to other patients but also to people without illness. When the
focus was on types of performance that patients found difficult (e.g.
writing, tying shoelaces) other patients disabled with RA were used.
When the performances concerned areas that patients had no difficulties with, other people without RA were used. Furthermore, if they
used similar others or those who were worse as comparators, patients
remained satisfied with their performance even where their perceived
ability was poor. Skevington (1994) reported similar findings in a qualitative study examining judgements about quality of life. Further support derives from a study by Affleck and Tennen (1991), who concluded
that RA patients compared themselves favourably with a 'typical' RA
patient, perceiving themselves as less severe than average and better
adjusted than average. Interestingly, those who believed themselves to

be better able to control their emotions, remain optimistic and keep physically active were also judged to be better adjusted by health carers.

Social network and relationships

People with arthritis can feel that others in their social network (i.e. family and friends) have little insight into the condition and the impact on the individual's way of living. People with arthritis often report that other family members have the same expectations of them in relation to family roles that they had before disease onset. Thus, family members seem to ignore the fact that the individual has a long-term, limiting condition that causes pain and restricted activities. People with arthritis talk of being expected to 'be there' for children and grandchildren regardless of their own wellbeing. Further, some suggest the full ramifications of their disease are largely ignored until they need hospital admission or are unable to carry out a social engagement so that their condition ultimately impacts on other family members. Paradoxically, many people are reluctant to burden their families, especially elderly parents, with arthritis-related needs. Friends are viewed in much the same light. Many people with arthritis find it difficult to communicate their needs and how they feel to either family or friends.

> I don't think friends really understand your problem. They tend to switch off, shut up or evade the subject if you talk about your problem. They feel embarrassed for you. It is very, very difficult. (Turner *et al.*, 2002)

The reluctance to seek emotional and practical support outside of the immediate family can be viewed as an attempt to minimise the threat to 'psychological tolerating' of the disease (Weiner, 1975). Eliciting assistance from non-family members may increase fears of becoming a burden (Weiner, 1975) or being rejected (Bury, 1991). Morgan (1989), in his examination of the relationship between social support and disability, found that the inability to foster support might result in further health deterioration and increased social isolation. Help-seeking tends to be focused on family and friends known to be responsive and understanding. The importance of receiving the right kind of support has been illustrated by Riemsma *et al.* (1998), who found that problematic social support (defined as lack of sympathy or understanding from social networks) was associated with higher fatigue levels among patients with RA. In recognition of the importance of social support, some arthritis education courses encourage family members to attend (e.g. J.H. Barlow & Barefoot, 1996). One of the hidden benefits of group interventions lies in the immediacy of an available social network whose members have an innate understanding of the demands of living with arthritis (J. Barlow, Cullen, Davis & Williams, 1997). Interview data from group interventions for people with arthritis illustrate this point:

> It was good to be able to talk about pain to people who could understand what you are going through … to find all the feelings, anger and frustration were normal. (Turner *et al.*, 2002)

Through the sharing of experiences with similar others, people with arthritis appear to find a way of normalising their feelings and moving forward to a more positive outlook. They realise that they are not 'odd' or difficult because they feel angry, frustrated or depressed. More importantly, through the sharing of experiences and coping strategies, group participants often find a way of breaking out of a negative cycle. Given that social isolation can be a common correlate of arthritis, finding an appropriate and easily accessible peer group is not always easy. This is where group education programmes have a valuable role to play as they offer an instant peer group with a commonality of experiences.

Resistance to Disruption

People with arthritis have a strong desire to live a 'normal life' despite their awareness of the potential, adverse consequences. Indeed, a qualitative exploration of outcomes perceived to be important by 10 women living with RA included perceptions of normality along with taking charge and the future (McPherson *et al.*, 2001).

The desire to live a normal life manifests in many ways. For example, at times of disease remission or mild symptomatology, people describe 'lunatic' days, doing valued activities, such as gardening or dancing at weddings, even though the pain next day can resemble 'torture'. A mood of 'sheer stubbornness' or 'not giving in' enables some people to keep going despite feeling unwell (Turner *et al.*, 2002). Weiner describes this phenomenon as 'normalising'; that is, the person proceeds with an activity as if it were essential and as if arthritis was absent. A few people appear to engage in 'supernormalising', vigorously capitalising on symptom-free periods as a means of denying incapacity or recapturing their identity before they developed arthritis. The desire to remain active demonstrated by people with arthritis was noted by Locker (1983), who used the term 'keeping going', whereas Weiner describes the phenomenon as 'keeping up'. The activity accounts reported by people with arthritis involve both private and persistent activities (e.g. housework – 'keeping going') and more public, social activities (e.g. social events – 'keeping up'). Regardless of terminology, the importance attributed to the maintenance of a semblance of 'normal' physical activities suggests a strong desire to maintain or regain control by not letting the condition totally dominate all aspects of life.

In keeping with resistance to disruption, people with arthritis rarely view themselves as 'disabled'. Indeed, use of the word 'disabled' provokes negative emotions such as feeling 'sad', 'depressed', 'scared', 'useless', 'angry', and 'embarrassed' (J. Barlow & Williams, 1999). However, being disabled is used instrumentally in order to obtain benefits or car-park badges, for example.

> I will never say to anyone that I am disabled unless the situation calls for it. I will only admit that I am disabled to official people. (J. Barlow & Williams 1999)

Self-management and finding hope

Over the course of disease, people begin to learn what helps their condition and what exacerbates it, developing their own unique approach to self-management. Kralik *et al.* (2004) view self-management as central to the process of transition, whereby people incorporate the consequences of their illness into their lives. They investigated how nine people living with arthritis constructed the notion of self-management through written autobiographies and telephone interviews. Participants viewed self-management as a process initiated to create order. Four key themes emerged:

- recognising and monitoring the boundaries;
- mobilising resources;

- managing the shift in identity;
- balancing, pacing, planning and prioritising.

People learned to self-manage through a process of trial and error.

Several interview-based studies have investigated the nature of self-management strategies used by people with arthritis who have not attended formal psycho-educational interventions. For example, 13 elders interviewed by Tak (2006) managed the stresses of living with arthritis through the use of three main strategies: cognitive efforts, distraction and assertive actions. Additional self-management strategies identified by Taylor (2001) in an interview-based study included ensuring personal comfort, using gadgets, planning ahead, trying alternative treatments, keeping a positive attitude, acknowledging feelings, having emotional support, and facilitating self-awareness. Similarly, we have noted a number of methods used to manage daily life including pacing, relaxation, religious worship and distraction techniques (Turner *et al.*, 2002).

> Since giving up work I have been able to pace myself so when I am tired I don't try to push on. I can now sit down and have a rest and I can now get through a whole day and a whole evening … (Turner *et al.*, 2002)

An insight into the perceptions of people with OA is provided by Hampson *et al.* (1994) in a study conducted in the US with data collected via structured interviews. The personal models of OA and their relationship to self-management activities were explored among 61 patients with OA (mean age 72, SD 7.8) who attended the clinic of one rheumatologist. Results showed that this group of older people believed their condition to be fairly serious and chronic, although amenable to control by one or more treatments recommended by their healthcare practitioner. Not surprisingly, patients who viewed their condition as more serious reported greater use of medical services and self-management activities and had a poorer quality of life. In accord with previous studies, patients viewed pain as the major symptom of OA and used it to assess the seriousness of their condition.

Ryan (1996) described the feelings of uncertainty that can arise among people with RA when families fail to respond positively to patients' attempts to adopt self-management strategies. For example, pacing activities involves acceptance of the need to alternate between periods of rest and activity. Other family members may interpret rest as being lazy. Such findings emphasise the need for patients and families to communicate effectively; part of being a successful self-manager is being able to express one's needs in a given situation and at a given point in time and to mobilise the support needed.

A different approach was adopted by Loffer (2000) in her examination of the views of women self-identified as 'thriving with the adversities of RA'. The journey to a better life encompassed five themes. First, women embarked on a journey of rediscovery whereby they examined their old belief systems and created new meaning and fulfilment. Second, women took control of what they could and educated themselves to make choices in their own best interests. Third, they made linkages and built themselves a support system of personal, professional and spiritual connections that counterbalanced the isolation of RA. Fourth, they achieved a perspective of their journey that allowed acceptance of life with chronic illness whilst still cultivating hope and optimism through the use of perseverance, humour, gratitude and aspirations for better lives. Finally, they shared what they had learned with others who also had chronic illness. This study is somewhat unique in seeking out women who felt they were thriving despite RA. Many of the emergent themes resonate with the approaches adopted in interventions for people arthritis discussed in Chapter 8. Of particular note is the concept of sharing with similar others, which is a recurrent theme through many evaluation studies in psychosocial rheumatology.

A naturalistic study of the nature, meaning and impact of suffering experienced by people with RA also found that there were positive outcomes. Dildy (1992) collected data from 14 people with RA via interviews, field notes, memos and socio-demographic data sheets. Using grounded theory and the constant comparative method, Dildy identified a social psychological process of suffering comprising three phases: disintegration of the self, the shattered self and reconstruction of self. During disintegration, participants felt intense fear about the future particularly of becoming 'a cripple'. During the second phase (the shattered self), participants dealt with suffering including pain, mental anguish, activity limitation and exhaustion. During the final phase of reconstruction, a more positive mindset was adopted, suffering and hopelessness were diminished, and acceptance was attained. Thus, although living with RA encompassed a struggle, lost dreams, restricted future and withdrawal, participants had found meaning through positive life changes including re-evaluation of their life trajectory, increased sensitivity and spiritual growth.

Positive mood was identified in an investigation of the role of daily spirituality. Data were collected via structured diaries over a period of 30 days among a sample of 35 people living with RA (Keefe *et al.*, 2001). Participants who reported frequent spiritual experiences, such as feeling touched by the beauty of creation or wanting to be closer to God, reported using more spiritual and religious coping strategies and also had a more positive mood and social support, and a less negative mood compared to those who did not report such frequent spiritual experiences.

Children with JIA and their Parents

Arthritis is not only an issue for the individual with the disease but also for other members of the family unit who 'live' with arthritis. When onset of disease occurs during childhood, the impact of arthritis quickly permeates the lives of parents, siblings and members of the extended family (e.g. grandparents, aunts, and uncles). However, there are few studies of JIA from the perspectives of children or their parents. One exception is a study based on focus group methodology reported in J. Barlow, Harrison and Shaw (1998) and J.H. Barlow, Shaw and Harrison (1999). Focus groups can provide access to the disability perspective of the whole family (Oliver, 1992) and offer insight into the world of those who live with the reality of chronic childhood disease. Hence, focus-group discussion was selected as a method that would enable participants to raise issues that they felt were important, rather than issues determined by the researchers. This approach ensured that the voices of children and parents could be given free expression in describing life with JIA.

Box 4.1 Methodological Note: Focus Groups

The focus group is described as a group interview that seeks to capitalise on communications between participants in order to generate data (Kitzinger, 1995). Since attitudes and opinions are both formed and articulated within a social context, focus groups provide an interactive dynamic for developing, challenging and refining ideas.

Box 4.1 (cont'd)

By actively engendering a permissive atmosphere, focus-group methodology aims to generate a situation whereby a more complete and thorough understanding of key issues is obtained (Vaughan *et al.*, 1996).

Compared to the normally passive role assumed by research participants, the focus group offers a more empowering experience for all involved (Harrison & Barlow, 1996). Focus groups typically consist of six to eight people who meet to discuss a topic of common interest. The discussion is guided by a moderator, who facilitates the flow of verbal exchange whilst maintaining the focus of discussants on the designated topic. Focus-group discussions are usually between 60 and 120 minutes in length, although duration can be shorter when the group is comprised of children. During the course of discussion the moderator seeks to ascertain the range of opinion held by the group.

A series of focus groups was conducted separately with health professionals, children aged between 8 and 15 years (one group had mild JIA and the other had severe JIA), and parents. The focus groups produced a wealth of rich data that provided the foundation for later quantitative studies, including the development of new measures (e.g. J.H. Barlow, Shaw & Wright, 2001).

Symptoms and functioning

Parents identify very closely with their child's condition and its treatment (J. Barlow, Harrison & Shaw, 1998), using terms such as 'our pain', 'our drugs' and 'we have blood tests', suggesting that the child's condition had become their condition as well. This phenomenon may help to explain the over-protective nature of many parents of children with JIA, who find it hard to 'let go' and allow their children to develop independence.

Children tended to use the term 'hurt' rather than 'pain' in describing symptoms and had developed their own conceptions regarding the nature of arthritis. For example, one child viewed arthritis as a liquid inside her and wanted to know if it 'would spread to other parts of the body'. Other children described their pain as 'a circle round my knee' or 'an achy fuzzy feeling', 'like being pressed really hard' and 'as though someone is thumping me'. In addition to pain, fatigue was a problem experienced by many children, particularly during a disease flare (J. Barlow, Harrison & Shaw, 1998).

Similar descriptions emerged from an interview study by Beales *et al.* (1983) based on the views of 75 children and adolescents (aged between 7 and 17) about their pain and JIA. Responses were classified into four categories, the first being subjective feelings such as 'my fingers ache'. Second, children used surface descriptions (e.g. 'it makes my knee red') and, third, loss of functional ability was described in terms such as 'I can't move my neck properly'. Finally, phrases such as 'it damages my bones' were used to describe internal disease pathology. Beales *et al.* found that children aged between 7 and 11 tended to use the first two categories, whereas two-thirds of the older children included descriptions of internal pathology and unseen processes. Despite this greater appreciation of the biological explanations of JIA, older children were more upset, worried, frightened and sad compared with the younger children in this sample. Beales *et al.* suggest that health professionals need to take account of these different conceptualisations of disease when talking to children in clinical settings.

Limited mobility and stiffness can interfere with instrumental tasks (e.g. getting dressed). The frustration that children can feel when meeting difficulties with daily task can manifest in their behaviour and emotions. For example, parents in the Barlow, Harrison and Shaw study reported that children lost their tempers, head-butted or kicked walls and doors and often directed their anger at parents and siblings.

He'll start trying to get dressed and then he starts 'I can't do this Mum' and 'I can't get my trousers on'. He gets very angry and then it's 'I wish I were dead – I wouldn't have to do it then. (J. Barlow, Harrison & Shaw, 1998)

She is angry towards things. You know, she's a very loving child but she wants to be the same as everybody else. (J. Barlow, Harrison & Shaw, 1998)

A qualitative survey of 50 adolescents by Shaw (2001) confirmed that JIA was experienced as aversive physical symptoms, treatment side effects, physical outcomes and psychosocial consequences. As in younger children and adults, JIA was described in terms of pain, stiffness and fatigue along with small stature, joint deformity, weakness, slow healing rate, loss of appetite, dizziness and loss of sight. Adolescents felt that the visible signs of illness made them appear different from their peers and were linked to negative evaluations of body appearance, self-confidence and social exclusion.

> The disease and the drugs seem to have stopped my growth, making me feel very self-conscious of my height. (Shaw, 2001)

Emotional consequences for children and adolescents

Both children and parents in the focus groups (J. Barlow, Harrison & Shaw, 1998) felt that every aspect of JIA and its treatment served to make children look, feel and behave differently from their peers. Consequently, their greatest hopes were for peer belonging and social acceptance. Parents felt that their children were subjected to bullying and experienced discrimination. Children reported being called names by classmates and siblings (e.g. 'sticklegs', or 'monkey', due to the hair growth associated with medication). Adolescence emerged as a particularly difficult time: children who developed JIA or experienced a return of active symptoms during this time appeared to have greater difficulties in adjustment compared with adolescents who had been diagnosed as toddlers and had 'grown up with it'. In the face of this suffering, parents perceived themselves to be helpless, inadequate and powerless. At least one couple had decided not to have any more children. Positive attributes emerged as parents felt their children were actually more 'quiet', 'loving' and 'insightful' as a result of JIA.

The majority of the 50 adolescents surveyed by Shaw (2001) mentioned the emotional consequences of JIA, using verbal descriptors such as 'depressed', 'lonely', 'isolated', 'frustrated' 'and 'upset'. However, the overwhelming feeling was that of being different from their peers, a feeling that was attributed to the visible signs of disease that led to negative evaluations of body appearance, self-confidence and social exclusion.

> The girls take no interest in me because I'm small and limited too. They just like to flirt with the big, tough, hunky guys. It's all because I'm different. (Shaw, 2001, p.60)

Having arthritis had some positive aspects such as meeting other people with the 'same problems' who in some cases had become special friends. This emphasises the importance of finding an appropriate peer group and developing a sense of belonging.

Social wellbeing

The foci of parents' concerns were to ensure that their children had similar opportunities for self-development as children without JIA and to provide a sense of 'normality' in children's lives (J. Barlow, Harrison & Shaw, 1998). When JIA was less visible, children and their families reported a lack of both institutional and personal support, and the failure of others to understand the nature of the condition, such as its unpredictability. Indeed, problems at school were often attributed to teachers' lack of understanding regarding the fluctuating nature of JIA, whereby a child is unable to walk in the morning but can run and play with classmates in the afternoon after stiffness has worn off and medication has taken effect. Although children want others to understand their needs, they find it difficult to explain the nature of JIA, particularly at school, as the following quotes illustrate.

> People ... think it's more older people that get it. They do not understand how I feel and what the pain is like.

> People don't understand that one day you can be okay and the other day, that you can't.

> Some of my friends don't understand that I can't do things as well as they can. I would prefer them (friends) to know a lot about it because then they'd know how I feel and they would understand more.

> ... when I have been playing a lot of games and when I sit out, everyone thinks that I'm doing it because I really don't want to do any of the games, but, it's because it's really hurting me and I can't.

The impact on education, vocation and peer involvement were major themes to emerge from the survey of Shaw (2001). Many adolescents felt that they missed schooling because of JIA and some found it difficult to keep up with schoolwork. As well as absence due to periods of being unwell, adolescents found the school environment did not cater for their needs. For example, writing with pens and pencils was slow and frustrating for those whose hands were affected. Some adolescents had the use of laptop computers, extra time during exams or the help from special needs assistants. Others, who were less fortunate, struggled to keep up with classmates and felt that their condition led them to becoming even more isolated.

> I could not get around at school and had to sit in an office alone and have work brought to me ... I felt JIA was holding me down and keeping me back.

Adolescents found participation in sports activities both at school and outside of school to be particularly difficult. For example, some adolescents lost points in house events because they could not run as fast as their peers. The lack of belief reported by younger children regarding symptoms of arthritis was evident in the lives of adolescents, whom teachers often accused of being 'too young to have arthritis – stop complaining and get on with the game'. Adolescents' social lives were limited by the dictates and consequences of JIA that hindered such activities as going to discos and parties, wearing fashionable clothes and keeping up with peers. Some felt that they were a 'burden' upon their friends.

One strategy used by children and adolescents appears to be that of withdrawal. Rather than feel a burden or be seen to be slow and restricted in their movements or bike-riding skills, both children and adolescents with JIA tend to withdraw from social activities. The social isolation experienced as a consequence of this strategy is effectively the same as being socially excluded. Thus, in efforts to protect themselves from being viewed as dependent or different, children and adolescents can became isolated, lonely and lacking in social contact with peers.

An interview-based study of 22 children with JIA aged 6 to 17 years identified a core category of oscillation between hope and despair (Sallfors *et al.*, 2002). Oscillation was linked to disturbed order, dependency, ambivalence and uncertainty about the future. Chronic pain was a major feature of children's lives and, together with the need for disease management, resulted in restrictions on children's social lives.

Parental involvement in the management of JIA

Caring for a child with JIA places enormous demands on the entire family. Where leg splints are worn at night, parents are not only responsible for fitting them onto their child's legs but are 'on call' all night just in case they are required to carry their child to the bathroom. Children rely on parents (especially 'Mum') for disease management.

> She always does thing for me. Reminds me to do my exercises, take my medicine. She, either my Mum or my Dad, always comes to the hospital with me. (J. Barlow, Harrison & Shaw, 1998)

In order to meet their children's needs, parents are forced to balance a number of equally important demands. Children's current physical needs have to be balanced with their long-term developmental needs, and the time constraints of children's health regimens have to be balanced with the needs of other family members and parents' need for time for themselves. Both parents and children experience difficulties in the management of JIA at home, particularly in relation to scheduling and carrying out various therapies. There is consensus that children's concordance was poor: children and parents admit that children do not 'do' exercises or use aids and appliances. Health professionals believe that disease education explaining the benefits of physical therapy would make children more 'compliant' (J.H. Barlow, Shaw & Harrison, 1999). In contrast, children feel that there is nothing that anyone could say that would influence their behaviour, particularly in terms of exercise, which they view as 'boring.'

The demands of JIA on parental time have to be balanced with the needs of the family, including other siblings. Parents are well aware that children with JIA not only receive more of their time but also are excused household chores because of their physical condition. Indeed, children with JIA admit that they sometimes use their condition as an excuse to avoid household chores. The imbalances in parental attention often manifest in siblings' feelings of jealousy and resentment.

> When John was first diagnosed … the teacher called me in and said 'What's the matter with Paula? (sister) … She's not as happy-go-lucky as she used to be' … We'd given more love to him (John). Paula will say, 'I don't love you, John. I love Mummy, I love Daddy, but I don't love you.' (J.H. Barlow, Shaw & Harrison, 1999)

In contrast, children with JIA often appear to be unaware that their condition may be impacting upon the lives of their family. Although, parents are aware that children with JIA can be often 'spoiled' and overprotected, achieving the right balance between safeguarding health and encouraging independence is fraught with difficulties. Health professionals believe that some children fail to develop independence because parents, usually the mother, continue to provide assistance even when the child with JIA is quite capable of carrying out tasks or activities. Health professionals recalled cases where adolescents still relied on Mum to help them get dressed and to brush their teeth. One nurse said:

> I think they [mothers] get stuck in a role. So mum's always dressed them and they're very passive about it and just let them carry on ... mum's happy to carry on. (J.H. Barlow, Shaw & Harrison, 1999)

Emotional consequences for parents

Parents report a wide spectrum of emotional reactions in relation to parenting a child with JIA, including anxiety, powerlessness, anger, frustration, and helplessness (J. Barlow, Harrison & Shaw, 1998). Many feel guilty that they had not immediately recognised the symptoms of JIA and blamed themselves for not responding quickly enough and not being able to secure immediate attention from healthcare services. Some parents feel guilty that they had caused JIA. Health professionals can find it very difficult to deal with parents' questions about hereditary factors or the influence of environmental conditions in the aetiology of JIA. In turn, parents feel guilty that they cannot answer all their children's questions about JIA and cannot reassure them that 'everything would be OK' in the future.

Anxiety is associated with the uncertain prognosis of JIA, the unpredictable disease course, and the 'harmful side effects' of medication. A further major cause of anxiety concerns children's future in terms of career potential and ability to have and raise a family of their own. In contrast, health professionals feel that parental concerns and anxieties about children's career prospects and future family life can be magnified and exaggerated.

The daily grind of managing JIA can be a cause of considerable stress for parents. As well as time-consuming and sometimes painful therapeutic regimes, parents (usually the mother) have to organise medical appointments, and take children for tests (e.g. blood tests). The last of these were disliked by some children and are considered painful. All of these demands have to be 'fitted in' with parents' other commitments (e.g. work). Parents feel that there is a cost to successful management of their child's condition in that peer activities are often curtailed.

> If my Mum says I can't do something because it will make me ill then I get annoyed with my Mum. I say, 'Oh, I can do it, my friends are doing it. (J.H. Barlow, Shaw & Harrison, 1999)

It seems that the same desire to resist disruption that is found among adults with arthritis can be found among children also. They want to appear 'normal', to be part of a group and to be the same as their peers, regardless of the consequences for their physical wellbeing. Thus, children appear to adopt a process of 'normalising' in much the same way as adults with arthritis. Equally, parents strive to give children with JIA a 'normal' childhood experience, although there is a tendency to become overprotective.

Most parents found it difficult to maintain the family's equilibrium and expressed concerns for the psychosocial wellbeing not only of the child with JIA but also for siblings. Again, guilt emerged as the main emotional consequence of not feeling able to devote equal time and attention to siblings without JIA. Parents were concerned about the cohesive nature of the family as a whole and also sibling rivalry and jealousy.

> I have felt real frustration, real anger that our family has been affected by this ... My ideal world has fallen in ... you can't plan lots of thing and can't do lots of things. (J.H. Barlow, Shaw & Harrison, 1999)

Chapter Summary

The picture painted by qualitative accounts of living with arthritis is in direct contrast to general concepts of healthy living (e.g. Blaxter, 1983). Using data from a survey of 9000 people, Blaxter (1983) identified three main ideas about the meaning of health. First, health was associated with the notion of fitness exemplified by energy, strength and an efficient or athletic body. People with arthritis do not appear to fit in terms of this conception. Second, health was viewed as ability to carry out various roles normally, reflecting beliefs about a hardy personality who is never ill. It is clear that arthritis can interfere with role functioning. Finally, Blaxter found that health was conceptualised in psychological terms as being unstressed, unworried, able to cope with life and being happy and 'in tune' with the world.

In contrast to these notions of health, living with arthritis is characterised by pain, fatigue, lack of vitality, and adverse bodily changes leading to limited physical functioning and, in some cases, visible deformity. Although people with arthritis do not always see themselves as 'ill' *per se*, they do experience considerable difficulties with performance of normal roles, such as parenting, work, housework, gardening and leisure pursuits. Many become dissatisfied with their perceived inability to carry out these roles according to their own expectations and societal norms. Determination to appear 'normal' leads to overcompensation and use of techniques such as 'supernormalising', whereby people take advantage of good days to accomplish as many valued activities as possible. This pattern of behaviour continues despite the potential adverse consequences for health status. The final conceptualisation of health identified by Blaxter (1983) focuses on psychological coping and adjustment. The majority of people with arthritis appear able to gradually achieve this state of being, experiencing a satisfactory quality of life. Some are able to thrive in the face of apparent adversity. However, many appear to struggle at various points in the disease course, and a minority continue to experience persistent psychological distress. Emotional reactions are typically described in terms of anger, frustration, and loss of control and are consistent across various types of arthritis. The uncertainty of arthritis hampers both the initial attainment and the maintenance of adjustment. For example, disease symptomatology can vary within the space of a day, let alone weeks, months or years. Equally, disease progression is uncertain and highly variable; some people have mild disease with little impact on functioning whilst others have a poor prognosis, may require major joint replacement and have a reduced lifespan. Uncertainty impacts on ability to plan valued activities and can threaten one's sense of control. In addition, people living with arthritis experience a number of losses throughout the disease course. Social isolation is common, particularly among the elderly. Given this state of affairs, people who manage to live happily with their condition are to be applauded on their substantial achievement. Researchers and health professionals can learn much from such experts and could better utilise this knowledge to assist those who are less fortunate and find life with arthritis to be a continual struggle.

One man's arthritis journey is presented in the Appendix.

5

The Psychological Impact on Person and Family

The unpredictable course of disease, allied to an uncertain prognosis, combine with painful symptoms and progressive disability to pose considerable challenges for people with arthritis. The incurable nature of most forms of arthritis necessitates long-term disease management, including maintenance of complex treatment regimes. Not surprisingly, the impact of arthritis is wide-ranging and pervades all areas of life, such as psychological wellbeing (J. Barlow, Macey & Struthers, 1993; Creed & Ash, 1992), ability to work (J. Barlow, Wright & Kroll, 2001; Callahan *et al.*, 1992; Lubeck, 1995), social relationships (Fitzpatrick *et al.*, 1991), and family life (J.H. Barlow, Cullen, Foster, Harrison & Wade, 1999; Reisine, 1995). Paralleling the medical literature, psychological studies have tended to focus on people with RA, thus less is known about the psychological wellbeing of people with other types of arthritis such as OA, AS and JIA.

Psychological Impact on the Person

Studies of psychological wellbeing in psychosocial rheumatology have focused primarily on understanding depression and its correlates. Much less attention has been paid to other forms of distress such as anxiety or low self-esteem. Depression among people with arthritis is an important issue as it can adversely influence associated health outcomes. For example, a World Health Organization (WHO) survey of 245,414 adults (aged 18+ years) across 60 countries (Moussavi *et al.*, 2007) showed that and 10.7 per cent of participants with arthritis also had depression. Furthermore, among participants with two or more chronic physical conditions, the prevalence of depression was as high as 23 per cent. Participants with depression co-morbid with one or more chronic diseases had the worst health, thus emphasising the importance of addressing depression as a public health priority.

Overall, there appears to be consensus that a considerable proportion of adults with arthritis is at risk of clinically depressed mood at any one point in time, with prevalence ranging from 10 per cent to 30 per cent (e.g. Blalock, DeVellis, Brown & Wallston, 1989; Dickens *et al.*, 2002; Hawley & Wolfe, 1993; Katz & Yelin 1993; Wells *et al.*, 1989), compared to 6.6 per cent in the general population (Kessler *et al.*, 2003). The proportion at risk of anxious mood tends to be higher, at around 50 per cent. Lifetime prevalence of psychiatric disorder has been reported to be 64 per cent among a community sample of arthritis patients with a recent prevalence rate (during last six months) of 42 per cent (Wells *et al.*, 1988). Variation in prevalence rates may arise from use of different measures and cut-off points for establishing 'risk', and may vary between participants recruited from community settings versus samples recruited via clinical settings.

Although the level of depressed mood is in accordance with other chronic conditions (Cassileth *et al.*, 1984), it is nonetheless a cause for concern and has been noted by healthcare professionals working in rheumatology clinics. Indeed, concern amongst healthcare staff provided the impetus for an investigation of depressed and anxious mood among outpatients with RA (J.H. Barlow, Cullen & Rowe, 1999). One intriguing finding was that pain featured in the prediction of anxiety but not depression. A 12-month follow-up revealed that levels of depressed and anxious mood remained stable over time (J. Barlow, Cullen & Rowe, 2001). These findings parallel those of Smedstad *et al.* (1996) and Uhlig *et al.* (2000), who also found levels of psychological distress among patients with RA to be relatively stable over two-year and five-year periods, respectively. Viewed in conjunction with the proportions of patients who score in the at-risk categories for both anxious and depressed mood, there appears to be a need for additional intervention, over and above standard care, specifically targeting psychological issues. This conclusion is supported by interview data suggesting that patients would value the opportunity to discuss emotional issues (J. Barlow, Cullen & Rowe, 2001). Interestingly, patients reported that they would be happy to enter a dialogue focusing on emotional issues with other patients who would have an innate understanding of life with RA.

Box 5.1 Methodological Note

The overlap between symptoms of depression and symptoms of arthritis can be problematic when attempting to identify cases to measure the severity of depressed mood or to determine prevalence rates. For example, fatigue is a frequent problem among people with arthritis (Belza *et al.*, 1993) and can derive from the disease itself, the extra effort needed to carry out activities, anaemia or depressed mood. Although the inclusion of somatic items on depression scales can inflate estimates of severity and prevalence in RA, Blalock *et al.* (1989) maintain that the level of inflation is modest.

Dickens and Creed (2001) maintain that depression in RA is mostly unrecognised and is under-treated, a point echoed by Nicassio (2008), who suggests that research findings on depression 'may not be penetrating clinical practice'. A study of 200 RA patients attending four rheumatology clinics in the US found that 21 patients (11 per cent) had moderately severe to severe symptoms of depression (Sleath *et al.*, 2008). Of these 21 patients, only four discussed depression during their clinic visit, and in each case it was patients who initiated the discussion. It is likely that this situation occurs among other types of arthritis. Psychological distress can often be overlooked in clinical settings where the primary focus is on the physical aspects of a condition. Furthermore, the potential for overlap between the symptoms of arthritis and symptoms of depression is great. For example, fatigue, sleep disturbance and lack of appetite can frequently feature in the presentation of both arthritis and depression. Dickens and Creed (2001) further suggest that under-treatment can also result from lack of familiarity with antidepressant medication. This is a pity, since the old-style tricyclics medications have analgesic effects at low dosage and thus could assist with both pain and depressive symptoms. Furthermore, there is evidence that integrating treatment for depression in primary care and other rheumatological medical care can be cost-effective and is associated with improvements in quality of life and function (Lin *et al.*, 2003; Parker *et al.*, 2003).

The importance of addressing the issue of depression among people living with RA has been highlighted in a unique study of 1290 consecutive outpatients (Ang *et al.*, 2005). Data were collected at each clinic visit over a 12-year observation period. Analysis of the first four years of data entry showed that clinical depression resulted in a twofold increase in the risk of mortality in RA. Similarly, Persson *et al.* (2005) documented the development of emotional distress over a period of four years among a sample of 158 early RA patients (64 per cent females; mean age 51.4 years). Emotional distress was assessed using the Symptom Checklist (SCL–90) and was found to decrease slowly for most patients. However, a minority (12 per cent) had continuously high and increasing levels of distress. Interestingly, disease activity indicators were poor predictors of distress.

Depression, disability, pain and fatigue

Given its persistence and pervasive nature, it is not surprising that pain has been identified as a correlate of depression in RA (Creed & Ash, 1992) and AS (J. Barlow, Macey & Struthers, 1993), and has been found to remain a significant correlate when controlling for disease activity (Callahan *et al.*, 1991). Graphic descriptions of pain (e.g. excruciating) have been associated with depression (Mackinnon *et al.*, 1994). The degree to which enduring pain interferes with ability to perform daily activities is known as 'pain disability'. Among a sample of 141 older adults with RA aged over 50 years, greater pain disability was linked to heightened psychological distress, poorer perceptions of overall health, more operations, higher unemployment, more intense disease activity, longer disease duration and lower disease self-efficacy (James *et al.*, 2005).

A key issue yet to be resolved concerns the direction of causality: does pain lead to depression or vice versa? Results from longitudinal studies in RA have been inconsistent. For example, Brown (1990) suggests a causal model in which pain predicts subsequent depression. Nicassio and Wallston (1992) extended this work in a longitudinal study of 242 RA patients, showing that prior pain predicted adverse changes in sleep problems and that the interaction between high sleep problems and high pain was independently associated with depression. In contrast, Parker *et al.* (1992) found that depression had more influence over pain than vice versa. Zautra and Smith (2001) found that depressive symptoms were associated with weekly increases in pain, negative events, perceived stress and negative affect for patients with RA (n = 87), whereas in patients with OA (n = 101) depressive symptoms were only associated with increases in pain and negative effect. The sample comprised older women aged 42 to 76 years, thus generalisability may be limited. The causal relationship between pain and depression is an important one that warrants considerable attention. The reality is that causality may operate in both directions simultaneously: pain may lead to increased depression and depression may lead to increased perception of pain.

There are indications that the relationship between depression and disability may also be reciprocal. For example, longitudinal studies have shown that increased functional disability, particularly in valued areas (e.g. going on holiday), is followed by increased depression. Katz and Yelin (1995) report a sevenfold increase in depression in the year following a 10 per cent reduction in ability to carry out valued activities among women with RA. Equally, depression has been found to precede increased physical disability (McFarlane & Brooks, 1988). Although there is evidence of a robust relationship between depression and per-ceived disability, the precise mechanisms through which depression influences disability and vice versa remain to be clarified.

Regardless of the direction of causality, it is easy to understand how negative cycles of pain, fatigue, loss of physical functioning, loss of valued activities and depressed mood can become established. The challenge for psychologists is to find effective methods to enable people with arthritis to break out of negative cycles or to avoid them. This endeavour would be facilitated if the precise mechanisms, through which depression influences pain and disability and vice versa, were more clearly understood. Although, there appear to be links between psychological distress and immune system functionality, there is no evidence that psychological distress increases inflammation (Dickens & Creed, 2001).

Depression may be a key factor influencing perceptions of disability among people with arthritis. Psychological factors have been shown to be better predictors of disability compared with traditional, medical indicators of disease activity in RA (Katz & Yelin, 1993; McFarlane & Brooks, 1988; Newman *et al.*, 1989; Wright *et al.*, 1996) and OA (Jordan *et al.*, 1996; Summers *et al.*, 1988). Among people with OA, anxiety and depression served to decrease pain tolerance thus leading to functional impairment (Summers *et al.*, 1988). Dekker *et al.* (1993) provided support for this finding by showing that negative affect among patients with hip or knee OA increased the tendency to avoid painful activities. This in turn led to muscle weakness, which in turn led to physical disability. In a study of knee OA (Jordan *et al.*, 1996), severity of pain was found to be more important than radiographic evidence in determining self-reported disability. Moreover, arthritis-related pain is a risk factor for future physical disability (Hughes *et al.*, 1994).

Taken together, these findings are consistent with anecdotal evidence from healthcare professionals suggesting that the degree of psychological distress is not always directly related to disease severity or to objective indicators of disability. There is evidence from one study in RA showing that pain and disability are not sufficient to cause depression except in cases of advanced disease (Mindham *et al.*, 1981). Other variables, such as social support, may play a contributory role.

Traditionally, much of focus of both treatment and research has been on the important issue of pain. Nevertheless, it has become clear that for many people living with arthritis, fatigue can be major problem. Fatigue can be a symptom of both arthritis and depression. In a comparison of individuals with RA (n = 122) and healthy controls (n = 122), Mancuso *et al.* (2006) found that fatigue was relatively stable over time and was common in both the RA and control groups. However among the RA group, fatigue was more closely associated with greater anxiety and disability, less social support and more social stress. There are likely to complex interrelationships between pain, fatigue and psychological wellbeing among people with arthritis. The pain of arthritis can result in disturbed sleep which in turn leads to feeling fatigued during the day. Analysis of a large data set (i.e. the Canadian Community Health Survey) showed that the prevalence of insomnia and unrefreshing sleep was twice as high among persons with arthritis compared to the general population (Power *et al.*, 2005). Regression analysis showed that pain partially mediated the effects of arthritis on sleep problems.

It is important to note that disability in arthritis is often measured by self-report questionnaires, both for research purposes and screening in clinical settings. Respondents are typically asked to rate their ability to perform a range of daily activities (e.g. dressing, eating). Thus, ratings of disability may be influenced by psychological factors such as depression, self-efficacy or helplessness. The role of depression may be one of mediation whereby higher levels of depression produce a downward bias in perceived ability to perform daily activities. There may be other mediating or

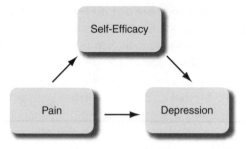

Figure 5.1

moderating variables operating in the relationship between the physical condition and psychological outcomes (e.g. social support). Furthermore, some variables may act as both mediators and moderators.

Although the terms moderator and mediator tend to be used interchangeably (Baron & Kenny, 1986), moderating and mediating effects can be distinguished conceptually in terms of the function of third variables. In a mediational model, the third variable (the mediator) functions as the mechanism through which the independent variable is able to influence the dependent variable. In a moderating model the third variable (the moderator) partitions an independent variable into areas of varying effectiveness in relation to a given dependent variable. Research attention has tended to focus on potential psychological mediations, with many researchers investigating mediation following the steps advocated by Baron and Kenny (1986). In health psychology, many variables act as partial rather than total mediators. For example, pain could influence depression both directly and indirectly through self-efficacy (see Figure 5.1).

Mediators and Moderators of Psychological Wellbeing

Helplessness

Appraisals, expectations and coping strategies have been investigated as potential mediators of pain, psychological wellbeing and disability. Feelings of helplessness can arise due to the uncertain disease course, lack of adequate pain control and the interference of arthritis on daily activities. People with high levels of helplessness tend to report high pain levels and greater depression. A cross-sectional study of 92 patients with RA revealed that perceived helplessness mediated the relationship between pain and depression in RA (T.W. Smith *et al.*, 1990). This finding has been replicated in a sample of people with OA (Wallston, 1993) and in a multi-wave study of patients with RA (C.A. Smith & Wallston, 1992). Similarly, longitudinal analyses have demonstrated that both helplessness and pain are significant mediators between disease activity (indicated by joint count) and future physical and psychological disability (Schoenfeld-Smith *et al.*, 1996). Affleck *et al.* (1987) found that positive mood and better psychological adjustment were associated with perceived control over symptoms in a cross-sectional analysis based on a combination of interview and questionnaire data. There is evidence that helplessness may also act as a moderator. Naidoo and Pretorius (2006) found that, among a sample of 186 adults with RA, helplessness moderated the relationships between swollen joint count and depression, tender joint count and pain, tender joint count and perceived disability and number of tender joints and functional ability.

Control cognitions

Given equal disease severity, some patients are incapacitated by their disease, whilst others continue to live full lives, are able to take an active role in the management of their condition and have good psychological adjustment. Concepts that may help in understanding variation in adjustment and perceived ability to self-manage are control cognitions, such as health locus of control, perceived control and self-efficacy.

Health locus of control
Health locus of control refers to generalised expectancies relating to one's health. 'Locus' means 'place' and thus health locus of control refers to the individual's perceptions of the location of control over reinforcements relating to their health. Health can be perceived as being controlled by one's own actions (internal locus of control), or by forces external to oneself (i.e. powerful others or chance). The role of health locus of control was studied among a variety of long-term conditions in the 1980s, much of it using the Multi-Dimensional Health Locus of

Control Scale (MHLC) designed by Wallston *et al.* (1978). The most adaptive pattern of control beliefs for people with long-term conditions is suggested to comprise strong internal control beliefs, strong beliefs in powerful others and weak beliefs in chance (Wallston, 1989). Supporting this proposition, RA patients with this pattern of beliefs were found to become less depressed over time regardless of their level of disease activity (Buckelew *et al.*, 1990). An alternative conceptualisation was suggested by Affleck *et al.* (1987), who proposed that surrendering control to others is adaptive where opportunities to exert personal control are limited and maintenance of internal control could lead to difficulties. Alternatively, people can search the situation for features over which they can exert personal control. An interview-based study of 92 RA patients (Affleck *et al.*, 1987) showed that those who viewed their condition as predictable also believed that they were in personal control of their symptoms and the course of disease. Interestingly, beliefs about controlling daily symptoms (e.g. fatigue, stiffness) were of greater import than beliefs about controlling the disease course. Furthermore, patients who believed they had more control over daily symptoms than their physicians tended to have a more positive mood than patients who believed physicians had most control. The relationship between vicarious control (through powerful others) and health outcomes is not well documented. Available findings have tended to be contradictory: some researchers report a positive relationship between vicarious control and psychological adjustment (S.E. Taylor *et al.*, 1984, in breast cancer) whereas others report a negative relationship (Reed *et al.*, 1993, men with AIDS). In the field of psychosocial rheumatology, internal perceptions of control have been related to better psychological wellbeing among patients with RA whereas vicarious control through health professionals has been related to poor psychological adjustment (J. Barlow, Macey, Pugh & Struthers, 1994).

Box 5.2 Methodological Note

There can be problems in assessing beliefs about general 'health' among people with a long-term condition. Respondents with arthritis are no exception. The meaning of 'health' for people with a long-term condition tends to vary.

Box 5.2 (cont'd)

Some respondents will give a rating of their health encompassing arthritis and all other illnesses, presumably in accordance with scale developers' intentions. In contrast, others do not consider 'arthritis' to be an illness *per se* and thus complete ratings of health only in terms of other conditions (e.g. colds, flu). Finally, a minority fail to complete such items, not knowing whether to respond in relation to arthritis or all other health matters. This problem can be encountered when using the Multi-Dimensional Health Locus of Control Scale among people with arthritis and may partly account for the low reliability that is sometimes reported for this measure.

Wallston (1992) argues that locus of control forms a relatively small component of the larger, more important construct of perceived control. The latter is defined as the belief that one can determine one's internal state and behaviour, influence one's environment and/or achieve a desired outcome (Wallston *et al.*, 1987). Hence, the concept of perceived control combines outcome expectancy (locus of control) with a behavioural expectancy (SE). An interview-based study examined the links between domain-specific and global perceived control, and health service usage among older people with arthritis (Chipperfield & Greenslade, 1999). Among people who reported that arthritis restricted activities, and after controlling for age and morbidity, people with low levels of perceived control were found to make greater use of health services (e.g. more physician visits, longer inpatient stays) compared to people with high levels of perceived control. There have been relatively few other investigations of perceived control in psychosocial rheumatology. More attention has been paid to the concept of self-efficacy.

Self-efficacy

Self-efficacy was introduced by Bandura (1977) to explain the effects of self-referent thought on psychosocial functioning. Self-efficacy refers to 'beliefs in one's capabilities to organise and execute the course of action required to produce given attainments' (Bandura, 1977, p.3). Once formed, self-efficacy beliefs influence not only the courses of action pursued, but also the effort expended, perseverance in the face of difficulties, the nature of thought patterns (i.e. encouraging or self-deprecating) and the amount of stress experienced in demanding situations (Bandura, 1977). The unpredictable nature of arthritis may result in decreased self-efficacy beliefs, with patients viewing their disease as uncontrollable (Taal *et al.*, 1996), a situation that may in turn exacerbate physical and psychosocial symptoms. Among patients with RA, several studies suggest that self-efficacy may be important for understanding psychological, cognitive and physical functioning. Wright *et al.* (1996) found that low self-efficacy for managing pain and distress contributed to predictions of depression. Similarly, Beckham *et al.* (1994) report associations between low self-efficacy, and psychological distress and worse physical functioning. Furthermore, self-efficacy and pain predicted physical functioning among younger women with a mean age of 43 and relatively short disease duration of six years and under (Dwyer, 1997). Dwyer concluded that learning to cope with pain might be the key to promoting improved health status. Although interesting, the study focused on the function subscale of the Arthritis Self-Efficacy Scales developed by Lorig *et al.* (1989), where higher scores indicate greater self-efficacy. Not surprisingly, the Arthritis Self-Efficacy Function (ASE: Function) scores were highly correlated with physical functioning ($r = -.82$); higher self-efficacy was associated with less impaired physical functioning. Lorig suggests that the overlap between ASE: Function and self-report measures of physical functioning is so great that use of the ASE: Function subscale adds little additional insight (Lorig, 1998).

Other studies have reported associations between high self-efficacy and improved health outcomes although many are based on cross-sectional rather than longitudinal data. One exception is a Norwegian study that investigated the relationship between self-efficacy at baseline and changes in health status over a two-year period among patients with RA (Brekke *et al.*, 2001a). The sample was relatively large comprising 815 RA patients with a mean age of 61.4 (SD 14.6) and mean disease duration of 12.8 (SD 11) years. High self-efficacy was correlated favourably with health status. For example, each unit increase in self-efficacy for pain was associated with an increase of 0.14 on bodily pain measured by the SF36. Similarly, for each unit increase on self-efficacy for other symptoms there was a decrease on a visual analogue scale for fatigue of 0.22. A further study by Brekke *et al.* (1999) showed that level of arthritis self-efficacy varied by socio-economic district, with those residing in less affluent areas of Oslo reporting lower self-efficacy and poorer health status. There were no differences in terms of joint counts, disease severity or number of joint replacements. Interestingly, a laboratory-based investigation found that OA patients with very high arthritis self-efficacy for pain had higher pain thresholds and pain tolerance compared with participants with very low arthritis self-efficacy for pain (Keefe *et al.*, 1997). Thus, people who felt confident in their ability to manage their pain were able to tolerate more pain and had higher pain thresholds. Self-efficacy has also been linked to fatigue among patients with RA leading, to the suggestion that self-efficacy enhancement may contribute to improvement on fatigue (Riemsma *et al.*, 1998). This suggestion is an important one, since fatigue is believed to be a predictor of work dysfunction and overall health status (Wolfe *et al.*, 1996) and emerged as a key factor among people with AS in relation to work disability and family life (J.H. Barlow, Wright, Williams & Keat, 2001). Moreover, fatigue management often relies on cognitive and behavioural strategies (e.g. planning activities, relaxation) and is an area where the application of psychological techniques has the potential to positively contribute to the quality of life of those living with arthritis.

Empirical tests have provided support for the mediational role played by self-efficacy. For example, Rejeski *et al.* (1998) found that self-efficacy mediated change in exercise behaviour among people with knee OA. Arthritis self-efficacy has been shown to mediate between disease severity and adaptation, protecting individuals with AS from the adverse effects of disease severity (J. Barlow, Macey & Struthers, 1993). Shifren *et al.* (1999) examined self-efficacy, cognitive functioning and mental health of 121 people with RA (aged 34–84). Cognitive functioning showed evidence of both direct and indirect effects on mental health. The indirect effects were mediated through self-efficacy and pain, with higher self-efficacy and less pain being associated with better cognitive functioning.

There is less evidence of moderation by self-efficacy. Appraisals of self-efficacy have been shown to moderate the relationship between coping and emotions in a longitudinal study of people with RA (Lowe *et al.*, 2008). A sample of 127 RA patients was recruited from 11 UK rheumatology centres; all patients had agreed to attend the education programme used in the routine clinical care at each of the 11 centres. Coping with RA was assessed using the medical coping modes questionnaire (Feifel *et al.*, 1987), which has three subscales reflecting three coping styles:

1. confrontation – primarily based on information-gathering;
2. avoidance – use of distraction and attention redeployment to avoid thinking about illness;
3. acceptance-resignation – submitting to the illness.

Self-efficacy was assessed using the pain and other symptoms subscales of the Arthritis Self-Efficacy Scales (Lorig *et al.*, 1989). Results showed that the association between change in anxiety and change in coping could be moderated by change in self-efficacy: anxiety was decreased in patients with reduced use of avoidance coping when self-efficacy for other symptoms increased. Self-efficacy for pain and other symptoms moderated the association between depression and coping: reduced depression was associated with increased acceptance-resignation coping among those whose self-efficacy for pain had increased, and reduced use of acceptance-resignation coping among those who reported an increase in self-efficacy for other symptoms. The authors suggest that, as pain can be difficult to control, there are situations when resting and being inactive can be adaptive. Thus, reduced depression may be evident despite an increased use of acceptance-resignation coping when this is accompanied by increased self-efficacy for pain.

Orbell *et al.* (2001) maintain that goal importance as well as self-efficacy is an important predictor of disability among people with arthritis recovering from either a hip or knee replacement operation. A prospective study assessed people before surgery and again at three months and nine months post-surgery. The final sample (n = 77) had a mean age of 67.77 (SD 10.17), were mainly women (58 per cent), and 42 per cent reported co-morbidity that was associated with greater disability throughout the study. Self-efficacy and goal importance were assessed using scales specifically developed for the study, covering a range of 32 activities (e.g. mobility, body care, recreation). Goal importance was defined as:

> the extent to which participants attached personal importance to the ability to perform activities of everyday living. (Orbell *et al.*, 2001)

Disability decreased at both 3 and 9 months post-surgery whilst self-efficacy increased. Pre-surgery goal importance and self-efficacy at

3 months were independent predictors of disability at 9 months, controlling for pre-surgery and 3-month disability. Patients who valued functional activities highly and had high self-efficacy for performance of those activities were less disabled at 9 months. There was evidence that pre-surgery goal importance moderated the impact of self-efficacy on disability at 9 months. Specifically, patients with low self-efficacy but high goal importance were less disabled at 9 months compared with patients who had low self-efficacy and low goal importance.

In contrast to the body of evidence suggesting that greater self-efficacy beliefs have a positive effect on health outcomes, one investigation of the impact of self-efficacy beliefs on adaptation amongst RA patients produced mixed findings (Schiaffino *et al.*, 1991). Cross-sectional and longitudinal analyses showed that greater self-efficacy was related to lower disability regardless of the level of pain. However, a different pattern of results emerged when depression was used as the criterion. Although self-efficacy was unrelated to depression in cross-sectional analyses, an interaction between initial level of pain and initial level of self-efficacy predicted depression one year later. For people with low levels of pain, depression did not vary with self-efficacy beliefs. In contrast, for people with high levels of pain, greater self-efficacy was associated with greater depression. People with arthritis who believed they were capable of controlling (or managing) their condition in the presence of high levels of pain reported greater psychological distress. Study participation was limited to patients with a duration of two years or less, thus the sample were in the relatively early stages of the chronic illness experience and consisted mainly of women (90 per cent), factors which may limit generalisability.

Strategies shown to enhance self-efficacy are mastery experience, role-modelling, persuasion and reinterpretation of physiological and affective states (Bandura, 1977). These strategies have been incorporated either singly or in combination, into a range of psycho-educational interventions developed for people with various types of arthritis (e.g. J.H. Barlow & Barefoot, 1996; Lorig & Holman, 1993) and are discussed further in Chapter 8.

Coping styles and strategies

In their seminal work of 1984, Lazarus and Folkman proposed that adaptation to stress is mediated by appraisal and coping. There are two types of appraisal. Primary appraisal concerns the degree of harm, loss, threat or challenge perceived by the individual. For example, a person with severe arthritis may be faced with the loss of a valuable activity such as gardening. Secondary appraisal concerns evaluation of the individual's coping options. Loss of ability to do gardening may be minimised by having structural alterations made to the garden, such as raising flower beds so that they are within easy reach, and ensuring there is flat, even paving around the garden thus enabling the individual to move safely around it.

There are several methods of classifying styles of coping responses. These can be summarised as follows:

- problem versus emotional coping;
- dispositional versus situational coping;
- attentional versus avoidant coping.

Problem-focused strategies involve defining the problem, generating alternative solutions, weighing up the costs and benefits of each alternative and then taking action. Emotion-focused coping focuses on dealing with the emotions associated with the stressor, and often involves cognitive processes such as avoidance, distancing, denial or wishful thinking. The earlier example of having the individual's garden altered can be considered problem-focused and is of course dependent upon the individual having appropriate resources to have structural alterations carried out. In the absence of such resources, the individual may resort to emotion-focused coping by trying not to think about the garden and how much she enjoyed gardening in the past (denial) or accepting the situation. Dispositional coping occurs when an individual uses similar coping strategies in response to different types of stressors (e.g. arthritis, relationships, work), whereas situational coping refers to the individual response to a specific stressor (e.g. the pain of arthritis). Attentional coping would involve an activity such as exercise to help relieve pain, whereas avoidant coping would involve restriction of activity (e.g. stopping exercise because of pain). Within the above broad classification, coping can also be categorised as active or passive, a categorisation that is sometimes used interchangeably with problem-focused and emotion-focused coping. An active strategy would be one that involves efforts to manage pain and continue with valued activities, whereas a passive strategy may involve trying to avoid pain by taking medication and limiting activities.

The lack of overall consensus regarding coping styles can be confusing when comparing the results of various studies. This situation is further confounded by the nature of the relationship between the individual and the environment, which is viewed as being dynamic and reciprocal. Thus, different coping strategies may be used by the same individual for the same or similar problem at different points in time. Equally, there may be high variability in the coping strategies used by people with arthritis for managing similar stressors (e.g. pain). The degree of control over the problem may influence the type of coping strategy used, with emotion-focused coping being used to deal with stressors that are not controllable (e.g. severe pain). Indeed, Tennen *et al.* (2000) found that when daily, problem-focused attempts to influence individuals' level of pain failed, greater effort was expended in the use of emotion-focused coping the following day.

Despite the complexity of coping and its measurement, there does seem to be a consensus that passive, avoidant, emotion-focused coping strategies are related to depression, negative affect and poor self-esteem, whereas active coping strategies are related to positive affect and decreased depression (Young, 1992). Wishful thinking has been associated with poorer psychological wellbeing, whereas cognitive restructuring and information-seeking are associated with better psychological wellbeing (Felton & Revenson, 1984; Manne & Zautra, 1989). Furthermore, passive coping strategies have been identified as mediators between pain and subsequent depression (Brown *et al.*, 1989). An interview-based study of 102 RA patients found that patients using self-blame or wish-fulfilling strategies had higher rates of depressive symptoms than patients who coped by using action-oriented coping strategies (Wilkins, 2000). In three independent samples of RA patients, Zautra *et al.* (1995) confirmed that coping mediates the relationship between disease variables and positive and negative affect. Drawing on the self-regulation model of Leventhal *et al.* (1980), Carlisle *et al.* (2005) tested the hypothesis that coping strategies acted as partial mediators between illness representations and illness outcomes in a cross-sectional study of 125 women with RA attending outpatient clinics. The self-regulation model purports that cognitive representations of illness (illness threat) influence selection and use of coping strategies, which in turn influence appraisal of illness outcomes. Coping strategies were assessed using the 36-item London Coping with RA Questionnaire (Newman *et al.*, 1990). Following a factor analysis, seven coping components were tested as potential partial mediators:

- active and information-seeking;
- avoidant and resigned;
- cognitive strategies and internalizing;
- faith;
- diet;
- rest;
- emotional expression.

The only significant mediating effects identified concerned avoidant and resigned coping, which was found to partially mediate between symptom identity and disability, and also between symptom identity and psychiatric morbidity. It is interesting to note that illness representations were not strongly related to coping strategies, and similarly, most coping strategies were not strongly related to illness outcomes. Thus, despite using a specific RA coping measure, results appear largely consistent with an earlier study by Scharloo *et al.* (1998) that failed to identify a mediating role for coping between illness representations and illness outcomes in RA.

The increasing importance of mediation by adaptation (defined as 'adjusted well and coping well') and self-esteem during the first four years following diagnosis has been highlighted by Nagyova *et al.* (2005) in a longitudinal study of 160 RA patients. High levels of pain were associated with risk of concurrent psychological distress (e.g. anxiety and depression). Moreover, high levels of pain were directly associated with a decrease in self-esteem and worse adjustment to the consequences of RA. One limitation of this study was that the measurement of adaptation relied on a single item rated from 1 to 5. Hence, a more detailed and reliable measure of adaptation may offer additional insight in future studies.

Although most studies in this area have focused on RA, there is a growing body of literature in OA with coping style identified as a key factor that determines pain and disability. A review by Dekker *et al.* (1992) concluded that catastrophising in response to pain was hypothesised to strengthen avoidance of pain-related activities. After controlling for demographic and medical status variables, coping strategies were shown to be important predictors of pain, health status and psychological distress among patients with OA knee pain (Keefe *et al.*, 1987). A later study confirmed that coping strategies were important for understanding pain 12 months after knee-replacement surgery (Keefe *et al.*, 1991). Recovery from knee-replacement surgery has been linked to purpose in life through two pathways: a direct association and an indirect association through active coping (Smith & Zautra, 2000). Finally, Keefe *et al.* (2000) found a gender difference in terms of use of catastrophising among 168 patients with OA of the knees (mean age 61.1 years). Not only did women have more pain and physical disability, but also catastrophising mediated the gender–pain relationship even controlling for depression. Keefe *et al.* focused exclusively on assessment of catastrophising in this study: no other coping strategies were included. It may be that women resorted to catastrophising because they had more severe disease. Another study focusing on women with OA (n = 107) aged ≥60 years found that more frequent use of emotion-focused coping strategies was associated with poorer functional ability and greater chronic, daily stress (Tak & Laffrey, 2003). Turner (2003) studied pain coping among 101 male ex-professional footballers with knee, hip, ankle or back pain, 58 per cent of whom had OA. The most frequently used pain-coping strategies were acceptance and active coping. The least-used strategies were substance abuse and behavioural disengagement. Perhaps of greater interest was the finding that 64 per cent of the sample coped with pain in other ways than those included in the coping scales: they used exercise, medication and relaxation, for example. Regression analyses showed that appraisal of the impact of pain on general health, emotional venting and active coping were the most significant predictors of psychological wellbeing. In addition, the effect of pain on psychological wellbeing was mediated through appraisals and coping. Overall, there is evidence that the way in which people with OA cope with their condition may mediate perceptions of pain, disability and wellbeing.

There may be a link between patients' coping style and the nature of their supportive environment. Griffin *et al.* (2001) showed that, among 42, middle-aged RA patients, punishing responses from others (e.g. anger or irritation when the patient is in pain) were infrequent. However, such interactions were associated with a patient coping style that typically focused on pain and vented negative emotion. Over time, patients experiencing punishing responses showed evidence of increased negative affect and were rated by rheumatologists as having more severe disease status. Similarly, Bermas *et al.* (2000) found that lower marital satisfaction among RA patients and spouses was associated with a passive coping style among patients. Thus the importance of taking into account not just the way in which the patient typically responds to pain and other symptoms of arthritis, but also how people in the immediate environment react, is highlighted. This point needs to be borne in mind when developing and delivering interventions designed to promote successful self-management and adjustment. The timing of interventions is also a key issue. The ideal scenario would be to provide appropriate interventions from the point of diagnosis onwards with the overall aim of preventing the onset of maladaptive coping styles. Furthermore, the importance of providing a range of interventions throughout the course of disease cannot be emphasised sufficiently. There is a tendency within health services to target newly diagnosed patients. This scenario is based on the erroneous assumption that those of longer duration know all there is to know about managing their condition. The chronic nature of most forms of arthritis necessitates living with the condition for long periods of time (e.g. 10 years, 20 years and more). Thus, introducing people to different methods of managing their condition and its wider consequences should become an integral part of a treatment plan from diagnosis onwards.

A unique approach was adopted by Danoff-Burg *et al.* (2000), who explored the concepts used by researchers in the context of coping measures and compared these with how respondents understood such concepts. Although in general patients' descriptions of coping matched researcher-derived definitions, there was some diversity in relation to cognitive and affective coping strategies. Furthermore, patients' descriptions of coping strategies often crossed multiple categories and therefore were not captured by most data-analytic techniques. This finding seems to reflect those of Newman *et al.* (1990) regarding a lack of distinctive coping style among many people with arthritis. Using cluster analysis, Newman *et al.* (1990) classified 158 RA patients on the basis of their coping strategies. Interestingly, the largest group (n = 105) did not demonstrate a distinctive coping style, but were found to utilise a range of strategies to limited extents. Although the four groups identified did not differ on demographic, clinical or laboratory measures, one small group (n = 14) characterised by lower levels of pain, stiffness and disability and greater psychological wellbeing, tended to use more open and active strategies to cope with their disease. These findings seem to reflect reality in that, over time, patients develop a repertoire of coping strategies from which they select the strategy that matches their given needs at a particular point in time. Given that the course of most forms of arthritis is variable, with periods of remission or lesser disease activity interspersed with bouts of exacerbation, it is likely that different coping strategies will be needed at different points in time. Thus, whilst broad generalisations about types of coping strategies (e.g. passive versus active) may be possible, it should not be assumed that all people with arthritis can be categorised by predominant coping style throughout the whole course of their disease (i.e. 10, 20 or 30 and more years). Whilst posing difficulties for researchers attempting to measure coping, adjusting and combining coping strategies and styles to suit given situations may serve to optimise desired outcomes for patients.

A different perspective is provided by Katz (2005) in an analysis of the self-management behaviours used by 511 persons with RA in response to five RA-related stressors: pain, fatigue, physical limitations, joint changes and symptom unpredictability. During telephone interviews, participants were presented with lists of self-management behaviours for each stressor and were invited to indicate which behaviours they had used over the previous 12 months. In relation to pain, factor analysis revealed four self-management strategies: accommodation (e.g. avoiding or limiting activities, resting); active remediation (e.g. applying heat or cold); social (e.g. asking for help, talking with a friend); and perseverance (e.g. pushing oneself to keep going). Similar factor structures were found for joint changes and physical limitations. A reduced set of self-management behaviour items was presented to participants in relation to managing fatigue and unpredictability. Thus, factor structure for these two stressors was slightly different and in the case of fatigue omitted the active strategy component. As noted by Katz, although this study focused on self-management behaviours rather than emotions and cognitions, there are some similarities to previously identified coping styles such as seeking social support, perseverance, and limitation of activities (Blalock *et al.*, 1993; Gignac *et al.*, 2000).

Satisfaction with abilities

As noted in the previous chapter, satisfaction with one's ability to carry out 'normal' roles and valued roles is important for people living with arthritis. In a series of studies, Katz and colleagues have focused on the mediating role played by satisfaction with abilities among people with RA. Firstly, it was noted that functional impairment preceded onset of new depressive symptoms among women with RA (Katz & Yelin, 1995). A distinction was made between types of functional activities. Specifically, there was little risk of new depression with loss of basic daily activities, whereas loss in ability to carry out valued, integrative life activities produced substantial risk of depression. Katz and Alfieri (1997) found that greater satisfaction with abilities was associated with lower depressive symptoms. Similarly, Blalock *et al.* (1988) reported that satisfaction with abilities in the areas of household activities, leisure activities and pain management was associated with psychological wellbeing. A longitudinal investigation among 373 RA patients (mean age 59.8, SD 12.9, 81.5 per cent female) showed that satisfaction with current abilities mediated the relationship between impact of RA on valued activities and depressive symptoms (Katz & Neugebauer, 2001). There were no gender differences in the findings. Finally, low satisfaction with abilities was found to be the most significant predictor of higher levels of depressive symptoms among a sample of 436 individuals with RA (Neugebauer *et al.*, 2003). Moreover, low satisfaction with abilities mediated the impact of physical impairment, valued activity disability and unfavourable social comparisons on depressive symptoms. A longitudinal study by the same team (Neugebauer *et al.*, 2004), found that low satisfaction with abilities was the most important predictor of a higher level of depressive symptoms and also acted as a mediator of the impact of physical impairment, valued activity disability and unfavourable comparisons on depression among people with RA. Thus interventions designed to enhance satisfaction with valued daily activities may have value in helping to 'protect' people with RA from the adverse impact of the condition.

Positive Aspects of Psychological Wellbeing

As noted at the beginning of this chapter, most research attention has focused on psychopathology, thus less is known about the positive aspects of psychological wellbeing among people with arthritis. There are of course exceptions where positive measures (e.g. positive affect) have been included alongside measures of psychopathology. For example, Curtis *et al.* (2005) included both positive and negative affect in their cross-sectional investigation of psychological stress as a predictor of psychological adjustment and health status in 59 patients with RA. Low perceived stress was associated with positive affect even controlling for disease status, age and disease duration. Zautra *et al.* (2005) collected an intensive data set over a period of 10–12 weeks for a sample of women (n = 124) with OA, fibromyalgia or both OA and fibromyalgia, including measures of both positive and negative affect. Higher weekly positive affect in addition to greater positive affect on average resulted in less negative affect both directly and in interaction with stress and pain. Higher positive affect overall predicted lower levels of pain in subsequent weeks. In contrast, weekly elevations of pain and stress predicted increases in negative affect and increases in weekly negative affect, and higher average negative affect was associated with greater levels of pain in subsequent weeks. Also focused on OA, Tak & Laffrey (2003) found that among older women (aged 60 years and over), perceived social support and an internal health locus of control contributed to the prediction of life satisfaction, controlling for demographic, illness-related and stress factors. The role played by purpose in life (PIL) was examined among 64 patients with OA who were recovering from knee-replacement surgery (Smith & Zautra, 2004). People with a sense of purpose feel that their lives have a direction and they possess goals for living. Regression analysis was used to predict changes in health six months following surgery. Results showed that PIL was related to lower anxiety, depression, negative affect, functional disability, stiffness and more positive affect. Even when optimism, pessimism and emotionality were controlled, PIL remained related to less anxiety, depression and negative affect, suggesting that PIL may be an important positive characteristic and could be a suitable target for psychological interventions.

Spirituality can be a source of strength and comfort and can be considered an important aspect of psychological wellbeing. For example, a diary-based study of 35 people living with RA (Keefe *et al.*, 2001) showed that participants who reported frequent spiritual experiences, such as feeling touched by the beauty of creation or wanting to be closer to God, also used more spiritual and religious coping strategies. In addition, they had more positive mood and social support compared to those who did not report such frequent spiritual experiences. The prevalence of daily spiritual experiences and how they were related to both physical and mental health was investigated by McCauley *et al.* (2008). The sample of 99 primary care patients had a mean age of 67.8 years, 50 per cent were African American, and 62 per cent were women. The most common co-morbid conditions were hypertension (74 per cent), arthritis (54 per cent) and heart disease (27 per cent). Women and people with arthritis had more frequent daily spiritual experiences than those with other conditions and men, respectively. Among people with arthritis in this sample, more frequent daily spiritual experiences were associated with increased energy, and less depression after controlling for age, race, sex, pain and co-morbid conditions. It is a pity that this study focused on assessment of depression and failed to include any measures of positive psychological wellbeing such as positive affect.

Children with JIA

Investigations of psychosocial wellbeing among children with JIA are limited in number, and findings are somewhat inconsistent. Whilst type of JIA appears to have little effect on psychosocial adaptation, an early study found children with arthritis to have a more negative self-image and lower than average achievement scores in school compared with a control group (McAnarney *et al.*, 1974). Similarly, Vandvik (1990) found that 64 per cent of a sample of 106 children with JIA had at least a mild level of psychological dysfunction and 50 per cent had a psychiatric diagnosis (e.g. anxiety, affective disorder). In contrast, many studies find psychological functioning of children with JIA to be within the normal range (Billings *et al.*, 1987; Huygen *et al.*, 2000; Ungerer *et al.*, 1988), or fail to find any difference in psychosocial functioning between children with JIA and their healthy peers (Shaw, 2001). In a traditional review of psychosocial factors, Miller (1993) concluded that, in general, children with rheumatic diseases do not show evidence of psychological or social dysfunction. This conclusion contrasts with findings of qualitative studies that revealed JIA and its treatment can lead to children feeling 'different' from their peers (J. Barlow, Harrison & Shaw, 1998). In addition, many children meet substantial barriers when attempting to participate in school and leisure activities, resulting in social exclusion, marginalisation and victimisation. It is difficult to believe that this state of affairs would not lead to some adverse emotional response at some point in time among some children. The likelihood is that JIA places some, but not all, children at risk of psychosocial problems. In accordance with adult rheumatology, given equal disease severity, some children may be incapacitated by their disease whilst others live full and active lives. Support for this assumption is provided by Shaw (2001), who found that poorer adaptation was related to higher levels of pain, stiffness, fatigue and functional disability, whereas better adaptation was related to greater hope and arthritis self-efficacy. Moreover, whilst the majority of the sample of 42 adolescents (aged 11 to 18 years) showed evidence of good adaptation, a small proportion appeared to experience considerable difficulty. For example, 40 per cent of adolescents with JIA were at risk of clinically anxious moods compared to 35 per cent of a comparison group of healthy peers. Similarly, 12 per cent of adolescents with JIA were at risk of depressed mood whereas none of the comparison group was at risk.

Support for the increased risk of psychological distress is provided by a Canadian study that adopted a population-based approach to investigate the effects of adolescent arthritis and rheumatism (AAR) using data from the 1996 National Population Health Survey (Adam *et al.*, 2005). Among the 26,012 respondents aged 12 to 19 years, 213 reported AAR. This group were compared to all other adolescents and a group of 9161 adolescents reporting other chronic diseases. Respondents with AAR were found to have higher rates of co-morbidity, depression and moderate or severe pain than adolescents without AAR. Compared with the chronic disease group, those with AAR made greater use of healthcare services and pain relief medications. Overall, the authors concluded that AAR affected mental health, health service use, school, work and home activities, suggesting considerable disease burden. A small study conducted in Bangladesh found evidence of psychiatric disorders in 35 per cent of participants with JIA (n = 40) aged 10 to 18 years compared with a frequency of 12.5 per cent among age- and sex-matched controls (Mullick *et al.*, 2005). In the JIA group, 15 per cent had depressive disorder, 12.5 per cent had somatoform disorder, 5 per cent had adjustment disorder and 2.5 per cent had mixed anxiety and depressive disorders. Muller-Godeffroy *et al.* (2005) assessed health-related quality of life (HRQOL) among a sample of 72 children and adolescents aged 8 to 16 years living in Germany. Results showed that participants with JIA or reactive arthritis had lower HRQOL compared to normative data. Almost 20 per cent of the sample reported problems such as social isolation and depression/anxiety. Indeed, impaired

HRQOL was predicted by functional limitations, social isolation and depression/anxiety.

The impact of JIA on psychological wellbeing may be long-lasting. One study traced and followed up 82 out of 101 patients who had attended a clinic for JIA (Foster *et al.*, 2003). The median age of respondents was 30 years (range 17 to 68) and data collected included both physical functioning and quality of life using the SF36 (Ware *et al.*, 1993). Compared to age- and sex-matched norms, the sample had significantly worse scores on a number of the SF36 dimensions: bodily pain, general health, physical functioning, vitality, emotion, and social isolation. Not surprisingly, the JIA group showed significantly worse mental health, and unemployment rates were three times higher than the norm.

Whereas single studies and traditional reviews provide a very mixed picture, with some authors concluding that chronic disease has no adverse effect on children's psychosocial wellbeing, systematic meta-analytic reviews can be useful, as they are designed to draw together findings from individual studies and to identify overall patterns in the pooled data. A meta-analytic review of 21 studies of psychological adjustment included children and adolescents (aged up to 20 years) with chronic arthritis (LeBovidge *et al.*, 2003). Searches for the meta-analysis were limited to Medline and Psychinfo and were conducted from the start of the databases to July 2001. Although the focus was on 'chronic arthritis', it should be noted that this term covers a group of heterogeneous diseases characterised by joint inflammation and stiffness resulting in wide variations in physical functioning and severity. Of the 21 studies identified, only five measured depression and only one measured anxiety. 'Internalising symptoms' was used to refer to anxiety, depression and social withdrawal, whereas 'externalising symptoms' referred to hyperactivity, oppositional body behaviour and aggression. Many studies used the Child Behaviour Check List (CBCL) (Achenbach & Edelbrock, 1983), a parent report measure that includes eight somatic items that may inflate problems among children/adolescents with physical conditions such as arthritis that are characterised by pain, stiffness etc. The meta-analysis found evidence of overall adjustment problems and internalising of symptoms compared to controls, although there was no effect on externalising symptoms or self-concept.

An overview of evidence from published reviews of children's psychosocial wellbeing across childhood chronic diseases including JIA concluded that children are at slightly elevated risk of psychological distress, although the numbers who fall within clinical parameters is relatively small (J.H. Barlow & Ellard, 2006). It is important to note that the precise proportion of children who experience psychological distress remains to be determined, not only in the context of JIA but also among other life-threatening and life-limiting conditions of childhood. Equally, risk factors for psychological distress require clarification.

The overview by Barlow and Ellard highlighted a number of measurement issues that need to be considered regarding the studies incorporated into both traditional reviews and meta-analyses. Not all studies assess key variables such as depression and anxiety, and standard measures, such as the CBCL, often include somatic items that could inflate psychopathology when used in the context of many chronic diseases of childhood. The failure of many studies to assess depression or anxiety is not surprising when one considers that child measures are often substantially longer than measures used for adults. Use of samples of convenience and single-site recruitment is linked to the problem of small sample sizes endemic in research on chronic diseases of childhood. Such measurement issues are equally applicable to studies of psychosocial wellbeing in JIA. Finally, ratings of psychosocial adjustment tend to differ by respondent (i.e. children, parents or teachers), with parents consistently providing the most negative ratings of children's psychological wellbeing. For example, Sawyer *et al.* (2005) found that parental ratings of children's HRQOL were consistently worse than children's own ratings. Similarly, Palermo *et al.* (2004) concluded that disagreement between parents' and children's reports of pain and function were common and were associated with depressive symptoms in the children. In contrast, April *et al.* (2006) concluded that there was generally good agreement between children's and parents' perceptions of quality of life, with the exception of ratings of fine motor functioning. This study does seem to be the exception to the general pattern evident in the published literature on children with other chronic diseases as well as JIA (see J.H. Barlow & Ellard, 2006).

Pain, disability and psychological wellbeing

Paralleling the literature on adults with arthritis, the relationships between disease severity, pain, disability and psychological wellbeing among children with JIA tend to be inconsistent. Some authors report an association between increased severity, including level of pain, and psychological adaptation (e.g. Billings *et al.*, 1987; Ungerer *et al.*, 1988) whereas others find no association (e.g. Vandvik, 1990). There are indications that those with milder disease and adolescent onset may be at increased risk of psychological distress (e.g. J. Barlow, Harrison & Shaw, 1998; Daltroy *et al.*, 1992). Ungerer *et al.* (1988) showed that level of self-concept was associated with adaptation among adolescents with JIA. Those with low self-concept had fewer close friends, dated less often, were lonelier, were teased more about arthritis, had worse health status and were keener to leave school. Interestingly, Palermo and Kiska (2005) found evidence to suggest a relationship between the experience of recurrent and chronic pain and sleep disturbance, with the latter being linked to mood disturbance and reductions in daily functioning and quality of life. Their sample comprised 86 adolescents with JIA, chronic headache or sickle cell disease. Few studies have addressed sleep disturbance or fatigue in JIA.

Box 5.3 Methodological Note

Many of the measuring instruments used to assess psychological wellbeing among children were developed over 20 years ago and have not been validated for use outside of the US. There may be cultural differences in the experience or expression of psychological distress. Divergence in the underlying structure of psychological measures developed in the US and applied in the UK has been noted among adults with arthritis (J.H. Barlow, Wright & Lorig, 2001). Also, the terminology used in scale items may not accord with that used by children growing up today. Paralleling the situation in adult psychosocial rheumatology, there are few measures of positive wellbeing for use among children. Hence, it is true to say that most studies rely on assessment of psychological morbidity rather than psychological wellness. Differences between children with childhood chronic diseases and their healthy peers may lie in the area of how happy they feel, rather than in degrees of sadness, for example. A further difficulty lies in finding a suitable control group with which to compare samples of children with JIA. Most studies of JIA are based on clinic samples and thus may not reflect those who are in remission or with mild disease.

Box 5.3 (cont'd)

Sample size is a problem, with many studies being based on samples of 30 and under, thus limiting generalisation. Small sample size is understandable given the relatively low prevalence of JIA. Where control groups are used, they often comprise siblings. Whilst siblings may be subject to similar family and environmental influences to the child with JIA, they may themselves be affected by the presence of a sick child within the family unit. A diversity of respondents is used to assess psychological wellbeing in JIA, including the child with JIA, their parents, teachers and health professionals. Few studies distinguish between children and adolescents, and age groupings used to categorise respondents as 'children' versus 'adolescents' tend to vary. Finally, findings rarely differentiate between age groups or developmental age.

Risk and resilience factors

Models of risk and resilience factors have been proposed in attempts to explain adjustment among children with JIA (Shaw, 2001). Family studies suggest a variety of risk factors, including parental dysfunction, high family stressors, scarce family resources and low family cohesion or harmony (Harris *et al.*, 1991; Ross *et al.*, 1993, Vandvik & Eckblad, 1991; Varni *et al.*, 1988; Wallander & Varni, 1989). Reciprocally, the child's psychosocial functioning can influence other family members. Indeed, it has been suggested that adaptation of both child and parents is as closely linked to the child's psychosocial wellbeing as to disease status (Timko, Stovel & Moos, 1992; Timko, Stovel, Moos & Miller, 1992). Overall, distinguishing between risk and resilience factors has shed some light on the process of adjustment, although the approach can be limited by the tendency to polarise factors as either protective or detrimental thus ignoring situations where a family's resources are scarce (risk) but cohesion is high (resilience).

As in the adult literature, the majority of studies of psychosocial wellbeing in JIA tend to focus on psychopathology and lack of adjustment.

There has been little investigation of opportunities for positive growth following childhood illness although a few studies incorporating positive factors are beginning to appear in the literature. Morrill (2004) included 'happiness' in her questionnaire-based investigation among parent–child dyads. Happiness was significantly correlated with approach coping, peer support and family support.

Parents' psychological wellbeing

Little is known about the psychosocial wellbeing of parents or siblings. It has been suggested that, whilst some parents experience severe psychosocial problems, the majority appear to cope well, with some actually reporting positive family changes (Konkol *et al.*, 1989). Understanding the variation in parental wellbeing is important for the development and implementation of interventions designed to enhance adjustment of the whole family unit. Attempts to identify factors that lead to variation in parental wellbeing have examined a number of variables, including characteristics of the child's illness (e.g. disease severity, functional status), social and environmental factors (e.g. demographic variables, family resources), family functioning, stressful life events and use of statutory service provisions. Much of this work has focused upon measuring 'objective' aspects of the child's health status based on medical records and laboratory data. However, the strength and direction of the relationships between these variables are often inconsistent and difficult to interpret (e.g. Daltroy *et al.*, 1992; Timko, Stovel & Moos, 1992; Timko, Stovel, Moos & Miller, 1992). In other chronic diseases of childhood, parental perceptions of the child's health status have been shown to be better predictors of adjustment than objective indices alone (e.g. Bradford, 1994).

The few studies that have focused on parental functioning in JIA suggest an increased risk of psychosocial symptomatology among mothers (e.g. J. Barlow, Wright, Shaw, Luqmani & Wyness, 2002; Timko, Stovel & Moos, 1992; Timko, Stovel, Moos & Miller, 1992; Vandvik & Eckblad, 1991). In the US, Timko, Stovel and Moos (1992), explored the adaptation of 159 mothers and fathers of children with JIA over a 12-month period and found that, despite reporting greater mastery over the stressors involved, mothers were more depressed than fathers. Poorer parental adaptation was associated with avoidance coping, the child's functional disability, pain and psychosocial wellbeing, spousal dysfunction and family resources. J.H. Barlow, Shaw & Wright (2000) also found that mothers (n = 115) were more depressed than fathers (n = 63), with 29.4 per cent and 22.3 per cent respectively, scoring above the cut-off point for risk of clinical disorder. The proportions at risk of clinically anxious mood were comparatively high for both mothers (45.9 per cent) and fathers (43.0 per cent). We found similar proportions of 'at risk' parents in a further study of 121 mothers and 82 fathers (unpublished data) using the same measure, the Hospital Anxiety and Depression Scale (HADS) (Zigmond & Snaith, 1983). Almost a quarter of mothers (24 per cent) and fathers (24 per cent) were at risk of depressed mood, and 54 per cent of mothers and 42 per cent of fathers were at risk of anxious mood (see Table 5.1). The proportion of those 'at risk' is less than is typically found among adults with arthritis but higher than the norms published by Crawford *et al.* (2001) (i.e. 13 per cent females and 8 per cent males; 38 per cent females and 26 per cent males at risk of depression and anxiety respectively). Of particular note is the relatively high proportion of fathers in the at risk group for clinically depressed mood. The increased levels of anxious mood noted among parents accords with qualitative data suggesting that parents perceive life with JIA to be stressful, particularly with respect to anxiety-provoking factors. The importance of parental wellbeing is emphasised by Reisine (1995), who concluded that where parents have better physical and emotional status and the family is characterised by greater cohesion, more harmony, and fewer stressful events, children demonstrate fewer adjustment or behavioural problems and report fewer symptoms.

Table 5.1. Proportions of mothers and fathers scoring above the cut-off point for risk of clinical disorder on the Hospital Anxiety and Depression Scale (Zigmond & Snaith, 1983)

	Mothers	*Fathers*	*Female norms**	*Male norms**
J.H. Barlow, Shaw & Wright (2000)	n = 115	n = 63		
Depression	29.4%	22.3%	13%	8%
Anxiety	45.9%	43%	38%	26%
Unpublished data	n = 121	n = 82		
Depression	24%	24%	13%	8%
Anxiety	54%	42%	38%	26%

* Published by Crawford *et al.*, 2001.

Elfant *et al.* (1999) adopted an original approach to understanding adjustment of adult children's arthritis by investigating the effects of parents' avoidant illness behaviours. A total of 49 patients (aged 29–85) described how their parents usually responded to minor illness. The sample was then divided into avoidant (avoiding routine activities when ill), non-avoidant or mixed (one parent avoidant and one parent non-avoidant). Disease severity was similar across all three groups. However, adults with avoidant parents had more behavioural restrictions, helplessness and depression compared with adults with non-avoidant parents. Hence, the authors conclude that the behavioural responses of parents can influence the way in which their offspring appraise illness, report symptoms and adjust to the presence of arthritis.

Mediators

An increasingly promising avenue of investigation concerns the role of intrapersonal factors as potential mediators of psychosocial functioning (e.g. the role of cognitive appraisals). In a study of 365 mothers of children with diverse chronic conditions including JIA, Silver *et al.* (1995) concluded that psychological distress might be reduced by interventions enhancing perceived levels of control and self-worth. In the context of JIA, Lustig *et al.* (1996) suggest that mothers' appraisals about the impact of disease upon the family might mediate between aspects of the child's condition and the mother's mental health. Thus, changing maternal appraisals using positive social support may serve to safeguard maternal wellbeing. Similarly, reduction of stress and maintenance of parents' self-esteem, psychological stability, and social support may foster parental wellbeing. Interventions targeting parents are likely to generate benefits for their children, since parental functioning is likely to have reciprocal consequences for the child's physical and psychosocial status.

In a review of juvenile arthritis, Miller (1993) suggests maternal competence is one of the most important influences on the psychosocial adjustment of children with the condition. The need to better understand variation in parental adjustment and the role of potential mediators was part of the rationale for developing a Parent's Arthritis Self-Efficacy Scale (PASE) (J.H. Barlow, Shaw & Wright, 2000) to assess parents' perceived ability to control, or manage, salient aspects of their children's JIA. Given that parents may use different courses of actions to control different aspects of JIA at different points in time and in different situations, the scale was designed at an intermediate level of generality. The scale covers 14 issues salient to parenting in the context of JIA, including parental management of children's pain, stiffness, swelling, sleep, fatigue, activity, sadness, loneliness, frustration, pleasure, participation in school activities and participation in activities with family and friends. Interestingly, the pattern of correlations between fathers' self-efficacy and children's wellbeing was generally weaker than that found for mothers, thus affirming the close bond that often seems to develop between mothers (usually the primary caregiver) and their children with JIA. Indeed, qualitative data suggests the identity of the mother becomes merged with that of the child as mothers recount the need for 'our blood tests', 'our exercises', and 'our pain' (J. Barlow, Harrison & Shaw, 1998).

A qualitative UK study highlighted the many stressors encountered by parents and the resultant impact on their wellbeing (J. Barlow, Harrison & Shaw, 1998). One dilemma that appeared to cause considerable anxiety concerned the use of medication. Parents felt that, although medication was necessary to alleviate symptoms (e.g. pain), it could have adverse side effects (e.g. stunted growth, increased body hair). Parents were faced with difficult decisions balancing benefits versus costs for their children. They were very anxious about the impact of JIA upon their child's development and were especially concerned about their child's future. Encouraging children to become independent was difficult for parents of children with impaired physical functioning. In these cases, parents felt compelled to assist their children with daily activities whilst at the same time worrying that they might be perpetuating dependency. Visibility of the child's condition appeared to influence both the way the child coped with the disease, and also the extent of social support and understanding received by the family.

Support for these qualitative findings was provided by a small survey of families (n = 31) attending outpatient clinics at a regional hospital (J. Barlow, Wright, Shaw, Luqmani & Wyness, 2002). The original intention was to include both mothers and fathers in the study. However, only one father accompanied his child to the clinic, thus supporting the notion that mothers have the primary care-taking role for chronically ill children. Mothers exhibited poorer physical function and poorer general health perceptions when compared to UK normative data on the widely used SF36 (Jenkinson *et al.*, 1993). In contrast, mean scores

Table 5.2.   Summary scores of maternal stressors associated with JIA

Variable (Visual analogue scales 0–10)	Mean	Standard deviation
How much do you worry about the side effects of medication?	7.49	2.86
How much do you worry about your child's future?	6.52	3.22
During the last 3 months how much have you worried about your child's health?	6.16	2.89
How much do you worry about becoming over-protective of your child?	5.03	3.48
Over the last 3 months how much distress has your child's health caused him/her?	4.62	3.07
How visible is your child's arthritis?	3.62	3.26
To what extent do your health problems interfere with your child's ability to lead a normal life?	3.53	3.43
To what extent do your child's health problems interfere with your ability to lead a normal life?	3.86	3.04

for energy/vitality and pain were consistent with population norms. The proportion of mothers at risk of anxious mood was 43 per cent, whilst 20 per cent were at risk of depressed mood: these proportions were slightly higher than female norms (54 per cent and 24 per cent respectively). Maternal ratings confirmed that the greatest stressors associated with caring for a child with JIA, concerned the side effects of medication, the child's future and becoming over-protective of the child (see Table 5.2).

There are some notable comparisons between this study and that of Bradford (1994), who explored the adaptation of families with children who had undergone a liver transplant. Mothers of children with JIA rated their children's health worse compared to mothers of children who had undergone a liver transplant. However, parents of both sets of children exhibited the same major concerns, worrying primarily about the side effects of medication, the child's future and becoming over-protective. Similarly, there was a robust relationship between maternal ratings of children's physical functioning and maternal wellbeing that has been noted by Bradford (1994), Walker *et al.* (1987) and Perrin *et al.* (1989) in relation to liver disease, cystic fibrosis and asthma, respectively. The direction of causality has yet to be determined: poor physical functioning of the child may lead to maternal psychological distress, or, alternatively maternal psychological distress may result in lower ratings of children's physical functioning.

Box 5.4 Methodological Note

Generalisability of findings of psychological studies in JIA is often limited by the relatively small sample sizes and recruitment through hospital clinics that may lead to samples of children with more severe disease. However, families attending regional hospitals tend live in a much wider geographical area and their experiences of the healthcare system are likely to be varied at the primary care level. The problem of small sample size is one faced by many researchers investigating chronic childhood illnesses. One solution is to collect data through multi-centre studies, although these are notoriously costly and time-consuming to organise. Furthermore, funding bodies are often cautious about supporting a study focusing on one medical condition that affects relatively few children and families. Hence, studies including children with different conditions (a non-categorical approach) might offer a way forward, particularly given the similarities noted between the JIA and findings from other chronic disease of childhood (e.g. liver disease). In addition, many studies are cross-sectional and therefore issues of causality remain to be examined.

Chapter Summary

Paralleling the medical literature, psychological studies have tended to focus on people with RA, thus less is known about the psychological wellbeing of people with other types of arthritis such as OA, AS and JIA. Furthermore, studies of psychological wellbeing have focused primarily on understanding depression and its correlates. Much less attention has been paid to other forms of distress, such as anxiety or low self-esteem. However, there is consistent evidence that people with arthritis are vulnerable to depression and anxiety. There appears to be a minority who become psychologically distressed early in the disease course and remain distressed throughout their arthritis journey with levels of anxiety and depression remaining fairly stable over time. There are indications that depression among people with arthritis is under-treated; one reason for this may be the overlap between symptoms of arthritis and symptoms of depression. For example, fatigue can be part of depressive symptomatology or can be a major consequence of arthritis. Not surprisingly, depression has been linked with pain and physical disability, although the direction of causality of the interrelationships between these factors remains unclear. A number of mediating and moderating variables have been examined in attempts to better understand the relationship between depression, pain and disability. These include helplessness, health locus of control, self-efficacy, coping strategies and satisfaction with abilities. Research attention has focused mainly on psychological pathology (particularly depression), although a few studies of positive psychology are beginning to emerge.

In the context of children with JIA, their parents and siblings, there is a need to extend the evidence base for psychosocial wellbeing. Children with JIA appear to be at slightly elevated risk of psychological distress, although the number of those who fall within clinical parameters is relatively small. Risk and resistance factors have been examined, and there are now a few studies reporting aspects of positive psychological wellbeing. Little is known about the psychological wellbeing of siblings or parents, although the few studies that have focused on parental functioning suggest an increased risk of psychosocial symptomatology among mothers. Developing a more informed understanding of the psychosocial needs of the child with JIA and the impact on their families will help in the development and targeting of interventions that are timely and effective, thus improving the quality of care in the future. An increasingly promising avenue of investigation concerns the role of intrapersonal factors as potential mediators of psychosocial functioning (e.g. the role of cognitive appraisals).

6

The Social Impact on Person and Family

Many people with arthritis experience a reduction of fine motor skills, restriction of mobility and an increased vulnerability to psychological stress (e.g. depression) that may interfere with family and social role functioning. For example, in RA the hands and feet are often affected, making it difficult to perform even the simplest of nurturant activities associated with childcare (e.g. cuddling a baby, playing). Equally, people with OA of the hip or knee may experience problems when attempting instrumental tasks such as moving about the kitchen when preparing meals or walking to local shops. Empirical investigations of these issues (e.g. Yelin, Lubeck *et al.*, 1987) show that over 50 per cent of people with RA and OA experienced loss in eight life domains, including household chores, leisure activities, work and social relationships. Furthermore, Reisine *et al.* (1987) found that, among women with RA, the most affected areas of social role functioning were shopping, cleaning and maintaining family ties. The importance of instrumental tasks, such as cooking, was highlighted in a study of women with RA that found a link between inability to carry out valued family activities and depression (Katz & Yelin, 1994). Clearly, interference with activities perceived as central to family roles can be a source of anxiety for many people with arthritis and their families. One area that has received increased attention from psychologists and healthcare professionals alike is that of parenting.

Parenting with Arthritis

Contrary to the popular belief that arthritis is a disease of old age, onset of many types of arthritis typically occurs between the ages of 20 and 40, thus coinciding with peak childbearing and childrearing years. As discussed in Chapter 2, RA is more predominant among women, has an early age at onset (i.e. typically under the age of 45) and is known to be associated with a remission of disease symptomatology during pregnancy. Unfortunately, this can be followed by disease exacerbation during the postpartum period (Spector *et al.*, 1990), therefore coinciding with the time that a new mother is faced with the demands of a dependent infant. Some women experience initial disease onset during the postpartum period, coinciding with hormonal change.

One perception of a 'good mother' is based upon the extent of participation in children's physical games and activities (Kocher, 1994). For parents with arthritis, meeting these social expectations may be difficult and feelings of guilt may develop. In addition, difficulties in meeting one's own expectations as a parent can lead to feelings of frustration and distress. Reisine *et al.* (1987) found that, of 142 mothers with RA, 29 per cent felt they did not meet their own expectations in the context of childcare. The unavoidable and persistent nature of childcare demands can add to feelings of inadequacy, already amplified by the nature of arthritis and its consequences. For example, mothers experiencing physical difficulties in holding their babies may be reluctant to seek assistance because of fears of being viewed as unfit to be a parent. Research on young mothers with arthritis (Geirdal, 1990) found that feelings of inadequacy in relation to the role of mother were far more painful to accept than feelings of inadequacy in relation to any other role (e.g. paid employment or housework).

Research into parenting has been dominated by the concept of 'homemaker', focusing primarily on women in 'mothering' roles. The importance of fathers and grandparents in the context of parenting has been largely neglected. One exception was a survey of 162 people with AS that encompassed mothers, fathers and grandparents (68 per cent male, 32 per cent female). Of these, 10 per cent had taken the decision not to have children, mainly because of the hereditary risk factors and the likelihood of 'passing on' the disease to one's offspring. One third of the remaining sample reported difficulties in some aspects of parenting (J.H. Barlow, Cullen, Foster, Harrison & Wade, 1999). The main areas of difficulty caring for babies and toddlers (aged 0–5 years) were breastfeeding, lifting, holding, bathing, bending to change nappies, putting to bed and inability to partake in 'rough and tumble' play. Typical comments were:

My neck was totally fused and I could not see where my child was feeding. (Mother)

Not being able to pick them up was a great drawback. (Father)

I had difficulty lifting without fear of dropping the children. (Grandparent)

The main problems reported in caring for children aged over 5 years were the inability to join in physical games and sporting activities with children. Many parents commented that they had 'missed out on the fun of being a parent'. As may be expected, a gender difference emerged, with women reporting more difficulties with babies and toddlers, whilst men experienced more problems as children grew older and became more active. Figure 6.1 illustrates the proportions of women and men reporting problems caring for children from babies to adolescents.

Mothers felt that lack of sleep whilst pregnant, pain, and sleepless nights after the birth had a cumulative effect which left them feeling exhausted. They felt guilty when they had to rely on older children for help with chores or a new baby. Mothers became less concerned with the physical impact of AS as children grew older, but this situation was accompanied by greater emotional distress as they felt they were not fulfilling their perceived role as a 'good mother'. The main problems reported by fathers concerned twisting and turning movements; thus,

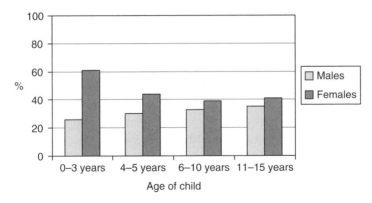

Figure 6.1 Proportions of women and men reporting problems caring for children from babyhood to adolescence

they had difficulty holding hands with small children whilst walking. Fathers found that fatigue was a major problem, particularly after a day at work which left them with little spare energy they could devote to playing with their children. Some fathers reported being short-tempered during times of disease activity. Several fathers feared the consequences of joining in with physical activity, feeling 'scared to death that I will be in agony the next day'.

Parents felt that the fatigue, pain, restricted mobility and the adverse emotional reactions (e.g. depression) associated with AS detracted from their perceptions of being a 'successful' parent. They reported being irritable and lacking patience with children because of their own health problems. Consequently, many parents felt deprived of the joys and pleasures that being a mother or father can bring, feeling overwhelmed by perceived inadequacies. Feelings of frustration, impatience, anger, irritability and depression were typically expressed:

I became irritable due to discomfort and stiffness. (Mother)

Being unable to join in physical activities left me feeling very frustrated. (Father)

I let my pain control my anger instead of understanding youthful behaviour. (Father)

A survey of parenting disability among 231 women with RA reports similar findings (Katz *et al.*, 2003). Separate sets of questions were asked depending upon the age of children (i.e. young – aged 0 to 5 years; older – aged 6 to 18 years). Not surprisingly, women reported more difficulties in parenting younger children. Greater parenting disability was associated with poorer general function, more severe pain, greater fatigue, greater parenting stress and greater psychological distress.

It is important that health professionals involved in the care of people with arthritis are aware of the potential impact on nurturant and caring roles. Some issues can be resolved using relatively simple techniques. For example, purchase of a cot with a side opening (like a door) rather than the traditional drop-down style can make life easier for parents who have difficulty in bending over. Similarly, baby clothes with velcro fastenings rather than poppers are easier to manage. Many of these techniques, resources and equipment have been collated into a handbook (Grant & Barlow, 2000) for use with parents and grandparents with arthritis. The handbook has been distributed among occupational therapists in the UK, who meet rheumatology patients.

Social Support

Arthritis not only affects the individual but also permeates through the whole family unit with variable effects. Whilst the impact of arthritis leaves some families feeling closer, others report no difference or adverse effects on family life (Pritchard, 1989). Family conflict has been linked to levels of arthritis pain, but not always in the expected direction. Faucett and Levine (1991) found that family conflict was associated with less pain, and concluded that spouses make an effort to reduce tensions during times of a disease flare in order to help reduce their partner's pain. As may be expected, living with a partner or spouse offers greater opportunity for support and thus appears to have a protective effect for the person with arthritis. For example, married people with RA perceived that they had greater access to assistance with instrumental tasks, more physical affection and expressed feelings of being needed by others, compared to those who were not married (Manne & Zautra, 1989). Similarly, Reisine (1995) showed that married RA patients felt more 'needed' than unmarried patients and suggests that this may have assisted them in maintaining higher levels of social and psychological functioning in order to meet the needs of others. In terms of physical functioning, a prospective study by Ward and Leigh (1993) found that marriage was associated with a slower rate of progression of functional disability. These findings are reinforced by results of a comparison of income, social support and psychological wellbeing among women with RA (Kraimaat *et al.*, 1995). Widowed or divorced women had a lower income, less potential support, and higher levels of depression and anxiety than women who had never married or those living with a spouse. One intriguing finding from this study was that pain contributed to depression and anxiety only in women living with a spouse. One potential reason for this finding is that patients' own perceptions of their ability to meet a spouse's expectation may influence their psychological wellbeing. For example, Bediako and Friend (2004) found a correlation between spouses' expectations and perceived inability to meet such expectations among 39 women with RA. Moreover, patients' perceived inability to meet spousal expectations contributed to the prediction of depressive symptoms.

As may be expected, longer disease duration has been associated with less problem-oriented instrumental support and high disability (Fyrand *et al.*, 2002). It is likely that opportunities for social support may decrease with advancing age and increasing disease duration. The appreciation of support received from loved ones was the most frequently reported benefit described by RA patients in a longitudinal study by Danoff-Burg and Revenson (2005). Indeed, 71.3 per cent of the sample reported interpersonal benefits whereas 16.2 per cent reported other types of benefit and 12.5 per cent found no benefits. These findings emphasise the importance of satisfactory support among people with arthritis.

Greater support reported by newly diagnosed RA patients has been associated with less anxiety and depression (Evers *et al.*, 1997), regardless of physician-rated disease severity (Revenson & Majerovitz, 1991). Following a longitudinal study of social support based on a large sample of early RA patients (n = 542) assessed over a period of three years, Demange *et al.* (2004) concluded that, whilst there may be cross-sectional relationships between specific social support/support network and functional limitations and psychological distress, there is no evidence of a longitudinal association. In contrast, Evers *et al.* (2003) found that among 78 early RA patients, social support and coping predicted disease activity at three- and five-year follow-ups, controlling for baseline disease activity, other biomedical and psychosocial factors and use of medication. Finally, one study reports less fatigue among people with RA who had higher levels of positive social support (Huyser *et al.*, 1998). This finding was independent of demographic and disease factors.

Arthritis can impact not only on the wellbeing of the individual but also on their close family, spouse or carer. A survey of the burden of care among informal caregivers of people with RA showed that 60 per cent of caregivers provided help seven days per week for an average of 33 hours (Riemsma *et al.*, 1999) and two-thirds of caregivers had other obligations (e.g. their own household, job or study). Given this typical scenario, it is not surprising that spouses of people with even mild RA have been shown to experience depression (Revenson & Majerovitz, 1991). Indeed, Walsh *et al.* (1999) found that there was no significant difference between RA patients and their partners in terms of level of distress. Both patients and partners had elevated levels of depression.

The relationship between communication (both verbal and nonverbal) of OA pain by wives and their husbands' wellbeing was examined by Stephens *et al.* (2006). Results showed that among women with severe pain, verbal and nonverbal expression of OA pain increased the likelihood of poor psychological wellbeing among their husbands and reduced the level of emotional support provided by husbands. This scenario is understandable given that it would be hard to provide emotional support to another if one is not feeling positive oneself. A unique approach to investigating concordance between patients' and spouses' reports of patients' pain severity and the relationship to support was adopted in a related study (Martire *et al.*, 2006). Patients and spouses independently viewed patients carrying out simulated household tasks and rated patients' pain. Interestingly, analysis showed that the most common type of non-concordance was an overestimation of patients' pain by spouses. Spouses who accurately rated patients' pain responded less negatively and provided more satisfying emotional support for their partners. In addition, such spouses reported less stress from providing such support and assistance.

Interestingly, a cross-sectional study found that optimism among carers and a lower level of caregiver burden was associated with high self-efficacy among patients with RA (Beckham *et al.*, 1995). In contrast, caregiver pessimism was associated with higher levels of physical disability among the patients. Clearly, causal inferences cannot be drawn from this cross-sectional analysis, but the associations are interesting and appear to warrant further investigation, particularly with a view towards developing interventions for both patients and carers.

The mechanism through which social support influences adjustment among people with arthritis has been investigated in terms of a direct effect, with more social support leading to improved mood and a buffering effect, whereby people with greater levels of stress derive greater benefit from social support. Hence, at times of disease exacerbation (i.e. high levels of pain, fatigue, and functional limitation), social support plays a greater role than at times of disease remission. Both direct and stress-buffering models have been examined in RA but have rarely been explored among people with other types of arthritis. Brown *et al.* (1989) found evidence of both direct and stress-buffering effects on depression among patients with RA in cross-sectional analyses, although only a direct effect was maintained longitudinally, at six

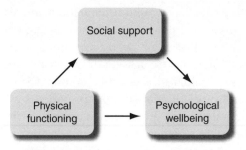

Figure 6.2   Diagrammatic representation of mediation by social support

months. Fitzpatrick *et al.* (1988) revealed that social support was associated with greater self-esteem and lower levels of depression, regardless of level of disability, thus providing support for the direct effects model in RA. There was no evidence of a stress-buffering effect. Similarly, Doeglas *et al.* (1994) failed to find support for the stress-buffering hypothesis among people with RA. A later study by the same group (Doeglas *et al.*, 2004), investigated patterns of relationships with social support over time in 264 early RA patients. Although large variations on functional ability, depressive feelings and social support were noted, mean scores remained fairly stable. Although depressive feelings were linearly related to functional ability, there was no evidence for a stress-buffering effect of social support. In contrast, Affleck *et al.* (1998) report a limited buffering effect for social support in the relationship between functional limitations and psychological wellbeing. One study examined the moderating effects of social support on the psychosocial adjustment of children with rheumatic disease (von Weiss *et al.*, 2002). Results were consistent with a main effect rather than a buffering model: fewer daily hassles and higher social support predicted fewer psychosocial adjustment problems. Support from classmates and support from parents were both significant predictors of adjustment. Overall, there appears to be more support for a direct-effects model of social support in arthritis.

Positive and negative effects of social support

The effects of social support may not be positive if the nature of the offered support fails to match the needs of the person with arthritis or if the nature of social interactions is negative. Positive support can affirm the value of the people with arthritis and their efforts to manage their conditions, thus encouraging positive adaptation. In contrast, support that is perceived in a negative light may interfere with coping efforts and may be associated with victim blaming and failure. The expression of negative support may reflect a lack of adjustment among spouses, family and friends in relation to the realities of life with a person with arthritis. Seeing a close relative in constant pain and not knowing how to respond could surface as adverse comments and criticism. Hence, a close relationship may be a double-edged sword in that positive and negative aspects of such relationships may detract from as well as enhance coping and adjustment. For example, the presence of RA can evoke negative responses among healthy spouses (Reisine, 1995). Furthermore, critical comments from spouses have been associated with maladaptive coping strategies and worse psychological wellbeing among people with RA (Bermas et al., 2000; Griffin et al., 2001; Manne & Zautra, 1989, 1990). A study of 103 women with RA and their husbands showed that positive support assisted cognitive restructuring and information-seeking whereas critical comments encouraged ineffective coping strategies (e.g. wishful thinking about a cure, fantasising). Similarly, a high degree of criticism from spouses has been linked to poorer psychological wellbeing among both men and women with RA (Kraimaat et al., 1995).

The relationship between both positive and negative aspects of social support and depression has been investigated among RA patients by Revenson et al. (1991). Positive support was operationalised as social interactions that provided affect, affirmation or aid, whilst problematic support was operationalised as support perceived as non-supportive regardless of the provider's intentions. Results showed that positive support was associated with less depression whilst problematic support was related to greater depression. There was no significant relationship between positive and problematic support, indicating that receipt of positive support does not preclude receipt of problematic support. Further, these two aspects of support appear to be independent. Indeed, an interaction effect between positive and problematic support upheld the notion of a stress-buffering model: positive support served to minimise the potentially adverse impact of problematic support. Subsequent investigation of the relative effects of positive and problematic support was conducted by Riemsma et al. (2000) using a sample of 197 patients with RA of over five years' duration. Findings confirmed the independence of positive and problematic support. In addition, hierarchical multiple regression analyses showed that the main predictors of depression were physical functioning and pain that together explained 29 per cent of the variance after controlling for sex, age and education. Positive and problematic support explained a further 6 per cent of the variance in depression. However, the majority of variance (58 per cent) remained unexplained. The authors suggest that other variables, such as fatigue, health beliefs and health behaviours, may contribute to the explanation of depression. Finally, a series of interaction effects were tested but failed to show evidence of a moderating effect for either positive or problematic support in the relationship between disease severity (physical functioning and pain) and depression. However, there was evidence of a weak effect for the interaction between the two types of support. Post-hoc analyses showed that for RA patients experiencing greater problematic support, the amount of positive support received influenced level of depression, suggesting a stress-buffering effect. However, it should be noted that the overall level of depression in this sample was low. Furthermore, the measure used, the AIMS-Depression scale from a Dutch version of the Arthritis Impact Measurement Scale (Meenan *et al.*, 1992), has not been validated in a clinical setting and does not distinguish between clinically and non-clinically depressed patients (Abdel-Nasser *et al.*, 1998). Finally, given the cross-sectional nature of the study, issues of causality remain to be addressed.

A related though slightly different approach was taken by Plach *et al.* (2003) in an examination of the mediating and moderating effects of social role quality among 156 women with RA aged 39–87 years. Hierarchical multiple regression analyses showed that role quality mediated the effects of physical health on depression and purpose in life, moderated the effects of health on depression, and moderated the effects of pain on purpose in life. In sum, women with high role quality and high pain had more purpose in life than women who were low on role quality and pain. Moreover, women with high role quality had better psychological wellbeing despite physical health problems.

Overall, satisfactory social support from family and friends appears to be consistently associated with less depression (Revenson & Majerovitz, 1991; Tsai, 2005), more life satisfaction (Burckhardt, 1985), less valued life disability (Neugebauer & Katz, 2004; Tsai, 2005), and greater self-esteem (Fitzpatrick *et al.*, 1988). Revenson (1993) concludes that the relationship between social support and psychological adjustment is a robust one. In terms of the mechanism of action, there is more evidence for a direct effects model than for a stress-buffering model. However, it is important to acknowledge that social support may not always be a positive factor in adjustment to arthritis and its consequences. People can receive both positive and problematic support, sometimes from the same person. This fact suggests that training family and friends to provide effective support may be beneficial for all concerned.

One limitation of the social support literature is the focus on people with RA. Although it is highly likely that social support plays a similar role among people with other types of arthritis such as OA, AS or JIA, caution is advocated in the generalisation of findings. Given the generally older age at onset of OA, the opportunities for social support may be more limited for people with this type of arthritis. Equally, AS is more prevalent among men, who are generally less willing to discuss health-related issues with family, friends and work colleagues and are concerned about denting their 'macho' image if they have to request help. Social support for children with JIA and their parents may raise different issues compared to adults and is discussed further below.

Children and Parents

The effects on children of having a parent with arthritis have received little attention. One of the few studies in this area suggests that adolescent children of parents with RA may have difficulty in maintaining self-esteem (Hirsch *et al.*, 1985). On the positive side, children of parents or grandparents with arthritis are perceived as developing a more caring attitude to others and often decide on a career in one of the caring professions (e.g. occupational therapy) (J.H. Barlow, Cullen, Foster, Harrison & Wade, 1999). However, some parents feel that adolescents are 'embarrassed' by arthritis-related aids (e.g. a raised toilet seat) in the house, and avoid inviting friends home.

Compared with many other chronic diseases of childhood (e.g. cancer), there is little published work regarding the impact of JIA upon parental functioning. When parents are included in studies it is often to provide ratings of their child's pain and physical functioning or to investigate the influence of family cohesion on the child. Nonetheless, having a child with JIA is likely to be a source of stress for parents, who are faced with the possibility that their child may experience pain, emotional distress and social limitations, and have limited life expectancy. The burden of care falls primarily on parents, who have to manage complex health regimens involving medication, physical therapy, specialised diets, avoidance of health-risk behaviours and frequent hospital attendance. Moreover, therapies can be associated with unpleasant side effects, may be painful and may not bring immediate relief or benefit. All of these demands have to be integrated with parents' other family, social, financial and career commitments.

Along with self-efficacy and parental competence, social support might mediate between parental stress and the impact of children's disease on the family (e.g. Lustig *et al.*, 1996; Miller, 1993), and could form the basis for psychological intervention. Similarly, the impact of a child's arthritis on siblings and grandparents, and vice versa, has received little attention but may be an important avenue of further enquiry in attempts to better understand the factors which promote family coping ability. One of the few studies in this area compared the relationships between 20 children with JIA and their siblings with the relationships of 20 control sibling pairs (Weiss *et al.*, 2001). The sample was aged between 7 and 21 years. There were no differences in perceived relationships or family structure between the JIA and control sibling pairs. However, among children with JIA, perceived conflict with siblings was positively associated with disease severity. This suggests that more severe disease is more difficult for children to cope with and may aggravate conflict. A qualitative exploration of having a sibling with JIA suggested that healthy siblings viewed their family as different from 'normal families (Waite-Jones & Madill, 2007). Healthy siblings felt that they forfeited time, which could have been spent with their peers. Social contagion was experienced due to having a brother or sister who was visibly disabled. In addition, healthy siblings were affected by emotional contagion through experiencing some of the emotional distress arising from JIA. Younger siblings were sometimes placed in the role of carer for their older brother or sister with JIA. Some positive aspects emerged, such as receiving extra treats and increased closeness within the family. However, this had to be balanced against the extra parental attention given to their brother or sister, especially during disease flares.

Adolescents with JIA were included in a descriptive study focusing on understanding the support networks of adolescents with chronic disease (Kyngas, 2004). Six categories of support were identified, including parents, peers, school, healthcare providers, technology and pets. Technology encompassed computers, mobile phones, television and videos. Interestingly, peers were divided into those with and those without a chronic disease. Opportunities for social interaction among children can occur in the context of play and leisure activities. A couple of studies have examined the important topics of play and leisure time among children with JIA. Hackett (2003) explored the perceptions of children aged 7 to 11 years via interviews. All children had difficulty with engaging in play and leisure activities irrespective of the level of disease activity. Symptoms, side effects of medication, treatment regimes and psychosocial factors combined to interfere with play and leisure activities. Moreover, play activities were often restricted by parents, teachers and even friends. Similarly, mothers in a detailed, qualitative study by Britton and Moore (2002a, 2002b) suggested that play for children with JIA became an 'armchair activity'. In this situation, JIA was believed to rob children of their childhood. Play is an important feature in children's lives that warrants more research attention.

Social Impact: Society

There is a tendency for health-related research to be framed within the medical model of disability, whereby 'the problem' is considered to be a deficit in adjustment, motivation or ability of the person with arthritis. This model construes professionals as the experts, who intervene with 'solutions' for those lacking in knowledge and expertise. In contrast, the social model of disability suggests that problems derive from the attitudinal, environmental and organisational barriers faced by people with arthritis (J. Barlow & Harrison, 1996).

There is a widespread myth that arthritis is an inevitable consequence of old age. This attitude derives from a lack of understanding in society, and is a constant source of frustration for young people and children who are told that they 'cannot have arthritis' because they are 'too young'. The effect of such attitudes serves to deny their personal experience and identity. Despite the widespread view that arthritis is usually a condition of old age, there does appear to be a general awareness of the painful nature of arthritis. A study of public attitudes (n = 503) by Badley and Woods (1979) revealed a consensus that the condition is very painful and is not just another name for aches and pains. Moreover, 16 per cent of respondents had experienced arthritis themselves and a further 40 per cent had relatives or friends with the condition. Arthritis was believed to be less serious than heart and kidney disease but more serious than bronchitis and migraine. Badley and Woods concluded that the public has a realistic idea about the nature of arthritis.

The bodily impact of arthritis can be visible or invisible, as well as permanent or temporary. Social expectations can vary according to the visibility or invisibility of disabilities (Stone, 1995). Hence, it is difficult to explain how one can be relatively free from pain one day, but in agony and unable to move the next. People with invisible or fluctuating arthritis can be accused of being lazy, malingering or using their condition as an excuse for failing to meet the expectations of others in their social network. When arthritis is visible there is an overwhelming propensity for people to see the arthritis (or its consequences) rather than the person, resulting in feelings of being different, marginalised and excluded.

Environmental barriers frequently derive from the inappropriate design of physical infrastructures that effectively limit not only access to buildings and public transport, but also freedom of movement once inside. Buses with high steps, the lack of ramps at the entrance to buildings, and the scarcity of disabled toilets are examples of environmental barriers frequently cited by people with arthritis of all ages (J. Barlow, Harrison & Shaw, 1998; J. Barlow & Williams, 1999). Restricted access to buildings and transport has major implications for leisure pursuits and establishing a social life. Everyday activities, such as shopping or going to the cinema, become significant feats of negotiation, endurance and even risk-taking.

A positive outlook, self-esteem and self-confidence become difficult to maintain. Feelings of isolation, anger and being different are common (J.H. Barlow & Cullen, 1996; J. Barlow, Harrison & Shaw, 1998). Finding a relevant peer group, through voluntary organisations or support groups, can enable people with arthritis to feel part of a community, a group with shared experiences and values (J. Barlow, Cullen, Davis & Williams, 1997; Shaw, 2001). Such feelings of belonging can also be engendered by attending psychological interventions based on group formats, which offer the opportunity for participants to meet with similar others and to discuss common concerns.

Young people and children can miss long periods of schooling, especially during times of an arthritis 'flare', for example. The choice between segregation, if steered down the special needs route, or isolation if left trying to cope in unsupportive and disabling institutions is a dichotomy faced by many young people. Institutional regulations frequently dictate inflexible working or school hours, causing difficulties for those who experience fatigue as an integral part of their condition. Fatigue can render the individual unable to muster the intellectual or physical capacity necessary to negotiate a day in education or work.

There appears to be some discordance regarding the impact of missed schooling on children's educational achievement, with some authors reporting no difference in performance when compared to healthy peers (e.g. Miller *et al.*, 1982), and others maintaining that children with JIA perform less well (e.g. Lovell *et al.*, 1990). A unique study by Shaw (2001) ascertained the views of 42 adolescents regarding the impact of JIA on their schooling. Results showed that adolescents felt that they missed more schooling than healthy peers and had more difficulty in completing schoolwork. Consequently, this group of adolescents was worried about their academic achievement and felt that the opportunities for further education and employment were limited by JIA.

There are few studies of the impact of JIA on educational attainment. In the study by Shaw (2001), adolescents with JIA (n = 42) were compared with their school peers (n = 21). Results showed that, although adolescents with JIA had higher absenteeism and met many functional barriers within the school environment, there was no difference between the groups in terms of psychosocial functioning. Further investigation showed that risk factors for poor adaptation included higher levels of pain, stiffness, fatigue and functional impairment whereas factors promoting resilience included greater hope and higher arthritis self-efficacy. In accord with other studies of psychological wellbeing (e.g. Miller, 1993), Shaw concluded that whilst the majority of adolescents were well adapted to their condition, there was a minority who experienced considerable problems.

It may be that the impact of JIA on educational attainment is more keenly felt as adolescents attempt to enter the employment arena. Whilst there is a dearth of published literature on the educational consequences of arthritis, there is a growing body of reports regarding work disability. This is discussed in the next section.

Working with Arthritis

Definition

Issues associated with work are often studied and considered under the term 'work disability', which is commonly defined as unemployment due to a health condition. Among people with arthritis, the persistence of chronic symptomatology (e.g. pain, fatigue, limited physical functioning and psychological distress) can lead people to reduce their working hours, to miss out on promotion opportunities, increase utilisation of sick leave, and to change jobs with greater frequency, as well taking early retirement on health grounds. This suggests that a broader definition of work disability may be called for in order to reflect its multidimensional nature. Indeed, a systematic review focusing on people with RA includes work disability as one of three measures of productivity loss, the others being work loss (e.g. absenteeism, short-term sick leave) and work limitation (reduction in productivity while at work) (Burton *et al.*, 2006). However, in the published literature 'work disability' is the term that appears to predominate.

The ripples that work disability can have through the lives of people with arthritis is illustrated in the following quote from a male with AS.

> A total change in my life. I had qualified as a Pharmacist, was studying for my Masters and then I had AS. My plans for developing my career were stifled. I could not move house and as a result I became dependent on my parents as I still live at home ... With my qualifications, I would now have been at a much higher grade. When I see other colleagues (who I trained with), taking on more managerial roles, I find it upsetting, but I am coming to terms with it. (J.H. Barlow, Wright, Williams & Keat, 2001)

Prevalence

Unless otherwise stated, prevalence of work disability is estimated using the narrow definition (i.e. unemployment due to illness/disability). Not all countries distinguish between types of disabilities and chronic conditions in terms of employment figures, and thus precise figures relating to the prevalence of work disability in arthritis are often absent. In general, the economic activity rate among people with disabilities is substantially less than half that of non-disabled people. For example, young people with disabilities are almost twice as likely to be unemployed as their peers, and even where young people with disabilities are employed, they tend to be on lower salaries (Hirst & Baldwin, 1994). In the US, arthritis has been cited as the main cause of work loss and work disability payments (Yelin, 1992).

The majority of work disability studies have focused on RA. The systematic review by Burton *et al.* (2006) found that a median of 66 per cent of employed people with RA experienced work loss due to RA in the previous 12 months for a median of 39 days. The time from RA diagnosis to unemployment ranged from 4.5 to 22 years. Consistent predictors of subsequent work disability were physically demanding work, more severe RA and older age. Equally, rates of RA-related work disability were similar in the US and Europe. None of the studies reviewed addressed work limitation from the employer perspective.

In the US, 25 to 50 per cent of people with RA will experience work disability; a figure that can rise to 90 per cent for individuals with longer disease duration (Wolfe, Anderson *et al.*, 1994; Yelin, Henke *et al.*, 1987). Work survival analysis on Canadian data showed a steady increase in work disability among people with RA over a 10-year period (Lacaille *et al.*, 2004). In England for a single year (1992), the economic impact of disability associated with RA alone has been estimated at £1.256 billion and is mostly accounted for by lost production (McIntosh, 1996). The fastest decline in employment rate is within the first three years after disease onset (Mau *et al.*, 1996). In the Netherlands, Doeglas *et al.* (1995) found 42 per cent of patients with RA, who were in paid employment before the onset of the disease, left their jobs within an average of two years due to RA. Also in The Netherlands, Albers *et al.* (1999) report that unemployment among people with RA is, on average, seven times higher than that found in the general population. One year after RA diagnosis 14 per cent became work-disabled. This proportion rose to 42 per cent after three years and 72 per cent after 5 years (Albers *et al.*, 1999) suggesting a similar picture to that found in the US.

Gender differences in the correlates of work disability among 960 RA patients (aged 18 to 64) were identified by De Roos and Callahan (1999). Compared to working females, work-disabled females were more likely to have less education, a non-professional occupation and more pain. Among male RA patients, there was little association with these variables. However, work-disabled men had higher levels of helplessness and were not married. Correlates of paid and unpaid work were examined by Backman *et al.* (2004) in a sample of 269 RA patients (81 per cent were female, mean age 50 years, disease duration 13 years). Regression analyses showed that more hours of paid work were associated with being male, psychologically demanding work, higher social function, and less pain whereas more hours of unpaid work were associated with more children in the household, greater perceived physically and psychologically demanding work, social support from family and post-secondary education.

There is relatively little information regarding work disability among people with other types of arthritis, although there have been a few studies focusing on AS, a type of arthritis with a relatively early age at onset (between 20 and 40 years). Thus the impact of pain, fatigue, and progressive disability on the individual's lifestyle, chosen career path, family and social life could be long-term and far-reaching. However, prevalence appears to be lower than that typically reported in RA. For example, in Finland work disability due to AS is reported to be between 10 and 15 per cent (Kaarela *et al.*, 1987). Studies conducted in the 1980s suggest that the majority of people with AS do not experience work dis-ability and do not change the nature of their work as a result of AS (Carette *et al.*, 1983; Lehtinen, 1981; McGuigan *et al.*, 1984). For example, Lehtinen (1981) found that 25 years after diagnosis, 66 per cent were still working full-time; of these 50 per cent had retained their original jobs.

However, work disability in AS may be masked (J.H. Barlow & Barefoot, 1996; J. Barlow, Macey & Struthers, 1993). Wordsworth and Mowat (1986) reviewed 100 UK patients with AS and found that, although 84 patients had remained in full-time employment, the career decisions of 41 patients had been influenced by AS. Thus, nine had changed to less satisfactory employment, 24 had changed jobs com-pletely and 33 per cent had been on sick leave for more than three months due to AS and/or associated conditions (e.g. inflammatory bowel disease). Wordsworth and Mowat concluded that, although 93 per cent remained in gainful employment, difficulties in work ability (e.g. changing jobs and roles, increased use of sick leave) were experi-enced. A later survey of 133 people with AS (mean age 49 years, mean disease duration 28 years) conducted in the UK (J.H. Barlow, Wright, Williams & Keat, 2001) found that 31 per cent were unable to work because of AS. A further 15 per cent reported changes to working life that were attributed to AS, including reduced hours, change to a less strenuous job, change to a more accommodating employer, loss of career opportunities or early retirement. This figure rose to 46 per cent when participants who had changed the nature of their jobs were included. Thus, findings suggest that the prevalence of work disability among people with AS in the UK may differ from that found in Scandinavia (e.g. Kaarela *et al.*, 1987). In a comparison with the Dutch population, Boonen *et al.* (2001) found that, after adjustments for age, labour force participation was decreased by 15.4 per cent in males with AS and 5.2 per cent in females. Work disability was 15.7 per cent and 16.9 per cent higher than expected in the general population for males and females respectively. Patients took a mean of 10 days' sick leave due to AS per annum compared with a national average of 12 days.

Risk factors and barriers to employment

Risk factors for work disability are present at both an individual and a societal level. Pain, fatigue, limited physical functioning, uncertainty, extensive treatment demands and vulnerability to psychological distress can be barriers that the individual with arthritis has to overcome when trying to enter the workplace or maintain their position in it. Among adults with RA, individual risk factors identified include advancing chronological age, disease duration and severity, functional disability, level of formal education, nature of employment (e.g. degree of physical strength and stamina needed), low job autonomy, depression and a desire to stay at home (Callahan *et al.*, 1992; Felson, 1994; Mau *et al.*, 1996; Reisine *et al.*, 1995). Indeed, Allaire *et al.* (2005) found that, despite being better educated, individuals with RA aged 55 to 64 years had lower employment rates compared with same-age individuals in the US. Interestingly, older individuals with RA took less sick leave than younger individuals. Among people with AS, work disability (narrow definition) has been associated with older age at diagnosis, manual jobs and lower educational level (Boonen, 2002). Similarly, J.H. Barlow, Wright, Williams and Keat (2001) found work disability was associated with advancing chronological age, longer disease duration, fewer educational qualifications, co-morbidity, lower self-esteem, greater physical impairment, pain, fatigue, stiffness and depressed mood. After controlling for age, education and gender, logistic regression confirmed the importance of depression and pain in predicting work disability in AS. Interestingly, interview data revealed unpredictability, pain, and limited mobility to be associated with work disability.

> Quite frankly, at times, it is a living nightmare. I am in a job where I can
> be lifting items or spending time on my feet. I then suffer extra pain in my
> neck, wrists and feet. I wish I could be in a job where I would not have to
> put pressure on my various joints. (J.H. Barlow *et al.*, 2001)

Fatigue appeared to be one of the main challenges for people with AS, who report that its effects flowed into many areas of their lives (e.g. home, family and leisure). Strategies used to cope with these factors include reducing working hours, changing to less physical jobs, working from home, becoming self-employed or taking early retirement. Changes to working patterns and the nature of work are largely viewed as negative, although some people experience such changes in a positive manner (e.g. more time for the family, less stress at work). However, most are anxious about having time off work because of AS and the future. This anxiety appears to manifest as guilt and a feeling of vulnerability in terms of job security. It is likely that these risk factors are equally applicable to people with other types of arthritis with an onset of symptoms typically occurring before retirement age. A self-fulfilling prophecy begins to operate, whereby people with arthritis have little confidence in their abilities, believing that they have little to offer, and therefore cease attempts to enter or remain in the employment arena.

As well as individual risk factors, people with arthritis face a number of attitudinal, environmental and organisational barriers at the societal level (J. Barlow & Harrison, 1996) that form risk factors for work disability. Arthritis is generally viewed as a condition associated with old age. This attitude derives from a lack of understanding in society and is a constant source of tension for young people, children and their parents (J.H. Barlow, Shaw & Harrison, 1998). People with invisible or fluctuating arthritis are often viewed as being lazy, malingering, or using their condition to vindicate their failure to meet the social expectations of others. Missed schooling during periods of being unwell can hinder educational achievement. Environmental barriers frequently derive from the inappropriate design of physical infrastructures that effectively limit not only access to buildings, but also freedom of movement once inside. Access to transport and restricted access to buildings can prove to be major barriers encountered by people with arthritis in their attempt to enter or maintain employment. The types of jobs available, employer practices and regulations, and the nature of disability benefits and pension plans may add to the impact of arthritis on work.

Among younger people with arthritis, the focus is on encouraging attempts to enter the labour market and enabling young people to fulfil their potential. A Scandinavian survey suggests that few young people with arthritis receive adequate vocational guidance or counselling (Kroll & Peake, 1996). Similarly, barriers to vocational readiness faced by young people with arthritis and other chronic illnesses in the US include a lack of knowledge about the availability of existing career and vocational services, the attitudes of health professionals who view young adults as 'children forever' rather than adults with employment goals, and a lack of self-advocacy skills (White & Shear, 1992). A parallel situation appears to exist in the UK, where young people with arthritis report a variety of barriers to employment, including lack of awareness, confidence and support (Straughair & Fawcitt, 1992).

A number of barriers directly related to employment and training emerged from a study by J. Barlow, Wright and Kroll (2001). Focus groups were used as a means of understanding the employment situation and perceived prospects of younger people with arthritis (aged between 19 and 40). Three main barriers emerged, and concerned the lack of understanding about arthritis in society, transport difficulties and fear about not 'being able to cope at work'. In accordance with the literature on unemployed adults in general, a number of focus group participants reported intra-personal barriers associated with a general lack of confidence in their own abilities, low self-esteem and negative thinking, as illustrated in the following quotes.

> Society looks at you as a person who's not capable of doing a 40 hour week and bringing a pay packet home at the end of it.

> If I am not feeling well I cannot go out. You do not want to explain it all the time.

> My biggest barrier, I suppose, is pain because I am dying to get back to work and I am worried about not being able to work full-time.

> It's been a blow to our self-esteem to not feel physically well. That lowers your confidence and creates barriers within ourselves ...

Similar barriers to maintaining employment emerged from a focus-group study of people with inflammatory arthritis (mainly RA) living in Canada (Lacaille *et al.*, 2007). Interestingly, fatigue was identified as the most limiting aspect of arthritis in a work context. Other challenges faced included invisibility of the condition, fluctuating disease course, fear of disclosure and loss of self-efficacy. Helpful strategies include flexible work arrangements, ergonomic assessment by a professional knowledgeable about arthritis and provision of information about treatment options and living with arthritis.

Impact on psychological wellbeing

Unemployment can adversely affect psychological wellbeing in terms of depression (Vinokur *et al.*, 1996) and poor self-esteem (Sheeran *et al.*, 1995). When unemployment is combined with the experience of a condition such as arthritis, the impact may be additive. Chronic symptomatology, vulnerability to psychological distress, an uncertain disease course (flares and remissions) and progressive impairment of physical functioning may pose additional problems in relation to gaining or maintaining employment. Furthermore, identity is often linked to work and feelings of independence. Indeed, participants with AS described the meaning of 'work' as 'independence', 'money' and 'essential to my life' (J.H. Barlow, Wright, Williams & Keat, 2001). Hence, it is not surprising that a loss of identity could result in feelings of depressed mood and lower self-esteem. The links between psychological distress, disease symptomatology and work are well illustrated by the following quote:

> Teaching was a struggle for me, especially during the last 5 years ... I found listening to children increasingly hard. I became depressed and anxious. My doctor put me on antidepressants, I got more stooped and my ribs kept cramping up. Willpower kept me going, but anxiety forced me to resign. (J.H. Barlow *et al.*, 2001)

Recent studies have considered the nature of individuals' jobs as well as the impact of their physical and psychological health on lost productivity. Fifield *et al.* (2004) examined how job structure and the daily experience of work influenced chronic pain among 27 employed people with RA, using diaries that were completed over 20 work days. On days with more undesirable work events, those in high-demand/low-control (job strain) positions had greater pain irrespective of neuroticism and negative mood. Along similar lines, Xin (2006) found that productivity loss among people with arthritis was associated not only with low or medium control over the work schedule but also with more severe symptoms, greater workspace limitation and higher depression. People with RA have reported that compared to their normal performance they are 78 per cent as effective when working with symptoms of RA (Kim *et al.*, 2001).

Instability of employment among people with RA has been associated with higher levels of pain and depression (Fifield *et al.*, 1992). Depression was associated with work changes (e.g. occasional work loss, changes in type/hours of work) among 492 people with RA or OA (Gignac *et al.*, 2004). Interestingly, a related publication showed that respondents were more likely to report that work interfered with caring for their arthritis than to report that arthritis interfered with their work performance (Gignac *et al.*, 2006), a finding which appears to contrast somewhat with those of Kim *et al.* (2001) (see above). Seventy per cent of respondents reported work changes with younger participants and those with greater workplace limitations being most affected.

Levels of psychological distress among samples of people with arthritis participating in interventions aiming to enhance employment prospects (e.g. J. Barlow, Wright & Kroll, 2001) tend to be higher compared with samples recruited onto educational and self-management interventions (e.g. J. Barlow, Turner & Wright, 1998a; J.H. Barlow, Turner & Wright, 1998; J.H. Barlow, Turner & Wright, 2000). Table 6.1 shows that the proportions of participants on employment-related interventions who are at risk of depressed and anxious mood are substantially higher and accord with the notion of unemployment being an additive risk factor for psychological distress. It should be noted that, in general,

Table 6.1. Proportions of participants enrolling on educational versus employment-related interventions at risk of depressed and anxious moods

Type of intervention	Depressed mood	Anxious mood
Employment-related intervention – INTO Work	40%	77%
Employment-related intervention – Working Horizons	63%	83%
Educational/self-management intervention – Arthritis Self-Management Programme	30%	60%

employment-related interventions tend to attract younger participants compared to those who enrol on educational/self-management interventions.

The importance of work for quality of life was investigated in a large-scale study conducted in The Netherlands focusing on people with RA and AS aged 16 to 59 years (Chorus *et al.*, 2003). The sample comprised 1056 patients with RA and 658 with AS. There were no differences between RA and AS patients in terms of pain, physical role functioning, social functioning, emotional role functioning, vitality or general health perception, fatigue or behavioural coping styles. However, physical health-related quality of life was worse and mental health-related quality of life was better among patients with RA compared to patients with AS. Regardless, work was positively associated with physical health-related quality of life in both groups and was the most important predictor after disease characteristics.

Prevention

Prevention of work disability is an important goal in the treatment of arthritis, especially where disease onset occurs relatively early in the life course. Several interventions aimed at enhancing the employment potential and personal development needs of people with arthritis have been initiated in the UK by Arthritis Care, the leading voluntary organisation working with and for people with arthritis. Evaluations have shown these to be successful in achieving their aims and are discussed in more depth in Chapter 8.

Given the paucity of interventions targeting arthritis, the majority of people with the condition have to negotiate their own workplace adaptations and modes of working. As indicated by participants with AS in full-time paid employment, adjustments can be made to the work environment involving minimal cost and disruption (J.H. Barlow, Wright, Williams & Keat, 2001). For example, flexible working hours can help with the management of fatigue. Being able to get up and move around frequently can help to ease stiffness; and the purchase of ergonomically adapted office furniture can help to ease pain and discomfort. Many people with arthritis become self-employed as a means of attaining a flexible working pattern. Others change to part-time work, taking sedentary jobs or retiring early. Such strategies are more in accord with adaptation or accommodating to their condition than with preventative measures. The following quotes from the J.H. Barlow, Wright, Williams and Keat (2001) study exemplify the adaptive strategies employed by people with AS in the context of work.

I now work 18–20 hours per week … Initially when I first changed to part-time I was very bitter that I had to downgrade and accept a less dynamic role. Looking back, it has helped me a lot, as going part-time has eased the stress. I do not have the responsibility pressures and I have four days to recover, which helps the AS.

Most physical work is not possible any more due to my wrists being badly affected by AS. I have been an engineer and a keen DIY enthusiast, but now I have to get other people to do jobs for me. I can't stand or walk now, so I work on a computer in a software company. I have been in engineering all my working life, but this is not possible now.

I have a job (self-employed) which allows me to work around the uncertainty. For example, one day I am very painful and fatigued and can only do limited office work. Another day, I feel good and can get out and about, and even concentrate for a full working day.

As noted earlier, change in working life or pattern of working is not always viewed negatively. A reduction in time spent at work can lead to more time to spend with partners and other family members, or maintaining a healthy lifestyle (e.g. going to the gym). The improved design of office work stations can facilitate range of movement whilst sitting at a desk, and exercise can be introduced into the working day (e.g. walking during lunch hour). Even an enforced change of occupation can have positive results.

I have now achieved, at work, all I need to feel fulfilled. I have no intention of qualifying further and no longer need to prove myself. Importantly, I now have the energy to dance, walk and play tennis, which makes me happy! (I was a tired and achy recluse before!)

I have had to rethink how and what I do for a living, and do find full-time work very demanding … However, I have found a job which I really enjoy and feel very lucky to have found a second career which I love. (J.H. Barlow *et al.*, 2001)

Despite the fact that some people find positive features emerge from changes to working life imposed by arthritis, there does appear to be a general lack of assistance available for those who seek to enter the employment arena, to maintain employment or to manage arthritis effectively in the work environment.

Chapter Summary

This chapter has considered the impact of arthritis on social roles such as parenting, and working life. Mothers, fathers and grandparents find that arthritis symptoms (e.g. pain, fatigue), impaired physical functioning and feelings of anger, frustration and irritability can adversely impact on nurturing activities such as lifting, holding or dressing babies and young children and joining in with physical play or sporting activities. The actual impact on performance of social roles compared with the individual's perceived impact is difficult to tease out, since expectations of concepts such as a 'good mother' are likely to be high.

Social support, particularly from spouses/partners, is generally reported to be beneficial for the person with arthritis, although the burden of care experienced by informal carers can place them at risk of depression. Nonetheless, the relationship between social support and psychological adjustment among people with arthritis is a robust one. In the arthritis literature, there is more evidence for a direct effects model of social support than for a stress-buffering model. Thus, greater social support is typically associated with lower levels of psychological distress. However, it is important to acknowledge that social support may not always be a positive factor in adjustment to arthritis and its consequences. People can receive both positive and problematic support, sometimes from the same person. Social support studies have focused on people with RA, and thus less is known about the effects of social support among people with other types of arthritis. Equally, little is known about the effect on children of having a parent with arthritis. The social impact of caring for a child with JIA appears to be similar to that experienced among parents of children with other chronic diseases of childhood. For children, the presence of JIA is felt in the domains of play, leisure activities and schooling.

Arthritis can interfere with the ability to obtain employment, maintenance of employment and long-term plans for retirement. Risk factors for work disability are present at both an individual and a societal level. Pain, fatigue, limited physical functioning, uncertainty, extensive treatment demands and vulnerability to psychological distress can be barriers that the individual with arthritis has to overcome when trying to enter the workplace or maintain their position in it. However, it is important to note that not all changes in working life or work pattern as a consequence of arthritis are negative. Reduced working hours can leave more time to spend on valued activities with partners, family and friends. Despite the fact that some people find positive features emerging from changes to working life imposed by arthritis, there does appear to be a general lack of assistance available for those who seek to enter the employment arena, to maintain employment or to manage arthritis effectively in the work environment.

7

Health Care and Patient Education

The Experience of Health Care

Patient and provider perspectives

Ideally, patients and providers work together in partnership to promote the best possible health outcomes. This means that patients need to be fully involved in decisions affecting their care and to be both knowledgeable and aware of therapeutic options. In addition, patients need to understand what their condition means for them and how they can contribute to their own care and wellbeing. Routes towards attaining successful partnerships in health care are many and variable.

Patients need to feel that their views are valued and their judgements about treatment options are incorporated into care plans (Charles *et al.*, 1999). If providers operate within these guidelines, patients should report high levels of satisfaction with the care received. However, there is scope for misunderstanding at various levels between patients and providers. Quite simply, each is viewing the same situation from a different vantage point: one founded on professional training and the other based on the lived experience of what it means to have arthritis. For example, pain is used as a touchstone by patients in deciding the nature and level of activities that they feel they can carry out at a given point in time. The fact that pain does not always correlate with the extent of OA when assessed radiographically (Dekker *et al.*, 1992) illustrates that the potential for a divergence of views between patient and provider in rheumatology is great. A survey of patient preferences for improved health among 1024 patients with RA in Norway found that 70 per cent of patients selected pain as their preferred area for improvement (Heiberg & Kvien, 2002). These findings need to be interpreted with some caution since the patients were not allowed to freely nominate their preferred area for improvement; rather, they were asked to select up to three areas from a list of 12, that included pain, work, mood, social activity and hand and finger function. Nonetheless, the results confirm the importance of pain management among people with RA. Interestingly, the authors conclude that pain management may fall 'in a vacuum' between health professions. They suggest that nurses may view pain as the domain of physicians (i.e. to be treated by pharmacological intervention), whereas physicians may focus on physiologic issues and disease progression as indicated by laboratory tests. The reality is that a collaborative approach to the management of pain drawing on patients' preferences and health status is needed.

Being seen and being believed emerged as two central themes from an interview-based study of two groups of patients: those with well-defined inflammatory arthritis (i.e. RA and AS; n = 12) versus those with no-inflammatory widespread chronic pain (n = 14) (Haugli *et al.*, 2004). Within the RA and AS group, 'being seen' in the context of medical encounters related to being viewed as an individual rather than a diagnosis, and 'being believed' related to acceptance of the level of pain and suffering reported. For the non-inflammatory group, 'being seen' and 'being believed' related to acquiring a somatic diagnosis. Ryan (1996) provides further insight into patients' views of their relationship with health professionals. Her phenomenological study revealed that the main concerns expressed by RA patients were that:

- too much emphasis was given to the physical manifestations of the disease;
- the patient was not always reviewed by the same doctor, thus making it difficult to develop a relationship between doctor and patient;
- consultations were not always interactive in nature.

Similarly, the tendency for consultations to focus on medical matters to the exclusion of the wider impact of disease and feelings of being kept in 'the dark' emerged in a study of 79 younger people aged between 19 and 40:

Doctors are not prepared to actually give you the full treatment or actual diagnosis. ... They would not tell me physically what was wrong and whatever was going to happen mentally after having to give up work and my hobbies. ... No-one worried about it. No-one got into your mind or even cared about asking what was going on in your head ... (J. Barlow, Wright & Kroll, 2001, p.210)

Past treatment policies are criticised for the degree of suffering that they can cause for the individual. One ex-professional footballer who was diagnosed with OA of the hip when aged 38 recalls the time spent waiting for hip replacement thus:

I suffered a great deal with OA from a young age, and because it was hos-pital policy in the 60s not to operate on people too young, I had to wait and suffer many years before they would operate on me. (Turner, 2003)

The theme of concentration on the biological parameters of disease to the exclusion of wider psychosocial issues continues in the context of JIA. Britton and Moore (2002a, 2002b) found that families were more concerned with the psychosocial consequences of JIA, which they felt went largely unaddressed. Similarly, parents of children with JIA have reported that health professionals tend to focus their attention on 'dis-ease activity' rather than the child as a person, or themselves as parents (J.H. Barlow, Shaw & Harrison, 1999). Children had difficulty in under-standing and remembering the verbal information received, both par-ents and children felt unable to voice their questions in clinical settings, and parents felt that health professionals did not understand their situation in the context of the home environment.

They really don't understand the problems you have at home ... The doctors see them for half-an-hour ... and examine the joints ... but, it doesn't just affect their joints. It affects them mentally and that's what we have to put up with. (Parent) (J.H. Barlow, Shaw & Harrison, 1999)

Following an investigation of differences in perceptions of quality of life between parents and paediatricians at diagnosis and thereafter, Janse *et al.* (2005) argue that the quality of life of paediatric patients, including those with JIA, may be misunderstood by health profes-sionals. Paediatricians provided consistently lower ratings of children's emotions, pain and discomfort than did parents. The potential for a divergence of views not only between health professionals and patients but also among patients is illustrated in relation to a video

(Southwood, 1992). Children with relatively mild JIA and their parents felt the video was pessimistic and even distressing in places. Paradoxically, more severely affected children and their parents felt that the same video was overly optimistic. However, regardless of disease severity, there was consensus that showing children talking about their own experiences of JIA helped both children and parents to feel less isolated and was seen as a major benefit of the video.

> The first time he watched it [the video] he got quite anxious because he wasn't particularly severely affected and he said, 'Is this what's going to happen?' So I went through it and picked out the bits that I thought were relevant. (Parent's view)

> I thought that it was going to go worse and I'm going to get it in most places. It was like the first time I went in to hospital. There was a load of old people there and mostly old people have it. I don't know anyone who has arthritis at school, except for a few teachers who have it. (Child's view)

> Sometimes I thought, 'Oh God! I'm the only one that has got it [arthritis] out of all my friends.' Then when I watched the video, I knew that quite a lot of other people had got it other than me. (Child's view)

Inpatients' experience of care

The importance of considering patients' perspectives and priorities has received greater recognition in recent years, although there are few studies investigating how consumer and provider views may be combined to provide optimal care. In relation to inpatient care, the organisation of services varies enormously. Some inpatients receive care in dedicated, specialist rheumatology wards whereas others find themselves admitted to general medical or surgical wards and receive non-specialist care. Early studies suggested that inpatients on non-specialist wards may receive a lower quality of care due to lack of experience among staff, whereas comparatively better outcomes were achieved for inpatients cared for in specialised rheumatology units (Duff *et al.*, 1974; Spiegal *et al.*, 1986). Given the growing emphasis placed on rheumatology nurse specialists (practitioners) and multi-disciplinary teams, it could be argued that care within a dedicated unit should be more widespread in the 21st century.

The care received in specialist versus general wards was explored in a phenomenological study by Edwards *et al.* (2001). Interviews were conducted with nine RA patients who had been admitted to a specialist, rheumatology ward or an internal medicine ward. Five themes emerged:

- the uncertainty and anxiety experienced by the novice inpatient;
- the progression through multiple admissions to becoming an expert inpatient;
- the positive and negative effects of meeting other inpatients;
- the comfort derived from experienced and knowledgeable staff;
- loss of privacy during inpatient care, particularly for younger patients.

During their first admission (novice inpatient), participants had experienced considerable uncertainty regarding the treatment that they might receive. Terms such as 'scared', 'panic' and 'frightened' were used as participants related their fears about having something 'done' to them. Of particular note was patients' fear of intra-corticosteroid injections in their joints. Eight of the nine patients had been admitted on several occasions. Thus, a sense of familiarity and 'belonging' had replaced their novice fears and uncertainty. They also expressed very positive expectations regarding the outcomes of admission and the ability of the staff. As patients evolved into experts, they mentored novice patients, a situation that may have influenced the feeling of comradeship that developed on the wards. Patients talked of supporting one another through bad days and becoming long-term friends not only with staff but also with other inpatients. Interestingly, there was no apparent difference between inpatients on the specialist ward compared to those on the general medical ward, where most patients had rheumatological disorders. The two younger patients felt constrained by the ward procedures (e.g. lack of privacy) and felt degraded by having to rely on nurses for the personal care of their bodies and assistance with instrumental tasks (e.g. eating). Overall, the two younger patients expressed a preference for being nursed in single rooms rather than on a ward. Generalisability of findings is limited by the small, purposive sample. However, this study is valuable in providing a rare insight into the views of inpatients regarding their admission to hospital.

Box 7.1 Methodological Note

Edwards *et al.*, 2001 set an excellent precedent in the report of their phenomenological study, by listing their own preconceptions before they commenced the interviews. Thus they expected to find that:

- patients would avoid inpatient care and view hospitals as an alien environment;
- all patients would be anxious on admission;
- patients would derive support from other patients with the same condition;
- joint injections would be a cause of distress;
- patients admitted to a general rather than specialised ward would be disadvantaged.

This process of transparency about researchers' preconceptions is known as bracketing and allows readers to make their own decisions regarding potential bias in the results. This study also included a clear report of the procedural steps taken in analysing the data making it very clear to readers how the authors' arrived at their conclusions.

Outpatient care

The majority of people with arthritis receive health care at the primary care level (e.g. general practitioner practices) or as outpatients in specialist rheumatology departments. There are few data regarding the experience of care at the primary level. One exception is a qualitative study of the experiences of 26 RA patients regarding the quality of care received in both primary and secondary care (Lempp *et al.*, 2006). The majority of patients (24) had visited their GP for an initial assessment following onset of symptoms; 11 of these patients complained of delays by GPs in making a diagnosis which they attributed to GPs' lack of knowledge and/or interest in the patients' presentation of symptoms. There were contrasting views regarding GP care following diagnosis, with 16 patients providing critical comments (e.g. 'GP knows little about RA') whereas 10 others were positive and had appreciated their GP's understanding, sympathy and long-standing knowledge of the patient. Regarding secondary care, clinic visits focused on regular monitoring, physical examination, assessment of the effectiveness of current treatment with additional support being provided when necessary, and degree of perceived understanding of patients' situation by healthcare staff. In terms of organisational issues, three patients expressed a preference for less frequent outpatient appointments and six female patients expressed a preference for discussing general health, emotional or gynaecological issues with female members of staff (doctors or nurses) rather than male staff. An innovative Canadian study aimed to improve the diagnosis and treatment of arthritis in primary care through provision of a two-day educational workshop ('Getting to Grips with Arthritis') for healthcare providers (Glazier *et al.*, 2005). The workshop was followed up with reinforcement activities and provision of a toolkit of written materials for providers and clients. A total of 21 multidisciplinary providers attended from five community health centres designated as intervention sites; two community health centres acted as control sites. The impact of the intervention was assessed via a mailed survey to clients. Results showed that clients from intervention sites had higher referrals to the Arthritis Society therapy programme and were more often provided with information on arthritis, medications and their side effects, disease management strategies and arthritis community resources. Results illustrate that it is possible to impact on arthritis management strategies at healthcare provider level using a short intervention.

There is an increasing literature regarding comparisons between nurse-led care and doctor-led care of hospital outpatients. As may be expected, there is consistent evidence supporting the variation in focus between nurse-led and doctor-led approaches. For example, Hill (1992) found that consultants' clinics emphasised diagnosis and medication whereas nurse practitioner-led clinics focused more on patient education and were more likely to refer patients to other members of the multi-disciplinary team. The coverage of wider areas of disease management is reflected in the comparative length of consultations, which tend to be shorter with consultants compared with rheumatology nurse practitioners (RNPs). Indeed, Wright and Hopkins (1990) found consultations with nurse practitioners were twice as long as consultations with doctors. The difference in time is reflected in patient throughput; Hill (1997) reported that consultants saw an average of 17 patients per clinic compared with an average of eight patients seen in nurse-led clinics. An observational component of a study by J. Barlow, Wright, Carr *et al.* (2001) confirmed the findings of Hill (1992) and showed that consultations with consultants tended to revolve around medical management with a focus on test results and RA treatment involving medication. In contrast, consultations with RNPs tended to cover wider issues of the consequences and management of RA, including strategies that patients could use at home to relieve fatigue and pain (e.g. rest activity cycling, pacing of activities) and lifestyle factors (e.g. diet). Further insight is provided by Ryan (1995), who showed that patients valued the extra time afforded in nurse-led clinics in order to discuss the wider implications of their condition. However, a later study highlighted two topics that RA patients rarely discussed with nurse practitioners: relationship problems within the family and the need to adopt self-management strategies at home (Ryan, 1996).

Although it was not set up to directly compare doctor-led approaches versus nurse-led approaches to outpatient care, the results of the study by J. Barlow, Wright, Carr *et al.* (2001) are of interest in the context of outpatient care. The study rationale was based on the premise that incorporating patients' views in the setting of treatment goals would enhance patient-centred and clinical outcomes. Thus, two packages of care were compared in a randomised, controlled trial. The first package was the traditional problem-orientated, doctor-led approach (the Control). The second was an individualised goal-setting approach delivered by an RNP (the Intervention). The sample comprised over 400 RA patients (median age 61 years; range 25–86 and median duration of 9.5 years; range 0–58) attending outpatient clinics at two hospital sites. Results failed to find any statistically significant differences in terms of biological disease parameters or patient-centred outcomes between the traditional problem-orientated, doctor-led approach and the individualised, goal-setting approach delivered by an RNP. Findings support the notion that management of RA outpatients by RNPs using goal-setting could be used as an alternative approach to the traditional style of patient management and would not have an adverse effect on patient outcomes. Indeed, patient satisfaction, expectations, health status (e.g. depressed and anxious mood, pain, fatigue) and clinical markers were remarkably similar regardless of the package of care received. A measure of arthritis self-efficacy was included in the study but failed to show any changes. Although the goal-setting package was designed to involve patients in priority setting and decision-making, it may have lacked sufficient efficacy-enhancing strategies to effect change on this set of expectations. For example, in a one-to-one consultation with a nurse there is no opportunity to observe similar others carrying out the target behaviour (role-modelling). Equally, translating the practice of new behaviours from a 'safe' clinical setting into the home environment may have been difficult for some patients.

It is generally accepted that there are variations in the receipt of resources by outpatients. Variation may be dependent upon the availability of local facilities, and factors associated with the knowledge and current practice of health professionals who act as gatekeepers to resources. A groundbreaking study conducted in The Netherlands, set out to assess variation in the daily practice of 27 rheumatologists on eight different rheumatologic conditions. Assessment of actual practice was operationalised using 'standardised patients' (i.e. real or healthy people who have been trained to play a role in a consistent and accurate way). A checklist was used to indicate the diagnostic and management process. The eight 'cases' included AS and RA. The results provided evidence of considerable variation in practice and the costs for laboratory and imaging investigations (Gorter *et al.*, 2001). Mean costs per rheumatologist ranged from US \$4.67 to \$65.36 per visit for laboratory costs and from US \$33.15 to \$226.84 for imaging tests. There was no significant association between resource utilisation costs and years of clinical experience or performance on checklist scores. However, those with longer clinical experience scored lower on the performance checklist. The authors suggest that similar variation in practice performance and costs would be found in other healthcare systems. One limitation is that the rheumatologists were aware that a study was being conducted and may have altered their practice accordingly (e.g. referred patients for more or fewer tests). Nonetheless, results provide valuable feedback that can be used in medical education and in the development of guidelines for care, and the methods could be used to identify areas in need of an injection of financial and service improvement.

A further study conducted in The Netherlands examined the prevalence of unmet healthcare demands among RA patients in terms of orthopaedic care, allied health care, home care and psychosocial care (Jacobi *et al.*, 2004). Indications of 'under-use' were ascertained by comparing the health outcomes of patients reporting unmet healthcare demands and patients who were healthcare users. Of the 679 RA patients,

28.7 per cent had an unmet need for one of the four services: 13.4 per cent for allied health care; 9.7 per cent for orthopaedic care; 9.4 per cent for home care and 6.2 per cent for psychosocial care.

Patient satisfaction with care

The growth of quality mechanisms and the increasing value placed on consumer views has led to greater use of patient satisfaction surveys. A key factor determining patients' satisfaction appears to be their interactions with health professionals (Rosenthal & Shannon, 1997). Satisfaction does not solely rest upon patients' perceptions of technical ability. Rather, skills such as ability to listen, to provide information and to involve the patient in decision-making are salient. In addition, the patient's prior experiences, expectations, norms and psychological wellbeing are brought to bear on ratings of satisfaction.

A postal survey conducted in Norway investigated satisfaction and involvement in health care (Brekke *et al.*, 2001b). The sample comprised 1024 patients with RA (mean age = 62.4, SD 14.8), 78.7 per cent females, mean disease duration = 12.7 years, SD 11.1). Satisfaction was assessed using one item scored on a five-point scale. Results showed that 11 per cent of the sample was dissatisfied with the health care received whilst 57 per cent were satisfied. Satisfied patients were better educated, had better health status and higher self-efficacy than dissatisfied patients. Logistic regression showed that satisfaction was independently associated with being female, having low pain, good mental health, high self-efficacy and high involvement in health care. In general, patients with poorer physical or mental health status tend to report less satisfaction with the care received (Hall *et al.*, 1998), and RA patients appear to be no exception. Given the positive associations between self-efficacy and psychological wellbeing, it is perhaps not surprising to find an association with satisfaction. Referral of patients to self-management programs known to enhance self-efficacy beliefs and psychological wellbeing may also lead to improved satisfaction with health care.

Brekke *et al.* (2001b) assessed involvement with care using three questions concerning receipt of information regarding diagnosis, information about self-management-style activities (e.g. exercise) and whether patients were asked for their opinion regarding therapeutic decisions. A total of 13 per cent reported that they had not received information at diagnosis and treatment, 21 per cent had not received information on self-management, and 33 per cent had not had the opportunity to inform therapeutic decisions. High involvement was independently associated with younger age, high education level, high disability, good mental health and visits to a rheumatologist during the last 12 months.

Much of the published literature on patient satisfaction in rheumatology compares patients' ratings of nurse-led versus doctor-led clinics. Findings are somewhat mixed: some show higher satisfaction among patients attending nurse-led clinics compared with those attending doctor-led clinics (Hill, 1997) whereas others find no difference in satisfaction (J. Barlow, Wright, Carr *et al.*, 2001). In the latter study, it is worth noting that not only was there no difference in satisfaction between nurse-led or doctor-led care, but also there was no difference in satisfaction between the two hospital sites used for the study. The latter was somewhat remarkable as there were a number of significant differences in patients' health status and medication usage between the hospital sites, with patients at one hospital demonstrating a significantly worse profile. There did not appear to be any major differences in socioeconomic profiles of the respective catchment areas; therefore such differences may arise from historical management issues or current inequalities in hospital resources for example.

The use of three control groups by J. Barlow, Wright, Carr *et al.* (2001) allowed investigation of the possible impact of highlighting patients' expectations and satisfaction through the assessment process itself. That is, completion of measures assessing patients' expectations and current satisfaction with care may serve to raise their future expectations and satisfaction levels. Thus, one control group completed a minimal data set only at baseline and the full battery of measures at 12 months. Subsequent analyses showed that assessing expectations and satisfaction at baseline did not appear to influence outcomes at 12-month follow-up. patients' expectations for relief from pain and fatigue were consistently related to their feelings of satisfaction with the care received, with greater expectation for relief from pain or fatigue being associated with higher ratings of satisfaction.

One study compared care provided by a clinical nurse specialist, an inpatient team and a day-patient team for patients with RA (Tijhuis *et al.*, 2002). Patients were randomly assigned to each type of care. The mean number of visits to the nurse specialist was three over a 12-week period; inpatient and day-patient care comprised nine treatment days over two to three weeks. Functional status, quality of life, health utility and disease activity improved in all three groups. However, with increasing age, greater improvements in physical function were found among the inpatient group. Although satisfaction levels were high among all patients, those receiving care from the clinical nurse specialist were slightly less satisfied. The authors suggest that this form of care was less intensive in terms of contact time, which may have been reflected in satisfaction ratings. This study is important, as it is the first randomised comparison of care by clinical nurse specialist and a multi-disciplinary team. The latter is often viewed as the optimal type of care for rheumatology patients. However, this study shows that care led by a clinical nurse specialist who could refer to other health professionals (e.g. occupational therapist, physiotherapist) can be just as effective as the more costly multidisciplinary inpatient and day-patient provision.

Pain already receives a great deal of attention in outpatient settings and is used by patients as a touchstone for determining the degree of severity of their condition (J.H. Barlow, 1998). However, pain management using psychologically based techniques in place of, or in addition to, medication may be worthy of greater exploration in rheumatology, especially as many patients express concern about the toxic side effects of the drugs used to treat their condition. Equally, fatigue tends to receive less attention than pain in clinical settings but clearly is salient for patients' satisfaction with life and ability to function. The precise mechanism leading to fatigue in arthritis remains to be clarified. It is known that there can be a tendency towards anaemia in some patients, and also the extra effort required to accomplish simple tasks can serve to place further strain on scarce resources (i.e. patients' energy reserves). Thus, after ruling out biological causes of fatigue (e.g. anaemia), instruction in techniques such as pacing and other self-management strategies may help patients to cope better with this symptom in the home environment.

Box 7.2 Methodological Note

It is notoriously difficult to obtain accurate ratings of patient satisfaction. Ceiling effects are common; that is most patients express high levels of satisfaction with the care received.

Box 7.2 (cont'd)

Data collection conducted in clinical settings or even mailed to respondents' homes may be biased by patients' concerns that reporting their true views may adversely influence their subsequent care or relationship with the healthcare team. Patients are often grateful for the care that they receive and can feel that marking satisfaction as low is somehow criticising the health professionals whom they have come to know and respect over the years.

There are very different approaches to assessment currently in operation, ranging from single-item global satisfaction ratings to more complex scales. A single item offers little opportunity for respondents to discriminate between aspects of health care which are good compared to aspects of care that could be improved. Focus groups can be used to gain greater insight into the patient experience and have the advantage of enabling patients to feel that their views are valued and worth consideration. If groups are conducted by facilitators who are independent of the healthcare team, participants can more freely express their views, both positive and negative.

Therapeutic concordance

As in all chronic diseases, responsibility for the daily management of arthritis gradually shifts from the healthcare team to the individual. Management of home-care regimens is often complex, involving adherence to a range of therapies, including medication, prescribed exercise, splint wearing, clinic attendance and the avoidance of health risk behaviours. For the person with arthritis, the benefits of behavioural strategies (e.g. exercise, use of splints), may not be evident in the short term, but these strategies are necessary to prevent further disability. Complex, long-term therapies are extremely difficult to maintain, and thus it is not surprising that concordance with treatment recommendations in arthritis is often poor and not only detracts from the individual benefits of various therapies but, on a wider scale, can result in increased health costs.

Several terms appear in the literature, the earliest being 'compliance'. Compliance is defined as the extent to which the individual's behaviour (e.g. taking medication) coincides with medical advice (Haynes *et al.*, 1979) and tends to be associated with the medical model that views the patient as a passive recipient of health care. The term 'adherence' has been used more recently and is linked with the notion of health professional and patient working in partnership to make decisions about health care. Adherence has been superseded by the term 'concordance'. Unless specifically reporting on a study that aimed to examine compliance, adherence or concordance, the term concordance will be used throughout this text. This area of study is complex. For example, concordance with medication involves taking the prescription to a pharmacy and collecting it, and taking the medication correctly (e.g. at the right time, with or without food, taking the prescribed dose, taking the full course of medication). Opportunities for non-concordance are many. The patient could take a higher dose than prescribed, take it more frequently, forget to take it, take it on a full stomach when an empty stomach is ideal or stop taking it too soon. Any one of these could lead to partial non-concordance. Assessment of concordance is further complicated by the difficulty of ascertaining objective and reliable data. Methods used to measure concordance include biological measures, direct observation of behaviour, electronic medication dispensers, pill counts, checking prescriptions and self-reports. Pill counts and electronic dispensers can be unreliable if tablets are removed from the container and not taken. Similarly, patients can take medication in the days preceding a biological assessment and then stop taking it. The result is an erroneous picture of concordance. Observation is costly to conduct and is usually only possible during delivery of a clinic-based exercise programme for example, rather than observation of medication use.

A review of treatment adherence in RA (Bradley, 1989) revealed that rates of cooperation varied from 33 to 78 per cent for medication and from 33 to 66 per cent for therapeutic exercises. Adherence to non-steroidal anti-inflammatory drugs among people with OA has been estimated at between 60 and 95 per cent (La Montagna *et al.*, 1998) using patient self-report or tablet counts during clinical trials. It is likely that adherence will be higher during a clinical trial where patients know they are being studied. In primary care, self-reported adherence in OA has been estimated at the lower rate of 60 per cent (Weinberger,

Tierney & Booher, 1989). Adherence to therapeutic exercise in OA has been reported at 70 per cent where exercise was defined as completion of 75 per cent of the exercise program (O'Reilly *et al.*, 1999). These findings parallel those reported in the wider literature on long-term regimens, particularly those with a behavioural component (Deyo, 1982). Attrition from exercise programmes is approximately 50 per cent in the first six months, declining even further over time (Dishman, 1982).

Generally, the factors related to concordance are of a psychosocial rather than demographic or disease-related nature. Factors that may influence concordance include patients' beliefs about their illness, beliefs about health in general, the treatment offered, alternative therapies, and the relationship with healthcare providers. Discrepancy regarding medication and its side effects was discussed earlier in this chapter with particular relevance to children with JIA and their parents. When prescriptions for new medication are issued, it is essential that patients understand when they can expect to feel an improvement and the nature of that improvement. For example, if a patient believes that a drug will bring complete relief from pain within two days, the likelihood of the patient continuing to take the medication will decrease after this time if pain is not considerably improved. Equally, patients can believe that they will develop a tolerance to analgesic drugs and thus over time would need to continually increase their dosage. If patients are concerned about the prospect of taking increasing doses of analgesic drugs, then they may defer commencing treatment. Investigations of patients' expectations of their treatment have shown that some patients hold unrealistic expectations. For instance, 20 per cent of RA patients in one study expected complete relief from pain (Daltroy *et al.*, 1995). Interestingly and in contrast to health professionals' beliefs, OA patients awaiting hip replacement surgery expected and expressed a preference for improvement in function rather than reduction in pain (Woolhead *et al.*, 1996).

Paradoxically, there are arthritis patients who hold pessimistic expectations for treatment outcomes, believing that arthritis is a condition of old age and that nothing can be done for it. Lack of faith in medical treatments, concern about side effects of powerful medications and failure to find a cure for painful, disabling symptoms may all contribute to the increasing numbers of people with arthritis who decide to try complementary and alternative therapies (see Chapter 2). Donovan and Blake (1992) found that 60 per cent of a sample of RA patients cited fear of side effects as a major influence on their decisions to adjust their drug dosage and frequency. Patients appeared to assess risk by offsetting costs (e.g. unpleasantness of taking drugs, regular blood tests, side effects and drug dependence) against potential benefits (e.g. relief from painful symptoms in the short and longer term). In reality, it is likely that, just as in other chronic conditions, patients with arthritis experiment with their drug dosage and frequency in attempts to individualise treatment according to need and lifestyle. In a qualitative study of older adults with OA, adherence to pain medication differed from adherence to other prescribed medication (Sale *et al.*, 2006). The authors noted that, although participants had 'obvious physical limitations' they minimised their pain and reported that they had a high pain tolerance. Not surprisingly, participants were hesitant about taking painkillers. Generally, when they did take painkillers they used a lower dosage or frequency than that prescribed. A survey of RA patients found that, although respondents believed that their medication was necessary for their health, 47.4 per cent were concerned about potential adverse consequences (Neame & Hammond, 2005). Interestingly, there was no association between RA knowledge and beliefs about medication. However, concerns about medication were associated with helplessness and non-adherence. It is likely that people with arthritis who are also depressed may hold negative beliefs (e.g. that they are helpless) and this in turn may influence their healthcare utilisation and concordance. It is known that RA patients who are depressed are more likely to report physical symptoms (Murphy *et al.*, 1999) and are less likely to take prescribed medication (DiMatteo *et al.*, 2000). These scenarios suggest that improving treatment of depression among people with arthritis may have positive consequences for self-management. There are a number of psychology-based approaches that could help in this respect; some of these are discussed in Chapter 8.

Patients' beliefs about their ability to carry out the required therapies may also influence levels of concordance. For example, level of self-efficacy has been shown to be a determinant of how well RA patients adhere to treatment recommendations (Taal, Rasker *et al.*, 1993) and take medication regularly (Brus *et al.*, 1999). Self-efficacy has also been implicated in concordance with prescribed physical exercise among rheumatic disease patients (Stenstrom *et al.*, 1997). The importance of establishing and maintaining a suitable regime of regular exercise for people with arthritis is widely recognised. Indeed, performance of moderate recreational physical exercise is associated with a decrease in the risk of knee osteoarthritis (Manninen *et al.*, 2001) and could therefore be considered a prophylactic. An interesting study by Focht *et al.* (2004) adds an intriguing insight into the 'expected' benefits of exercise among older, obese people with OA of the knee. An experience sampling procedure was used to collect data on feeling states that occurred either on non-exercise days or before and after scheduled exercise activity. As may be expected, physical exhaustion was higher immediately following exercise. However, the older adults in this sample did not experience improvements in feeling states that are typically observed among younger, more physically active populations. This suggests that one of the benefits of exercise (i.e. feeling more positive) may not be available to older, obese people with knee OA and thus cannot act as a motivator to continue with the exercise schedule. This finding certainly warrants further exploration given the age profile of the majority of people with OA, the most common form of arthritis.

For conditions such as AS, exercise can form the mainstay of the therapeutic approach. Given the relatively early age at onset of this type of arthritis, the prospect of exercising every day for the remainder of one's life can be daunting for even the most enthusiastic of individuals. For example, a young woman diagnosed with AS at the age of 20 who exercises each day will have carried out over 18,000 exercise sessions by the time she is 70. Indeed, regular exercise and the monitoring and correction of posture have to become an integral feature of everyday life. Moreover, home exercise has to be maintained despite limited contact with health professionals. Psychological interventions can offer a useful means of enhancing home exercise concordance that have not been fully exploited in the field of arthritis. There are a few exceptions such as the interventions of Basler (1993) and J.H. Barlow and Barefoot (1996), which are discussed in greater detail in Chapter 8.

Differences between AS patients who habitually exercise (n = 30) and those who do not (n = 38) were examined by Lim *et al.* (2005). Exercising patients had significantly less pain, greater family support and better quality of life compared with more sedentary patients. It is important to remember that, from a lay perspective, pain is the body's way of signalling that there is something wrong, and this usually means that the individual has to rest. Patients need to learn when it is safe for them to continue to exercise and when they need to stop and rest. Although the symptoms of AS fluctuate over time, exercise needs to be continued regularly in order to prevent deterioration of posture and loss of physical function. The person with AS can make the most of the relatively pain-free periods by exercising vigorously and maintaining a good general fitness level. It is important to note that this strategy differs somewhat from that advocated for most other types of arthritis (e.g. RA), where patients are advised to pace themselves so as not to aggravate their symptoms during times of low disease activity. Adherence to a regular AS exercise regime has been associated with rheumatologist follow-up, belief in the benefits of exercise, and a higher education level (Santos *et al.*, 1998). A long delay between onset of symptoms and medical diagnosis is characteristic of AS and is associated with greater disease severity and functional impairment (J.H. Barlow & Barefoot, 1996) and greater adherence to home exercise. Receiving a diagnostic label for one's condition several years after onset of symptoms may increase motivation to carry out treatment recommendations. Alternatively, those with greater disease severity and worse functional outcomes may be more motivated to exercise compared with peers with a lesser degree of symptomatology. In accord with this proposition, Falkenbach (2003) found that AS patients with less disability exercised less than their more disabled peers. Other barriers to exercise among people living with AS include boredom, lack of short-term gains, poor body image, lack of knowledge, aversion to exercise, and denial.

Adherence to medication and exercise in OA has been shown to be independent of age, gender or disease severity (Kraag *et al.*, 1994; Rejeski *et al.*, 1997). In order to better understand the motivational factors that influence exercise, Damush *et al.* (2005) studied a sample of community-dwelling older adults at two points in time 12 months apart. A diagnosis of knee OA (53 per cent of the sample) was associated with motivation from an organised exercise opportunity and efficacy or outcome expectations. Knee pain was positively associated with motivation deriving from social support and experience with exercise. Also focusing on patients with knee OA, Hendry *et al.* (2006) conducted a qualitative study examining views about exercise. Exercise behaviour was found to depend upon physical ability to exercise, beliefs about exercise and factors such as enjoyment, social support, priority setting and context. Participants who had stopped exercising had done so because of worsening symptoms and the belief that exercise was damaging their joints. The authors of a review of exercise adherence in OA noted that almost all studies in this area are short-term and do not use validated measures of adherence (Marks & Allegrante, 2005). They suggest that interventions designed to enhance self-efficacy, social support and the long-term monitoring of disease progress are needed in order to foster exercise adherence among people living with OA.

Patient Education

From diagnosis onwards, people with arthritis require the necessary knowledge, understanding, skills and confidence to make informed decisions concerning treatment options, to carry out complex treatment regimens, to cope with the psychosocial consequences of their condition, and to perform self-care activities. In order to meet these needs, patient education has rapidly grown into an integral and important speciality within rheumatology, where it is often used as an adjunct to medical care. Moreover, it is an area where psychologists and psychological theories and methods have a vital role to play. Interest in patient education is illustrated in a study showing that approximately 50 per cent of a sample of older people with knee OA (n = 86) (none of whom reported having received education or advice), cited educational interventions as a priority for research (Tallon *et al.*, 2000). The authors suggest that patients were actually asking for education to assist them in feeling more in control of their condition.

Nurses, especially rheumatology nurse practitioners, play a key role in hospital-based patient education and are often the first point of contact following diagnosis. In addition, nurses are often responsible for running telephone helplines, and organising and delivering group education interventions. Other allied health professionals (e.g. physiotherapists, occupational therapists) also become involved in the educational aspects of care for people with arthritis, either during one-to-one consultations or as part of a multi-disciplinary team approach to care or as guest speakers on group education programmes.

In relation to children with JIA and their families, the picture reflects the general situation within the field of paediatric health care where the need for improved provision of educational intervention has been highlighted (Beresford, 1995; Diehl *et al.*, 1991). Most hospitals and relevant voluntary organisations offer some form of educational intervention for JIA, although the level and effectiveness of provision is difficult to determine. A review of psycho-educational interventions for children with

JIA (J. Barlow, Shaw & Southwood, 1998) identified only nine published studies, most of which were conducted in the US and concerned specific interventions (e.g. increasing medication 'compliance') among small, selected groups of children. None of these interventions was suitable for widespread distribution in a range of settings, such as outpatient clinics, general practitioner surgeries, schools or the home environment.

Definitions

In the field of rheumatology and health care in general, the terms 'health education' and 'patient education' are used interchangeably. Health education has its foundation in health promotion, which is concerned primarily with improving health and preventing disease, whereas patient education is firmly based in the context of patient care. Patient education grew out of acute health care and was based principally on provision of information either verbally, during a consultation, or as written materials (e.g. leaflets, information sheets). This information-giving model was based on the assumption that knowledge alone was sufficient to promote a lasting change in feelings, beliefs and behaviours. Both patient and health education have advanced over the past two decades, drawing on expertise from a number of disciplines, including education, health promotion, behavioural psychology and health psychology. Such advances are reflected in the definition of both health and patient education. Tonnes (1990) defines health education as 'any planned activity which promotes health or illness related learning; that is, some relatively permanent change in an individual's competence or disposition' (Tonnes, 1990, p.2).

Traditionally, health education aimed to change behaviour (e.g. smoking or exercise) assuming contingency between behaviours and health. More recently, the importance of psychological, social and environmental variables that may act as mediators of health outcomes has received recognition. A number of social cognition models have been proposed and tested with varying degrees of success in predicting behaviours in healthcare settings including the health belief model (Sheeran & Abraham, 1995), locus of control (Wallston, 1992) and self-efficacy (Bandura, 1977).

In the US, a National Arthritis Advisory Board (NAAB) has been established and has produced standards for arthritis patient education (Burckhardt *et al.*, 1994). These define patient education as:

planned, organised learning experiences designed to facilitate voluntary adoption of behaviours or beliefs conducive to health. It is a set of planned educational activities that are separate from clinical patient care. The activities of a patient education program must be designed to attain goals the patient has participated in formulating. The primary focus of these activities includes the acquisition of information, skills, beliefs and attitudes which impact on health status, quality of life, and possibly health care utilisation. (Burckhardt *et al.*, 1994, p.2)

Content, format, delivery settings, and recipients

The NAAB standards maintain that arthritis patient education programmes should ideally include:

1. specific objectives oriented to each individual or group;
2. content tailored to meet these specific needs;
3. education processes which deliver the content in a manner which enables the patient to achieve the set objectives.

Educational interventions can be provided in a variety of formats, modes of delivery and settings according to the needs of the target patients and availability of resources. The NAAB produced a comprehensive set of standards covering needs assessment, planning and management, curriculum, instructors, evaluation and documentation that serve as a useful guide for practitioners, educators and researchers.

The content of interventions is highly variable and largely dependent upon the delivery format. For example, written materials tend to focus on describing the disease and its treatment, whereas multi-component group programmes cover a much wider range of topics. These can include symptom management, dealing with psychosocial consequences, lifestyle (including exercise), social support, communication, other strategies (e.g. goal-setting) and making appropriate use of medical services. Interventions can also vary with the type of arthritis targeted. For example, educational interventions for OA tend to focus on exercise and other lifestyle factors (e.g. weight loss), sometimes in combination with social support. Similarly, interventions designed specifically for people with AS tend to focus primarily on exercise, which is the mainstay of treatment for this condition. Education for people with RA often places greater emphasis on joint protection. Examples of interventions are presented in Chapter 8.

Psycho-educational interventions for people with arthritis are delivered in clinical locations, the individual's home or the community. Interventions can be group-based (usually 6–10 participants), individualised (e.g. manuals, multi-media programmes), or a combination (e.g. group sessions supplemented with written materials). Learning formats are highly variable and can include booklets, lectures, role-plays, contracting, goal-setting and sharing experiences. The various types of patient education available are summarised in Table 7.1.

Recipients of educational interventions

Most patient education targets patients as the primary recipients. The education of others in the patients' network has received much less attention. Partners and other family members have a crucial supportive and guiding role in the motivation and reinforcement of behavioural change, but rarely receive specific educational intervention. Some programmes allow a limited number of partners to attend, or invite partners to attend the final session. In the case of children with arthritis, parents usually assume the main responsibility for day-to-day management and are the main recipients of information. However,

Table 7.1. Summary of patient education interventions

Type of intervention	Format	Location
Written materials: leaflets, books, manuals, internet	Individual	Home
Videos	Individual	Home
Computer multi-media programs	Individual	Home
Cognitive-behavioural therapy	Individual or group	Hospital or home
Self-management programmes	Group	Hospital or community setting
Workshops	Group	Residential, hospital or community setting
Summer camps	Group – usually children alone or children and parents	Residential setting

they often feel that they lack sufficient knowledge and relevant skills to effectively manage their children's condition. Indeed, unique video footage of parents taking their children with JIA through an exercise regime (Britton, 2000) serves to emphasise the need for high-quality education designed to prepare parents and other family members in their disease-management roles. However, it has to be acknowledged that social support can be a double-edged sword (Revenson *et al.*, 1991) if the support received is not wanted or does not match the needs of the patient. For example, a person with arthritis may need to discuss their anxieties about pain in their knee, whereas their partner may feel more comfortable providing practical support, such as doing the housework and gardening. Equally, some health professionals may need training in the precepts of self-management in order to avoid patient dependence on the healthcare team.

Finally, there are many myths that pervade the general public's perceptions about arthritis. For example, there is a widespread belief that arthritis is an inevitable consequence of getting older. Such a belief serves to deny the identity of children, adolescents and young adults with arthritis, and also the reality of their lives (J. Barlow & Harrison, 1996). Furthermore, with the increasing knowledge of risk factors for certain types of arthritis, prevention could become a focus for intervention. For example, adopting a healthy lifestyle, such as keeping active and avoiding obesity, may prevent or delay the onset and progression of OA. Therefore, education designed to increase public awareness, knowledge and reduction of risk factors certainly warrants greater attention.

Acquisition of information

Provision of information is an integral aspect of clinical encounters and often forms the opening section of many psycho-educational interventions. The successful transfer of information not only represents a useful first step in the process of empowering individuals to perceive themselves as capable of controlling their arthritis, but may also go some way towards satisfying patients' desire for information.

Patients' information needs may change over the course and duration of disease, which for many comprises 10, 20, 30 or even more years. The focus in the early years after onset is likely to be on understanding the disease itself and how it is treated, with a shift to understanding more about the impact on psychosocial dimensions over time. Educational strategies may be most effective if tailored to match the needs of the target population, although the optimal time for presenting patients with disease-related information (i.e. at diagnosis, after several years, or at repeated intervals throughout the disease course) has yet to be identified. Nonetheless, providing education early in the disease course is generally advocated as good practice and is aimed at providing patients with a firm foundation for managing their condition. However, there are indications that patients in the early stages of their disease can feel that they are given more information than they can cope with (Lineker *et al.*, 1995).

It is generally believed that patients with longer disease duration will possess greater knowledge of their condition than those more recently diagnosed, and therefore will not benefit from further disease-related education (J.H. Barlow, Bishop & Pennington, 1997). However, studies of patient knowledge among RA patients have failed to find an association with duration (J.H. Barlow, Cullen & Rowe, 1999; J. Barlow, Pennington & Bishop, 1997). This is despite the fact that those with more established disease tend to have fewer educational qualifications, and to have greater physical disability and higher co-morbidity.

An assessment of knowledge among outpatients with RA using the RA patients' Knowledge Questionnaire (Hill *et al.*, 1991) showed that patients were most knowledgeable about aetiology, symptoms and the tests used to monitor their wellbeing. They knew least about medication and its side effects (J.H. Barlow, Cullen & Rowe, 1999). Findings were independent of disease duration and age. Equally, unmet informational needs appear similar across short and longer duration, with over 80 per cent of RA patients believing it is very important to receive information and advice on the following topic areas:

- understanding of RA and its treatment;
- how to manage RA on a daily basis;
- how to deal with the pain of RA;
- how to deal with 'disease flares';
- how RA may affect their future.

Over 60 per cent of participants felt it was very important to have access to easily understood information leaflets and receive information and advice on the following topic areas:

- physical therapy;
- joint protection;
- aids and adaptations to help in the home;
- the effect RA may have on energy levels;
- the effect RA may have on employment and family relationships;
- the effect RA may have on self-image;
- how to deal with emotions.

Additional information needs concerned nurturant activities (e.g. childcare) and work (e.g. aids and adaptations for the workplace). These issues are not salient for all patients due to variation in age at onset (e.g. after raising a family or retirement from paid employment) and individual circumstance (e.g. nature of employment).

The needs of patients with RA, OA, back disease, systemic lupus erythematosus and systemic sclerosis were explored, and 20 areas of concern and 12 learning interests emerged that were largely independent of diagnosis (Neville *et al.*, 1999). The majority of respondents expressed most interested in learning about disease-specific topics; the physician was the preferred source of information; the preferred format was written material. The 20 concerns were reduced to the following five factors: psychological, coping, medication, social and financial. In terms of learning interests, three factors were identified: the illness, traditional health management and non-traditional health management topics. A study conducted in Finland found that most arthritis patients (70 per cent) were satisfied with the amount of patient education that they had received and felt they were knowledgeable about the disease, its treatment, symptoms and the results of X-ray and other investigations (tests). The major problem area reported by patients concerned the need for mental support and the opportunity to discuss their feelings. Most wanted one-to-one education. They believed that patient education resulted in increased ability to cope at home, perform self-care and have a better quality of life.

Greater provision of accessible, high-quality information about arthritis, its treatment, self-management strategies and the wider psychosocial issues is clearly needed by a majority of patients and seems to be independent of age and disease duration. An early study by Silvers *et al.* (1985) showed that, in North America, patients' interest in learning more about RA does not decrease with increasing disease duration. Furthermore, a UK-based study found that RA patients with longer duration demonstrated similar increases in knowledge following receipt of written materials compared with patients of short disease duration (J. Barlow, Pennington & Bishop, 1997) despite the scepticism expressed by health professionals that people with established disease already know all they need to know. However, it is possible that patients with longer disease duration 'forget' aspects of information on RA that are not relevant to their individual, clinical problems. In addition, knowledge of disease and the treatments used can change, especially over the long durations (e.g. 20+ years) typically experienced in arthritis. It is important to ensure that patients are kept up to date with the latest advances if they are to make informed decisions about their care.

Most hospital clinics have an array of written materials accessible to patients, although provision at primary care level may be more variable. Health professionals have an active role to play in information distribution. Kay and Punchak (1988) found that only 46 per cent of patients with RA reported that they had received information about their condition from health professionals. Nevertheless, these patients were keen to find out more about their disease, its management and drug treatment, and believed information on these topics would help them to cope better with their everyday lives. A survey of rheumatology outpatients revealed that 55 per cent had sought further information about their condition outside of the clinic setting (J. Barlow & Pennington, 1996). People wanted to know more about their condition (e.g. the cause, symptoms) and disease management, particularly self-care. Information-seeking behaviour was associated with a diagnosis of RA, being female and having educational qualifications.

Acknowledging that education and information are critical aspects of arthritis management which may be suboptimal, Adab *et al.* (2004) conducted a needs assessment of stakeholders including both patients (n = 201) and healthcare professionals (n = 232) as a precursor to establishing a community-based arthritis resource centre in the UK. Most patient responders (58 per cent) were currently on medication, but only 38 per cent reported having received written information about arthritis. The majority of both patients and professionals agreed that written information would be useful. However, patients placed higher value on information on benefits, diet and alternative therapy and symptom management. Non-Caucasian patients placed higher value on provision of written materials in different languages and also multilingual volunteer staff.

Information and JIA

There appears to be a gap between the information that children with JIA and their parents need and the amount of information that they actually received. In general, health professionals, voluntary groups and parent-oriented leaflets are cited as the main sources of information, for parents and children (J.H. Barlow, Shaw & Harrison, 1999). Parents appear to be the main recipients of educational interventions, with the emphasis being on the provision of factual information regarding disease (e.g. disease pathology, incidence of disease), and hospital attendance as either inpatients or outpatients. Educational provision has rarely addressed the wider aspects of JIA (e.g. psychosocial impact), although the situation is beginning to change with production of excellent child-centred booklets such as *Children Have Arthritis Too* (CHAT) distributed by voluntary organisations (such as Arthritis Care). The CHAT booklet contains contributions from a range of health professionals and young people themselves. The latter helps make it easier for young people to identify with the information presented.

The apparent scarcity of child-centred interventions means that children tend to rely on their parents for information. Unfortunately, parents can feel helpless and ill equipped to answer their children's questions. This situation becomes particularly fraught as children enter adolescence, a time when many begin to ask more questions and to voice their own anxieties about the future, as the following quote illustrates.

> Since the hip-replacement he isn't coping so well mentally … He's asking me lots of questions about the future and I just can't answer them. (Parent of adolescent with JIA; J.H. Barlow, Shaw & Harrison, 1999)

Leaflets and written materials

Leaflets offer a low-cost method of reaching large numbers of people, and can be viewed as a useful means of bridging the gap between the amount of information patients' desire and the amount they actually receive and are able to assimilate in a clinical setting. However, leaflets and other written materials are not always freely available in clinics but are distributed by health professionals, who adopt a gate-keeping role in this respect (J.H. Barlow, Bishop & Pennington, 1996). For example, a survey of 249 outpatients with various types of arthritis found that only

41.8 per cent of patients recalled receiving an information leaflet (J. Barlow & Pennington, 1996). Distribution of leaflets was controlled by health professionals, many of whom felt that allowing patients free access may cause more harm than good despite a lack of evidence to support this notion (Ong *et al.*, 1995; Weinman, 1990).

Leaflets are an effective means of improving knowledge among osteoarthrosis patients (Moll, 1986) and patients with various types of arthritis (Maggs *et al.*, 1996). Extending this work, a randomised, controlled study found that leaflets produced by the Arthritis Research Campaign were effective in increasing knowledge, decreasing pain and improving depressed mood among RA patients at three-week follow-up (J. Barlow, Pennington & Bishop, 1997). Furthermore, assessment of psychological wellbeing and telephone interviews found no evidence that patients found the leaflets worrying or anxiety-provoking. On the contrary, leaflets appeared to have a positive effect on patients' feelings and beliefs, generating a sense of reassurance, reducing isolation and helping them to 'come to terms' with their condition. A follow-up study showed that the positive changes on knowledge and depression were maintained at six months. However, it is not clear whether maintenance of such improvements among the intervention group was influenced by participation in a telephone interview following the three-week questionnaire follow-up.

Despite the positive reception that leaflets generally receive, a qualitative study revealed that parents of children with JIA felt leaflets were 'too little too late' and did not satisfy parents' need for detailed discussions of their children's condition with health professionals (J. Barlow, Harrison & Shaw, 1998). Furthermore, parents felt that socially orientated interventions (e.g. summer camps) were of greater educational value than any written or audiovisual materials and had the added advantage of allowing opportunities for discussion with professional experts as well as other parents. Moreover, family camps acknowledged the fact that JIA affects all members of the family, as is illustrated in the following quotes.

> Mary's benefited by groups ... like the summer school session and things like that where she's actually been with children with the same problems. (Parent)

> I ended up crying in a discussion because for two years that he'd had [arthritis], I'd never spoken to anybody, apart from my husband and the doctor. (Parent)

With regard to written information, parents do not limit their reading to relevant sections of leaflets but appear to examine 'everything' (i.e. the full spectrum of rheumatic conditions). This situation tended to result in more anxiety rather than less, as parents read about conditions that had 'worse symptoms and a poor prognosis'. In accord with the situation in adult rheumatology, parents seek information from libraries, saying 'The only way you can learn about it is by reading up on it yourself. We've had to go to libraries.' Unfortunately, library books can be outdated, and thus may be more of a hindrance than a help. Furthermore, the increasing use of the internet has facilitated increased access to a wide range of information regardless of its quality or accuracy. The common practice of restricting leaflet distribution to the point of diagnosis may be limiting the potential for positive change to those in the early stages of their disease.

Internet provision of information
There is an assumption that the written word is a universally acceptable medium for communicating health-related information. The effectiveness of alternative educational media, such as audiotapes, videos, computer multi-media programs and the internet, is certainly worthy of further exploration in the context of arthritis. Studies of internet provision are in their infancy though proliferating rapidly. For example, the contents of Web-source arthritis information and its influence on both patients and medical practice were examined in Korea (Kim *et al.*, 2004). A total of 138 Korean-language websites on 'arthritis' were assessed: 18.8 per cent were advertisements and 44.9 per cent had financial interests (e.g. promotion of products). Of 257 arthritis patients surveyed, 28 per cent had searched the Web for information on arthritis. Such patients tended to be younger, employed, with a higher income and higher education. Only 16.1 per cent of physicians felt that patients understood internet content accurately. The information needs and search behaviour of people accessing a US-based, health-education website for arthritis, orthopaedics and sports medicine analysed 793 free-text search queries (Shuyler & Knight, 2003). The five most frequent reasons for searching the site were:

1. information about a condition;
2. information about treatment;
3. information about symptoms;

4. advice about symptoms;
5. advice about treatment.

In 140 out of 178 cases, the person conducting the search was the patient. Queries were submitted from 34 nations, with most arising in the US, Australia, the UK and Canada.

At present there are few controls over the quality and reliability of internet-based arthritis information. Ansani *et al.* (2005) examined this issue using well-known search engines (e.g. MSN, Yahoo, Google and Lycos) using the search terms 'arthritis' and 'osteoarthritis'. Sites designated 'unique' were rated for disease and medication information content, website navigability, required literacy level, and currentness of information. The most highly rated sites tended to be '.gov' sites or '.edu' sites; however, none of the sites was rated as understandable by sixth-grade reading ability. In an attempt to provide high-quality and accurate web-based, arthritis information, Ansani *et al.* (2006) established a Drug Information Centre Arthritis Project comprising three content areas: an interactive ask-a-pharmacist component with a satisfaction survey; a health-assessment tools impact survey for RA and OA; and disease and drug information. Of 1800 OA and RA patients invited to use the secure internet site, 56 patients actually accessed it in 128 visits over a six-week period. Results showed that 85 per cent of these patients rated the site as useful/very useful, 83 per cent would use the site again and patients had slightly higher scores on physical and mental health compared with US norms for arthritis patients.

Internet provision is often believed to be the preserve of younger people. However, one US study has shown that among adults aged 80+ years, 28 per cent had a home computer and of these 95 per cent had internet access (Tak & Hong, 2005). Furthermore, 39 per cent had searched for arthritis information on the internet and these were likely to be those with higher education levels. Age and functional disability were not associated with internet use.

Delivery setting
The setting for information-giving may influence its impact on patient outcomes. One unique study examined this question, comparing the same information-based intervention delivered by telephone only, in person at the clinic, and using a combination of telephone and clinic (Weinberger, Tierney, Booher & Katz, 1989). The content of the

information included a review of medications, pain, gastrointestinal symptoms, early signs of other diseases such as heart disease, outpatient visits, barriers to keeping appointments and telephone availability of a general medical practice. Each patient received specific suggestions regarding questions that he or she could ask healthcare practitioners at the next appointment. Trained, non-medical interviewers delivered the intervention. A randomised, controlled trial with a sample of 439 patients with OA (mean age = 62.3) showed that pain and physical disability improved in both groups contacted by telephone, whilst physical disability worsened in the clinic group. The more positive effects of giving information by telephone rather than in a clinic setting have to be balanced against the increased number of contacts received by participants in these groups, and hence the increased effectiveness of the intervention. Furthermore, generalisation may be limited by the predominantly black (70 per cent) and female (88 per cent) sample. Further studies exploring the apparent preference of receiving information outside of the clinic setting may be worthwhile, as would a replication of the study in more heterogeneous samples.

Chapter Summary

The chapter began by considering the experience of health care where, ideally, patients and providers work together in partnership to promote the best possible health outcomes. However, the reality is that patients and providers may sometimes hold different perspectives in terms of what should be the main focus for treatment. Pain, being seen and being believed, as well as the wider impact of arthritis in patients' lives, are perceived as important from a patient's perspective. Although the tendency of providers to focus on biological parameters is understandable given their area of expertise, it can be interpreted and experienced by patients as a restricted perspective that fails to acknowledge the whole person. There are few studies of inpatient care from either patient or provider perspectives. Equally, there are few studies of the experience of care provision in primary care. Regardless, patient satisfaction with care tends to be high, although reports focus mainly on RA patients.

Levels of concordance with medication and therapeutic exercise are often less than optimal and can be influenced by patients' beliefs about their illness, beliefs about health in general, the nature of treatment offered, alternative therapies, the relationship with healthcare providers and presence of depressive symptomatology. Commencing and maintaining exercise among people with arthritis can be hindered by levels of pain and fatigue, which are both commonly experienced symptoms. Lack of adequate social support, poor body image and boredom are additional factors that can hinder performance of exercise.

Patient education has become an integral aspect of disease management for people with arthritis and is an area where psychologists can have a useful input. Patient education can be provided in a range of formats, modes of delivery and settings. Educational strategies may be most effective if tailored to match the needs of the target population, although the optimal time for presenting patients with disease-related information (i.e. at diagnosis, after several years, or at repeated intervals throughout the disease course) has yet to be identified. Greater provision of accessible, high-quality information about arthritis, its treatment, self-management strategies and the wider psychosocial issues is clearly needed by a majority of patients, and desire to learn more appears to be independent of age, disease duration and type of arthritis. It is important that people with arthritis are provided with updates of the latest developments and therapeutic strategies. Thus, education at one point in time (e.g. at diagnosis) is not sufficient. Written information in the form of leaflets offers a low-cost method of reaching large numbers of people, and can be viewed as a useful means of bridging the gap between the amount of information patients desire and the amount they actually receive and are able to assimilate in a clinical setting. Internet provision of written information has the advantage of being available 24/7, although the quality of internet sites is not always assured since at present there are few controls over the quality and reliability of internet-based arthritis information. Although information and written materials can provide a valuable mechanism to help inform people about their condition, additional techniques may be necessary to ensure that information is translated into action. Providing information and increasing knowledge alone do not guarantee positive changes in health behaviours. This issue will be discussed further in Chapter 8.

8

Psycho-Educational Interventions

The essential task of ensuring that patients have information about their condition and its treatment was a key driver underpinning the development of educational interventions in rheumatology. Many educational interventions developed in hospital settings were built around lecture-style programmes delivered by health professionals. The underlying ethos is that of an expert professional imparting their knowledge to passive recipients and is based on the assumption that patients will use their new knowledge to make changes in their behaviour. Whilst most educational programmes lead to change in knowledge, that knowledge is not always translated into action. Fortunately, the benefits of including cognitive-behavioural techniques and providing social support have been recognised, and they now feature in many successful interventions.

The increased range of learning techniques encompassed within interventions has been accompanied by a growing acknowledgement that the patient is more than a biological entity. A holistic approach to psycho-educational intervention views participants with arthritis as the experts, with unique insight into their own condition and its pervasive consequences. Interventions can build on the expert knowledge of participants to develop the self-determination needed to successfully manage arthritis. Self-determination is defined as a combination of autonomous behaviour, self-regulation and psychological empowerment (Wehmeyer *et al.*, 1997). A self-determined individual acts independently according to his/her own preferences, interests and abilities and practises self-regulation whereby goals are set and goal attainment is monitored and evaluated. Psychological empowerment (Zimmerman, 1990) includes cognitive, personality and motivational domains. Psychological empowerment occurs when people believe that they have control over important circumstances in their lives (e.g. internal locus of control), feel able to apply the relevant skills to achieve desired outcomes (e.g. self-efficacy) and believe that such skills will be effective in achieving desired outcomes (outcome expectations).

A wide range of interventions has been developed for people with arthritis. For the purpose of presentation, I have broadly categorised interventions under the following headings:

- cognitive behavioural interventions;
- interventions based on emotional disclosure;
- social support interventions;
- multi-component interventions focusing primarily on exercise;
- multi-component self-management interventions;
- personal development interventions;
- interventions for enhancing employment potential;
- interventions in JIA.

Examples of interventions and associated research are presented, although it is important to note that this does not necessarily imply that all such interventions are implemented outside of a research setting. The chapter ends with an overview of effectiveness of psycho-educational interventions for people with arthritis, drawing on relevant systematic reviews.

Cognitive Behavioural Interventions

Cognitive behavioural therapy (CBT) for people with arthritis tends to focus on pain management and comprises three components:

1. rationale for treatment – usually an educational component in which participants are introduced to the biopsychological model of pain;
2. training in coping skills;
3. application of CBT skills in real-life situations and training for maintenance of coping skills and setbacks.

A range of coping skills can be introduced, including relaxation, guided imagery, activity-rest cycling, pleasant activity scheduling, distraction, problem-solving, goal-setting and cognitive restructuring. The last of these involves the identification and monitoring of negative thoughts and encouragement of alternative positive thoughts and reattributions. Interventions are usually delivered by health or clinical psychologists (or other suitably qualified health professionals trained in CBT techniques) to groups of 5 to 10 people. Sessions typically last for two hours and are delivered on a weekly basis for 6 to 10 weeks.

Cognitive behavioural interventions have been shown to be effective for people with RA. Compared with patients in a social support control group, patients with RA receiving CBT reported significant reductions in pain, pain behaviour, anxiety and depression (Bradley, 1996; Bradley *et al.*, 1987). Other controlled studies have shown CBT to be an effective method of improving coping and function (Applebaum *et al.*, 1988; Parker *et al.*, 1988). Moreover, such improvements appear to be maintained in the longer term (Bradley *et al.*, 1988), particularly among patients who continue to practise coping skills on a regular basis (Parker *et al.*, 1988). Cognitive behavioural therapy has been shown to enhance perceived self-efficacy among patients with RA (O'Leary *et al.*, 1988); the degree of self-efficacy enhancement correlating with the magnitude of improvement on pain, joint inflammation and psychosocial functioning (e.g. depression). Although interesting, generalisability of findings is limited by the very small sample (i.e. 15 in the control and intervention groups respectively). Family support has been combined with CBT for people with RA (Radojevic *et al.*, 1992). Four conditions were contrasted to assess potential benefits: CBT with family support, CBT without family support, family support only, and a no-treatment group. The CBT interventions were found to provide more benefits compared with the other two conditions.

Most studies have examined the effects of CBT among people with RA: research on CBT in other forms of arthritis is sadly lacking. One exception is a study by Keefe *et al.* (1990) showing that CBT is more effective than arthritis education and standard care in reducing pain and psychological distress among people with OA. A trial of CBT among people with AS found improvements on depression and self-efficacy, but failed to show evidence of a reduction in pain or a decrease in disease severity (Basler, 1993). In accordance with other chronic conditions, CBT appears to offer benefits to people with arthritis, particularly in relation to improvements on pain, and psychological wellbeing. CBT is often used in combination with other forms of educational intervention, particularly self-management skills training.

Interventions Based on Emotional Disclosure

Use of emotional disclosure as an intervention in rheumatology is gradually increasing. In a unique study of verbal emotional disclosure in the context of a group psycho-educational intervention (the Arthritis Self-Management Program – see later in this chapter), MacFarland (2007) showed that emotional disclosure was a process that motivated participants to change their behaviour. Used as an intervention in its own right, emotional disclosure involves asking participants to disclose difficult or traumatic events and the emotions they experienced during these events. Typically, such interventions comprise three or four sessions and can focus on written or verbal disclosure. In the latter scenario, participants usually talk into a tape recorder rather than to another person or a group. The aim is to increase emotional awareness and enhance overall health and wellbeing. In the context of arthritis, emotional disclosure may work by reducing levels of stress, which in turn may have a positive influence on disease activity.

Most studies of emotional disclosure have focused on patients with RA. One such study compared verbal emotional disclosure of stressful events with talking about neutral topics (the control condition) and showed that, at three-month follow-up, RA patients who talked privately about stressful events had less affective disturbance and better physical functioning in daily activities (Kelley *et al.*, 1997). The effects of writing about stressful events compared with writing about neutral topics were examined by Smyth *et al.* (1999) among patients with asthma (n = 51) and RA (n = 49). At four-month follow-up, RA patients who wrote about stressful events showed improvements in overall disease activity. Similarly, improvements on disease activity at 10-week follow-up among RA patients participating in a written and verbal disclosure intervention were reported by Wetherall *et al.* (2005). In addition, reductions in fatigue, tension, anger and mood disturbance were also noted. Interestingly, Wetherall *et al.* found that, immediately after disclosure, RA patients reported deterioration in mood which may have been linked to the recall and disclosure of their negative memories. Given that positive mood ensued, it seems that this initial deterioration was followed by a reduction in mood disturbance as a process of cognitive restructuring and integration of such memories occurred. Further insight in to the processes involved in emotional disclosure is provided by Danoff-Burg *et al.* (2006), who showed that among RA and lupus patients, emotional writing was most effective at reducing pain among those with low trait anxiety. A benefit finding condition was used as a comparator and showed that this was most effective for participants with high trait anxiety. Danoff-Burg *et al.* suggest that emotional disclosure may be perceived as too threatening by patients with high trait anxiety.

Written emotional disclosure has been examined in a randomised controlled trial of 68 people with AS (Hamilton-West & Quine, 2007). The Ethics Committee that reviewed this study was concerned about asking participants to write about their 'most upsetting experience'. Thus, the intervention was adjusted to focus on 'stressful experiences during the last month or any worries/concerns that are currently troubling you'. The control group were asked to write about plans for the next day. At three-month follow-up there was a statistically significant improvement on physical functioning for the disclosure group, although this improvement was not clinically significant. Analysis of the words used during written disclosure showed that improvements in physical functioning were associated with increased use of positive emotion words for disease activity combined with a reduction in the use of words relaying sadness or depression.

One issue arising from studies of emotional disclosure is the relatively low take-up by arthritis participants. For example, Smyth *et al.* (1999) received expressions of interest from 243 RA patients; of these, 35 were not eligible, 49 were not interested due to other time commitments, 87 were not interested but did not give a reason, 16 were not contactable, five dropped out before commencing the writing intervention, and two failed to complete. Hence, 49 RA patients completed the writing disclosure intervention. Similarly, in the study of people with AS, Hamilton-West & Quine (2007) had 133 expressions of interest and, of these, 107 returned consent forms and were randomised. However, 27 in the disclosure group and 12 in the control condition dropped out before commencing the intervention; 30 completed the disclosure intervention and 15 completed the control condition. It may be that emotional disclosure, whether written or verbal, does not have immediate appeal to some arthritis participants. This is a pity as there does seem to be some benefit among those who complete the intervention, particularly in terms of disease activity in RA patients and physical functioning in AS patients. If this type of intervention is to be offered outside of a research project, then due consideration needs to be given as to how the intervention is marketed in order to attract participants who may benefit, and the potential link between disclosing emotions and physical wellbeing needs to be made explicit.

Social Support Interventions

Group interventions offer an opportunity for mutual social support with similar others. Indeed, some critics suggest that getting people together in a group is the primary mechanism of action underlying group psycho-educational interventions and there is no added value in providing a structured learning environment; simply enabling people to meet for a 'chat' is sufficient. The beneficial effects of social support forms the rationale for many group interventions, although results are not always as expected. One example is an intervention aimed at teaching people with rheumatic diseases to cope actively with their problems (Savelkoul *et al.*, 2001). The rationale for the study was that coping can be classified on two dimensions:

1. as active coping (managing the stressful situation) versus passive coping (avoidance);
2. as emotion-focused coping (e.g. wishful thinking) versus problem-focused coping (changing the cause of the stressful situation).

Active coping can be emotion-focused, encompassing techniques such as positive reappraisal and cognitive restructuring, whereas problem-focused coping involves changing the situation through seeking social support for example. Passive coping is always emotion-focused. A randomised, controlled trial compared the effects of a coping intervention with a mutual support group and a waiting-list control group, thus avoiding some of the criticisms of waiting-list controlled trials (i.e. absence of an equivalent group receiving attention). The coping and mutual support groups met for 10 sessions, each led by two supervisors and accompanied by a manual that described homework assignments. A nurse and a social worker led the coping intervention. Special attention was paid to action-directed coping via problem-solving and seeking social support. The mutual support intervention was led by two appropriately trained patients and followed the guidelines developed by the Federation of Patient and Consumer Organisations in The Netherlands. Participants selected the topics of group discussions.

The 168 participants were a highly selected group (i.e. aged between 35 and 65, with disease duration of over one year, higher than median scores on functional status and one other dimension of rheumatic disease impact such as loneliness). As may be expected, intention-to-treat analysis showed an effect of the coping intervention on action-directed coping (a small effect size .18) at immediate post-intervention only; there was no effect at six-month follow-up. Interestingly, there were no effects on coping by seeking social support, although this was one of the main aims of the coping intervention. Indeed, although a small improvement on functional status was noted among the coping intervention participants immediately post-intervention (a very small effect size of .08), this change was not maintained at six months. There were no significant differences between groups on loneliness, life satisfaction or negative social interactions at follow-up. Savelkoul *et al.* (2001) suggest that maintenance sessions are needed to ensure that changes in action-directed coping and functional ability are sustained. No cost information was presented. However, given that the coping intervention involved two professionals, the financial cost of running the intervention and proposed maintenance sessions would appear to outweigh the fairly limited short-term improvements reported.

One study compared a social support intervention with an educational intervention and combination of education and social support (Cronan *et al.*, 1998). The educational intervention comprised lectures from professional health educators on coping, diet, exercise and making appropriate use of medical services. The social support intervention involved group discussions around coping strategies and setting weekly task assignments. No staff members were present during the meetings. The combination intervention split each two-hour session equally between education and support. Participants attended 10 weekly two-hour meetings followed by 10 monthly two-hour meetings. The materials were adapted from the *Arthritis Helpbook* (Lorig & Fries, 1990). The sample comprised 363 health maintenance organisation members with OA, who were randomly assigned to receive either social support, or education, or a combination intervention or no intervention (control group). All three interventions reduced healthcare costs, without any adverse effect on health status. The increased costs among the control group were attributed to a greater number of days spent in hospital. In terms of the relative costs of the interventions, the social support intervention was least costly owing to the absence of a paid health educator. Interestingly, there was least attrition from the combination of education and social support, suggesting that participants liked the combination of social support and learning more about their condition. Respondents in the social support group rated this intervention lower than either the education or combination group, thus adding further support for the desire of people with OA to learn more about their condition and its treatment.

Online support groups are on the increase and have the advantage of not being limited by geographical barriers; they are accessible 24/7, can be anonymous, and offer opportunities for 'lurking' until the participant feels comfortable with the group and its norms. Interviews with online support group participants living in The Netherlands investigated empowering and disempowering processes that occurred as a result of taking part in such groups. The 32 interviewees had accessed online support groups for three conditions: arthritis (n = 11), fibromyalgia (n = 11) and breast cancer (n = 10) (van Uden-Kraan, Drossaert, Taal, Lebrun *et al.*, 2008). Empowering processes included exchanging information, receiving emotional support, finding recognition, sharing experiences, helping others and amusement. Disempowering processes were rarely mentioned but centred on being uncertain about the quality of information, being confronted with the negative aspects of disease and the presence of complainers. In contrast with the authors' expectations, there were few differences between the three disease groups and no clear or consistent pattern emerged. However, it was noted that breast cancer patients were more likely to mention being confronted with the negative aspects of disease whereas arthritis patients were less likely to mention amusement than fibromyalgia or breast cancer patients. A related study by the same authors explored the potential disadvantages of online support, such as lack of control of the quality of information exchanges and concern about group members making socially inappropriate remarks (van Uden-Kraan, Drossaert, Taal, Shaw *et al.*, 2008). The authors analysed a sample of postings from eight groups, including two for people with arthritis, using content analysis. Most postings were posted on weekdays (80 per cent) and in the daytime (59 per cent). Among the 172 arthritis participants, 85 per cent were female, the mean age was 36 years, 73 per cent had been diagnosed for more than one year, and 87 per cent were patients (rather than family member, friend, healthcare professional). Members of the online support groups used emoticons (35 per cent), excessive punctuation (38 per cent), and capitals (6 per cent) to compensate for lack of non-verbal cues. Postings from arthritis patients tended to be 'on-topic' focusing on regular treatment, regular medication or restrictions on daily life; there was less 'chit chat' (i.e. off-topic, everyday talk) than was found in the other two conditions. Arthritis patients posed more questions and focused mainly on exchanging personal information, suggesting greater use of self-help strategies than in the other two groups. Negative feelings about their condition were mentioned in 12 per cent of arthritis postings; these mainly concerned sadness but also included fear and anger. Given that few disadvantages were found, online support could be a viable option for some people with arthritis.

Multi-Component Interventions Focused Primarily on Exercise

Changing behaviour is a key theme of many psycho-educational interventions for people with arthritis, and many interventions draw on the principles of CBT to assist with lifestyle modifications such as increasing exercise. For people with OA, lifestyle modification often focuses on walking, which can improve physical functioning and is well tolerated without exacerbating pain or involving increased use of medication (Minor *et al.*, 1989). One excellent example of an intervention that drew on psychological theories and empirically tested intervention strategies is the Sidewalkers Walking Program for patients with OA of the knee. In contrast to much of the published work in the educational field, Allegrante *et al.* (1993), provide an excellent detailed description of the developmental process of this programme. Without a full description of content, delivery mode and format, it is difficult to make comparisons across the growing number of interventions. Also, it is useful for intervention developers to share good practice (i.e. what works and what does not) to prevent continual 'reinvention of the wheel'. Allegrante *et al.* provide a detailed description of the goals, objectives, process and impact on functional status and arthritis-related self-efficacy beliefs of the Sidewalkers Walking Program. The rationale for selecting self-efficacy as the main theoretical foundation of the programme is discussed, and the operationalisation of the major sources of self-efficacy information is described. Finally, the features of the literature on patient compliance, patient education, exercise compliance, behavioural psychology and relapse prevention that were incorporated in the intervention are outlined. Relapse prevention is a very useful component for inclusion in psycho-educational interventions aiming to modify lifestyle. Many participants find that they have to stop exercising, going on holiday, having friends to stay, etc. during times of disease flare. It is much better for participants to prepare for such interruptions to their exercise regime than to fail to restart their programme. Parts of the Sidewalkers Walking Program were modelled on an early version of the Arthritis Self-Management Program (Lorig & Holman, 1993) and the Rockport Walking Program (Rockport Walking Institute, 1988). The end-product, the four-phase Sidewalkers Walking Program, is a systematically developed walking programme with firm foundations in the theoretical and empirical literature. The programme is a hospital-based, educational, support and walking intervention that aims to teach participants how to manage OA pain and other symptoms through walking. It is delivered over eight weeks (three meetings per week) to groups of 10–15 patients with moderate to severe OA of one or both knees. Each session includes instruction by a trained interventionist, social support, light physical activity and walking. The format includes behavioural contracting, goal-setting, monitoring, feedback and reinforcement. A manual, a video, a cassette and a diary for recording daily physical activity accompany the programme.

A randomised, controlled trial of the Sidewalkers Walking Program showed that immediately following the eight-week intervention clinically meaningful improvements were noted in functional status with no increase in levels of pain or increased use of medication (Kovar *et al.*, 1992; Peterson *et al.*, 1993). Participants were followed up again at one year by telephone interviews (n = 29 of the original 47 intervention group, and 23 of the original 45 control group). No significant differences were found between the groups at one year (Sullivan *et al.*, 1998). Furthermore, the initial gain in physical activity and walking distance had returned to baseline among the intervention group. However, participants' anecdotal comments suggested that they attributed changes in confidence, posture, ability to walk and decreases in pain and stiffness to the programme. Thus, although based on a thorough review of both empirical and theoretical literature, change in walking behaviour was not sustained. Part of the Sidewalkers Walking Program was based on the theoretical proposition that past behaviour (i.e. walking) is the greatest influence on participants' current perceived ability to walk. Whilst this may be the case for healthy adults, there are indicators that typical features of arthritis (e.g. pain) play a part in behavioural expectations. Contrary to theoretical predictions, investigation of exercise self-efficacy among people with AS has shown that self-efficacy expectations are based on concurrent pain and concurrent psychological wellbeing rather than past exercise experience (J.H. Barlow, 1998). In other words, it does not matter how much or how often people have exercised in the past, the greatest influence on perceived ability to exercise today is the individual's concurrent physiological and psychological state (e.g. pain, depressed mood). This finding confirms that pain is a key aspect of arthritis and is used as a touchstone for determining level of severity (J. Barlow, 1997). It should also be noted that the self-efficacy scales used by Sullivan *et al.* were at a moderate level of generality and were not specific to walking. Outcome measures more closely linked to the aim of the Sidewalkers Walking Program may have been more sensitive to change.

The importance of establishing exercise as a regular habit among people with AS was the guiding factor underlying development of a group intervention, the Self-Management Course for People with Ankylosing Spondylitis (SMC-AS). This intervention emphasised promotion of home exercises and self-monitoring, both essential aspects of disease management in AS. The course comprised 12 hours of intensive tuition spread over two consecutive days and was delivered in rehabilitation facilities with a hydrotherapy pool by a physiotherapist (Jane Barefoot) and myself (health psychologist). Course content is summarised below:

- information about AS and its treatment;
- exercises in a hydrotherapy pool;
- exercises on land (in a gym);
- home checks for monitoring mobility;
- home checks for monitoring posture;
- exercise motivation (barriers and problem-solving solutions);
- living with AS (feelings and beliefs).

The SMC-AS was examined in a pre-post test design with an intervention group and a matched control group receiving standard care (J.H. Barlow & Barefoot, 1996), and was found to be effective in terms of enhanced self-efficacy and improved psychological wellbeing, with moderate effect sizes of .45 and .59 respectively at six-month follow-up.

Although significant increases in the range and frequency of exercise were evident at three weeks, these changes were not maintained over time. Similarly, disease severity had improved at three weeks post-intervention, but was not significantly different between the groups at six months. The positive association between disease severity and exercise at baseline suggests that people with greater perceived severity are more likely to carry out therapeutic exercise. Hence, as group participants began to 'feel better', their motivation to exercise may have declined. This finding illustrates one of the main challenges facing people with arthritis and those involved in their care. Motivation to maintain therapeutic regimens needs to be consistent throughout the disease course, regardless of disease severity. Although gentle exercise can be substituted for more vigorous activities during disease exacerbation, it is vitally important that exercise is maintained for the remainder of the individual's life. It should also be noted that fate appeared to play a part in the failure to maintain exercise among intervention participants. Several participants reported major life events following attendance on the course (e.g. birth of new son, moved house, bereavement). Thus, it was somewhat understandable that the routine performance of exercise would suffer.

The intervention format of the AS course (i.e. two consecutive days) may have contributed to the failure to maintain exercise in the longer term. Unlike interventions that are delivered over several weekly sessions, the SMC-AS did not allow for contact between participants and tutors after the end of the course. Thus, opportunity for reinforcement techniques such as encouragement, advice, support and positive feedback were limited. We attempted to address this issue by opening the course to both people with AS and their partners, based on the assumption that the partner could not only learn how to carry out the exercises with the person with AS but could also be trained to provide motivation and feedback. In addition, later courses included individual goal-setting and development of an individualised home exercise plan.

A home-based exercise intervention package for people with AS was tested in a randomised controlled trial (Sweeney *et al.*, 2002). The intervention was mailed to participants and comprised an exercise/educational video, a booklet and an exercise progress wallchart and reminder stickers. The video was introduced by a consultant rheumatologist, and contained an exercise regime designed for all levels of severity. The video concluded with a discussion led by a health psychologist, a physiotherapist and a patient. The discussion covered similar topics to those included in the intervention of J.H. Barlow and Barefoot (1996) (i.e. barriers to and benefits of exercise, and methods of planning exercise adherence). Participants were recruited from a self-help society database. There were 75 completers in the intervention group and 80 in the control group. At six-month follow-up there were significant improvements on exercise self-efficacy, and self-reported AS mobility exercise and aerobic exercise in the intervention group. There were no changes on disease activity, function, global wellbeing, or self-efficacy for pain or function. The last of these is perhaps to be expected with an intervention that focused primarily on exercise rather than pain management. This study is interesting in showing that an easily distributed, mailed programme can encourage people to exercise at home.

Given the demise of AS exercise classes in my local area (Coventry), I recently organised and piloted a one-day intervention for promoting exercise among people with AS. The COAching for eXercise in AS (COAX-AS) Day was held in Coventry University Sports Centre, thus taking the intervention away from a hospital or rehabilitation environment. The day was developed in liaison with a rheumatology physiotherapist and Coventry University Sport Centre's physiotherapist, and was delivered to 17 AS patients with additional input from a consultant rheumatologist and health psychologist with coaching expertise The programme content was as follows:

- short talk on AS and recent advances in knowledge and treatment;
- stretches for AS (whole group);
- trying out equipment in fitness suite (gym area);
- mat and ball exercises;
- coaching and goal-setting for exercise;
- question-and-answer session.

Undergraduate physiotherapy students assisted with the day, and this meant that each AS participant received individual coaching.

Several of the 17 participants had not been inside a fitness suite or gym area before or had attended a gym in the past but had stopped due to being teased about their posture or lack of mobility. With encouragement from the physiotherapists and students, the AS participants were able to learn more about which exercise-related activities would benefit their needs. The day ended with a coaching and goal-setting session designed to encourage participants to continue exercising after the course. The COAX-AS Day was observed and evaluated by a researcher (Lorraine McFarland), who was independent of course development and delivery.

The AS participants reported that they had learned a great deal more about AS, including how to exercise at home. The opportunity to talk to other people with AS provided an opportunity for social comparison, and participants found it helpful and encouraging to discover that there were people with worse disability than themselves who were determined not to let AS control their lives. Participants judged the event to be very successful and well organised, and there were many requests for a fortnightly or weekly class.

The course evaluation included the physiotherapy students who assisted on the day. Overall, the students reported little previous experience of working with people with AS, and were surprised to find that participants found exercise 'challenging'. The students had expected participants to be 'middle-aged' or 'old' but came to realise that AS had an early age at onset. Furthermore, the AS exercises presented on the day differed from the students' expectations, and they felt that prior to COAX-AS they had not considered how management of the condition had to be tailored to the individual's level of motivation as well as to their disability. Students felt that the Sports Centre was preferable for learning and trying out exercises because it removed AS participants from the 'caring stigma' associated with hospitals and located them in an environment where they were encouraged to self-manage. Prior to COAX-AS, students perceived their role as a physiotherapist to encompass leading, motivating, encouraging, and educating. After the event, students were aware of the psychosocial aspects of AS and the need to empower people to help them live as normal and active lives as possible. They were surprised by the participants' level of knowledge of and expertise in their condition. The students recognised the need to consider the whole person when promoting the benefits of exercise, and felt that the group involvement promoted encouragement between the participants. The very experienced physiotherapists who led the COAX-AS Day helped build confidence among both AS participants and the student helpers through their positive approach.

These findings are interesting as they demonstrate how the opportunity to work with people with AS in a supervised setting helped to raise awareness of key features of living and managing AS among physiotherapy students.

Multi-Component Self-Management Interventions

Many multi-component interventions are labelled as 'self-management'. The terms 'self-care' and 'self-management' tend to be use interchangeably. Clark *et al.* (1991) suggest a useful distinction whereby self-care is viewed as a preventative strategy (i.e. tasks performed by healthy people at home), and self-management is concerned with the daily tasks individuals undertake to control or reduce the impact of disease on physical health status. In addition, individuals have to cope with the psychosocial consequences of arthritis and must manage daily living according to their financial and social conditions. Successful self-management requires sufficient knowledge of arthritis and its treatment, performance of arthritis-related management activities, and performance of the necessary skills to maintain adequate psychosocial functioning. Thus, self-management can be defined as the individual's ability to manage the symptoms, treatment, physical and psychosocial consequences and lifestyle changes inherent in living with arthritis (J.H. Barlow, 2001). Efficacious self-management encompasses the ability to monitor one's condition and to achieve the cognitive, behavioural and emotional responses necessary to maintain a satisfactory quality of life. Thus, a dynamic and continuous process of self-regulation is established. The key messages of psycho-educational interventions should aim to assist people with arthritis in these self-management tasks in partnership with their healthcare providers.

Recognition of the need for self-management ability amongst people with arthritis has led to the development of interventions designed to enhance relevant skills and coping strategies as well as providing information and a supportive environment whereby participants can share their experiences. The current popularity of 'self-management' has led to many existing educational initiatives being relabelled, although it is not clear whether the content has been adjusted accordingly. Self-management interventions typically draw on a range of methods to assist change in behaviour, cognitions and emotions.

The leading exemplar of a holistic approach to arthritis self-management is the Arthritis Self-Management Program (ASMP), developed for people at the mild to moderate end of the disease spectrum (Lorig & Gonzalez, 1992). The ASMP is targeted at people with arthritis in the community, on the assumption that people attending hospital clinics tend to be better served in terms of educational provision. It comprises six weekly sessions of approximately two hours in length delivered to groups of 8–15 people in community settings (e.g. church halls, libraries and shopping malls). As well as being community-based, a second unique aspect of the ASMP is that it is delivered by pairs of lay leaders who themselves have arthritis. This feature of the ASMP emphasises the important role that people with arthritis can play in managing their own condition and educating their peers. In the UK, lay-tutor training for the ASMP is organised by Arthritis Care, a voluntary organisation, and is supported by a quality assurance system designed to ensure standards of programme delivery are maintained. In the US, cost savings of between $40 and $600 per ASMP are reported if lay rather than professional leaders are used, with no difference in outcomes (Cohen *et al.*, 1986; Lorig *et al.*, 1986).

The programme itself is very structured, with tutors following a comprehensive manual to ensure consistency across time and groups. Topics covered include information on arthritis and its treatment, exercise, cognitive symptom management, managing emotions and communication with health professionals. A variety of learning formats are used, including lecturettes, role-plays, problem-solving, and contracting. The last of these involves each participant learning to set a realistic goal for the forthcoming week and making a contract to achieve this goal. Progress in goal achievement is monitored each week during the session, with feedback and support provided by tutors and other participants. Tutors are trained to advise participants to contact their healthcare providers regarding specific queries about their condition and its treatment. All participants receive a copy of the *Arthritis Helpbook*. Many educational interventions draw upon this seminal programme and its accompanying manual.

A central aim of the ASMP is to increase participants' perceptions of arthritis self-efficacy, defined as perceived ability to control or manage various aspects of arthritis such as pain, fatigue or depressed mood. Self-efficacy became the theoretical foundation of this programme when investigation revealed that change in health outcomes was not necessarily correlated to change in use of self-management behaviours (Lorig, Seleznick *et al.*, 1989). Structured and open-ended interviews with ASMP participants found that those who did well believed that they could make a difference to the impact that arthritis was having on their lives, whereas those who did less well held the opposite beliefs (Lenker *et al.*, 1984). These findings suggested that expectations of self-efficacy for managing arthritis were mediating the outcomes of the ASMP and led to the development of an arthritis self-efficacy scale to measure change (Lorig, Chastain *et al.*, 1989) and subsequent modification of the ASMP to incorporate efficacy-enhancing techniques.

Change on health outcomes for the enhanced version of the ASMP confirmed its greater effectiveness (Holman & Lorig, 1992). Thus, drawing on the basic tenets of self-efficacy theory (Bandura, 1977), the current ASMP aims to enhance perceived ability to control various aspects of arthritis through skills mastery, modelling, reinterpretation of symptoms and persuasion. Skills mastery is the most effective efficacy-enhancing strategy, and involves learning and practising appropriate behaviours. New behaviours are broken down into smaller, manageable ones, ensuring that each is successfully performed. Participants on the ASMP often choose personal goals associated with increasing exercise behaviours, which can be tried in the 'safe' environment of the group setting and practised at home. Personal goals serve to provide a greater incentive for task accomplishment (Gonzalez *et al.*, 1990). Modelling involves observation of positive role models who are successfully managing their condition and therefore act as a source of inspiration for participants. In the context of the ASMP, course tutors with arthritis are positive role models. In addition, observing change among fellow participants and sharing knowledge and coping strategies offer further opportunities for increasing self-efficacy through modelling. Persuasive communication is most effective when it involves encouraging participants to attempt a little more than they are currently doing, and is used in combination with other techniques. Evidence suggests that group members can motivate reluctant participants to initiate and carry through actions (Gonzalez *et al.*, 1990). Finally, reinterpretation of physiological symptoms is an important aspect of managing the impact of arthritis. Participants learn how to distinguish between physiological disease-related symptoms (e.g. pain, fatigue, muscle soreness) and similar symptoms that can arise from therapeutic exercise or carrying out too many activities on 'good' days (e.g. pain-free days). In addition, participants learn that cognitive symptom management techniques can be used to overcome feelings of helplessness in response to pain, for example. Using these techniques, the ASMP encourages participants to become active agents in the care of their arthritis, confident in their ability to select the self-management strategies that best suit their individual needs at a given time.

Given equal disease severity, perception of arthritis self-efficacy may differentiate between those who are incapacitated by their disease and those who continue to live full and active lives. Moreover, theoretical propositions (Bandura, 1997) suggest that self-efficacy will mediate changes in behaviour and physiological wellbeing among people with arthritis. However, apart from the work of Lorig and colleagues, the potential mediational role of self-efficacy has rarely been tested in relation to health outcomes following self-management interventions. One exception is a study by J.H. Barlow, Williams and Wright (1999), who found that, among a sample ASMP participants in the UK, improvements in arthritis pain were mediated through change in self-efficacy rather than use of cognitive symptom management.

Insight into the participants' experiences of attending the ASMP and its perceived impact is provided through a series of qualitative studies conducted by myself and colleagues in parallel to quantitative studies (e.g. J.H. Barlow, Williams & Wright, 1999; Turner *et al.*, 2002). Below is a selection of typical quotes following course attendance:

'The Course gave me the strength to fight the pain and get on with life.'

'I found the Course enlightening. It let you discuss your problems with people who know exactly what you are suffering. I was relieved that I was not the only one. The Course opened me up and I blossomed from it.'

'I thought the Course was absolutely wonderful ... It helped me to get out of the house. What I found about other people was that most of them had had arthritis much longer than I had and they were great at giving tips. Not only did you learn from the people who were doing the official course, there was a lot of interaction between people.'

'Meeting people that were in the same boat as I was ... I suppose when you're in one room with other people that suffer from it you don't feel quite so bad.'

'Because before you didn't have any future. It was blank. Automatically, I use quite a lot of them [self-management techniques] now. I still get depressed but I realise why now, and I know that if I don't get myself motivated then I'm going into the pain cycle. It gave me a set of goals. I'd never set myself goals in my life before.'

'I try to ensure that I do some exercise, eat more healthily. I know my medication, I have a better rapport with my GP. I mean he regards me as an expert on arthritis as opposed to him being an expert.'

'Don't let arthritis decide what you're going to do, YOU decide, you take control. I came away thinking "right, get on with it, let's sort it" and I do to the best I can.'

'When you go to a group that's suffering from the same illness then you can compare notes and you can see that things do get better … it makes you look towards other people rather than inwardly all the time.'

'It really gave you an insight into the condition you were suffering and you could understand it a bit so, therefore you were more likely to accept it … and that's a very hard things to accept, because it's a major change in your life.'

'Interviews consistently show that ASMP participants enjoy meeting similar others in a structured learning environment. They appreciate the problem-solving sessions that enable the exchange of ideas and provide the opportunity to learn new ways of perceiving situations and communicating with others. Participants feel that their arthritis experiences are valued, and the sharing and receiving of advice is considered both helpful and empowering. They feel reassured that they are no longer alone; rather, they have a ready-made peer group that has an inherent understanding of the problems encountered in living with arthritis. Social comparisons with other participants and with ASMP tutors are common and can lead to a response shift. For example, downward social comparisons can result in a positive health re-evaluation, as participants' perspectives of the severity and burden of their own condition change after seeing others whom they perceive to be more severely affected. Equally, participants can gain hope and inspiration from those whom they perceive to be coping well with their problems; this is described as upward social comparison (Buunk, 1995; Turner *et al.*, 2002). Many participants refer to greater confidence in their ability to manage their arthritis, feeling more in control, and use of the techniques learned to help manage pain, fatigue and depression. Arthritis no longer dominates their lives. These qualitative findings point to a number of factors that may be implicated in facilitating improved outcomes including peer belonging, social comparisons, respect, goal-setting, problem-solving, emotional disclosure, disease acceptance and modelling.

Randomised, controlled trials of the ASMP in the US have been based on samples recruited through community sources (e.g. adverts in the media, libraries, shopping malls, healthcare provider practices). Results have shown the ASMP to be effective in terms of increasing arthritis self-efficacy, decreasing pain, reducing depressed mood, and leading to fewer visits to physicians at four-month follow-up (Lorig & Holman, 1993). Moreover, longer term follow-ups, at 21 months (Lorig & Holman, 1989) and four years, showed that, despite a slight increase in disability, reductions in pain and visits to physicians remained evident and there was a marked increase in self-efficacy (i.e. 17 per cent). Levels of depression remained fairly stable. Results were independent of type of arthritis. A cost-benefit analysis (Lorig *et al*, 1993) reported that the unit cost per participant of attending the ASMP as $54, with net savings per participant with OA over four years of $189 and of $648 for each participant with RA. This saving is largely due to a reduction in medical consultation. Lorig *et al.* (1993) estimated that if 1 per cent of the patients in the US with moderate to severe OA of the hand (103,000) attend an ASMP and achieved the same results as suggested in previous studies, then the total discounted savings over four years would be $19,491,720. Similarly, estimated savings for 1 per cent of patients with RA are $13,601,070. Other estimates of cost savings associated with the ASMP are provided by Kruger *et al.* (1998), who assert that for patients with RA, the savings are in the order of 10 times the cost of the course.

The first evaluation of the ASMP in a UK context (J. Barlow, Williams & Wright, 1997a) focused on older people with arthritis (i.e. over 55 years of age) using a pre-post test design. Results showed that, after four months, participants demonstrated significant increases in arthritis self-efficacy, positive affect, cognitive symptom management, communication with doctors, exercise and relaxation. In addition, significant decreases were found in terms of pain, depression and visits to primary care practitioners. It seems likely that the benefits of attending an ASMP are wide-ranging and may influence perceived ability to cope with the environmental demands faced in everyday life as an older person with arthritis. Thus, a measure of generalised self-efficacy beliefs was included and showed a small but significant improvement. Interview data across a number of studies has confirmed that participants generalise many of the techniques learned to other areas of their lives. Despite the group approach that facilitated meeting with similar others and sharing experiences, there was no change on satisfaction with social support. It may be that any change on social support is short-lived and is not maintained after the end of the six-week course, unless the participants establish their own supportive network. This problem of termination of support at the end of an intervention is not specific to the ASMP but is an inherent aspect of many short courses.

The ASMP has since been subjected to evaluation in a range of populations and delivery settings in the UK (e.g. adult education, community settings) (J. Barlow, Turner & Wright, 1998a, 1998b; J.H. Barlow, Williams & Wright, 1999) including two randomised, controlled trials (J.H. Barlow, Turner & Wright, 2000; Buszewicz *et al.*, 2006). In Barlow, Turner and Wright's randomised, controlled trial the sample comprised 189 in the control group and 241 in the intervention group with mean ages of 57 (SD 13.2) and 59 (SD 12.3). Participants' diagnoses were confirmed by their GP (J.H. Barlow, Turner & Wright, 2000). An intent-to-treat analysis revealed that at four-month follow-up, the ASMP had a significant effect on arthritis self-efficacy, use of self-management behaviours and depressed mood. Effect sizes ranged from .43 for arthritis self-efficacy to .27 for communication with physicians and depressed mood. This study extended previous research by including a measure of positive mood, which showed a significant increase among the intervention group at four months. At 12-month follow-up, the intervention group had maintained these improvements, and there were significant decreases in pain and in number of visits to GPs. Apart from a small improvement on physical functioning at 12 months among the intervention group with OA, results were independent of type of arthritis. An eight-year follow-up of the original intervention group participants (n = 125) suggested that improvements on self-efficacy, positive and negative affect, anxious and depressed moods, pain and fatigue, cognitive symptom management and communication with physician had been maintained in the longer term. There was one exception: Health Assessment Questionnaire scores had increased at eight years, indicating a decline in physical functioning, as may be expected over a long period. Interviews revealed that some participants continued to have problems with disease acceptance at eight-year follow-up. An unexpected and striking finding was the remarkable recall of the ASMP experience shown by participants. Such recall has been linked to emotionally salient events (Pashler, 2002), suggesting that, for some, ASMP attendance was a significant event; this was indicated in the data, where some participants talked about not having a future before the ASMP, for example.

Box 8.1 Methodological Note

Effect sizes are a way of representing the impact of an intervention on outcome variables in a standardised manner. The following formula is often used:

$$\text{effect size} = (x_2 - x_1)/SD_1$$

x_2 = mean score at follow-up, x_1 = mean score at baseline, and SD_1 = standard deviation at baseline. Small, moderate and large changes on outcome variables are indicated by effect sizes of 0.2, 0.5, and 0.8 respectively (Kazis *et al.*, 1989).

The randomised, controlled trial conducted by Buszewicz *et al.* (2006) focused on patients with OA aged 50 years or over (n = 812) recruited through 74 GP practices across the UK. The intervention group received the ASMP and an education booklet, whereas the control group received the booklet alone. At 12-month follow-up, there was a significant impact of the ASMP in terms of improvement on anxiety and arthritis self-efficacy for pain and other symptoms. A significant difference on depression was noted at four-month follow-up but was not evident at 12 months. There was no difference in GP visits at 12 months. Approximately 30 per cent of the intervention group failed to attend any of the ASMP session. Telephone interviews with a sub-sample of these revealed that the main reasons for non-attendance were the timing of the course or difficulties associated with accessing the venue.

The impact of the ASMP on physician/GP visits is the main area of difference between studies conducted in the US and those conducted in the context of the UK system of health care. In countries where health care is free at the point of delivery, raising patients' awareness and confidence could result in an increased number of patient-initiated visits to the GP. However, this does not seem to be the case. Indeed, studies show that visits tend to decrease at 12-month follow-up (J. Barlow, Williams & Wright, 1997a; J.H. Barlow, Turner & Wright, 2000), or do not change. The cost of attending the ASMP in the UK was £30.51 per participant in 1998, and compares favourably with other direct health-care costs, such as a home visit by a GP (£54.09) or a visit to a GP surgery

(£18.41). Moreover, in contrast to medication there are no known harmful side effects of attending psycho-educational interventions.

One of the other differences between UK and US participants concerns the level of physical functioning as indicated by scores on the Health Assessment Questionnaire. Typical mean scores for UK participants range between 1.4 and 1.7, suggesting a greater degree of impairment of physical functioning compared with the US where typical mean scores range between 0.6 and 0.9. This difference may be accounted for by the greater proportion of people with RA that enrol on the ASMP (e.g. approximately 40 per cent) in the UK compared to the US (approximately 14 per cent) (Lorig & Holman, 1993).

The ASMP has been adapted and delivered in a range of countries, languages and cultures. One programme based on the ASMP was evaluated in The Netherlands by Taal, Riemsma, Brus, Seydel, Rasker and Wiegman (1993). This programme differed in that it focused solely on patients with RA and used health professionals as tutors. Furthermore, the group practice of exercise was excluded, although RA patients received information about exercise, were encouraged to exercise at home, and could discuss any problems they were having with their exercise regime. Each patient received individual guidance from a physiotherapist regarding exercise. Evaluation comprised a randomised, controlled trial with 27 patients in the intervention group and 30 in the control group. The authors aimed for a homogeneous sample of RA patients with relatively good health status so that they would be able to cope with the exercise components. At four-month follow-up, the programme had significant positive effects on disability, exercise and knowledge. At 14-month follow-up, there were significant positive effects on exercise, self-efficacy for physical function and knowledge. There were no significant effects on pain, disease activity or psychosocial health. The additional input from physiotherapists seems to have influenced participants' exercise behaviour. However, compared with most studies of the ASMP led by lay tutors, results of this small study show few other long-term effects and no impact on psychological wellbeing. The role-modelling aspect of lay-led programmes may be important for promoting self-efficacy and psychological wellbeing. The aim of recruiting a homogeneous sample may have led to exclusion of those with more severe conditions and any associated psychological correlates. In addition, the 13 drop-outs were found to have fewer social contacts and were more anxious. Following on from this work, Riemsma *et al.* (2003) developed a revised group programme for RA patients who could participate with a significant other (usually a spouse). In addition, three booster sessions were provided at three, six, and nine months. The programme was delivered in five weekly sessions each of two hours to a group of eight patients with or without a significant other. The tutors were both arthritis nurses. Seventy-nine participants received education with a significant other, 80 received group education for patients only, and 79 were assigned to a control group who received a self-help guide. At 12-month follow-up, self-efficacy was significantly increased for the patient-only education group and was significantly lower for the patient-plus-significant-other education group. Furthermore, fatigue had also significantly increased in the patient-plus-significant-other group. No other significant effects were identified. This study has addressed two important issues in the arthritis self-management field, namely the potential value of including partners and also that of booster sessions. Logically, it may be expected that training partners may assist the patient in maintaining behaviour change in the home environment. Equally, it is logical to expect booster sessions to assist with behaviour change. However, results of the Riemsma *et al.* (2003) study suggest there may be no added value in either of these approaches.

A randomised, controlled trial conducted in the US for Spanish-speaking participants has shown the outcomes to correspond with other ASMP studies (Lorig *et al.*, 1999). The Spanish Arthritis Empowerment Programme was evaluated using a pre-test post-test design among 118 participants who completed the six-month follow-up (Wong *et al.*, 2004). There were significant improvements on self-efficacy, pain, self-care behaviour, arthritis knowledge and general health. Similarly, Yip *et al.* (2007) evaluated the effectiveness of the ASMP with an added exercise component for people with knee OA (88 intervention and 94 controls) living in Hong Kong. Results showed a significant effect of the intervention at 16-week follow-up on pain, fatigue, duration of weekly light exercise, and knee flexion.

The ASMP was the forerunner of the generic Chronic Disease Self-Management Course (CDSMC) (Lorig *et al.*, 1999). Both the ASMP and CDSMC have become major programmes for the delivery of self-management interventions in the UK, US, Australia, New Zealand and Canada. In the UK, the CDSMC was adopted as the foundation of the Department of Health's Expert Patient Programme (EPP) that was rolled out across England via primary care trusts. The programme was established as a Community Interest Company in 2007 and aims to increase its capacity from 12,000 course places to over 100,000 places by

2012 (see the 'Expert Patients Programme' homepages on www.dh.gov. uk/en/AboutUs for more information).

The ASMP has tended to remain the preserve of voluntary organisations in the UK and elsewhere. Given the widespread availability of both ASMP and CDSMC in the community, the relative merit of each programme for people with arthritis is a key question. This issue was examined by Lorig *et al.* (2005) among patients whose primary disease was arthritis using typical outcomes including self-efficacy, health distress, disability, pain, health behaviours and healthcare utilisation. It should be noted that anxiety, depression and positive psychological wellbeing were not measured. Comparison at four months showed effect sizes of at least 0.2 (i.e. a small effect size) on six outcomes for the ASMP versus three outcomes for the CDSMC. At 12 months, ASMP participants had effect sizes of 0.2+ on five outcomes compared to four outcomes for the CDSMC participants. The authors concluded that the disease-specific ASMP has advantages over the generic CDSMC, although these advantages decline over time. However, both interventions require an adequate number of participants to be viable in terms of delivery. Thus, it may be more cost-effective to run the CDSMC where patient numbers are low.

The relative merits of the ASMP and the CDSMC for people with arthritis have been further examined by Goeppinger *et al.* (2007) in a group randomised controlled design. After completion of baseline questionnaires and allocation to community coordinated workshops, researchers randomly assigned workshops to deliver the ASMP or CDSMC. The sample comprised mainly African Americans (365 out of 416 participants) with a mean age of 64 years; the mean number of chronic conditions was four and 75 to 80 per cent of the participants in each workshop were female. At four-month follow-up ASMP participants had significant improvements on self-efficacy, exercise, and general health, and CDSMC participants had significant improvements on self-efficacy, disability, pain and general health. There were differences between the groups on pain and disability, with the CDSMC producing stronger results. However, improvements had attenuated over time, and at one-year follow-up the only statistically significant improvement to be maintained was on self-efficacy for ASMP participants; no statistically significant improvements were maintained for CDSMC participants. The authors conclude that, for people with several co-morbid conditions, the CDSMC may be viewed as being more relevant due to its generic nature.

Results are interesting in that they show that these lay-led, community-based interventions can be effective for African Americans. However, this also may limit generalisability to other participant groups. Indeed, both the ASMP and CDSMC used in this study had been slightly modified following preliminary work evaluating the cultural acceptability of both programmes for African Americans living in the south-eastern area of the US. Revisions included the addition of a sentence to each of three activities to strengthen cultural dimensions to healthy eating, to address dietary fat and salt intake and to emphasise the two-way nature of communication with healthcare professionals. One cognitive symptom management strategy (using one's spirituality) was added to both programmes. Recruitment was via a community coordinator (a third lay tutor) who was known and respected by the community.

The apparent stability of pain following self-management interventions is worthy of comment. In accordance with studies of similar cognitive-behavioural-type interventions (e.g. Basler, 1993; Slater *et al.*, 1997) participants feel better able to manage their pain but do not necessarily experience a reduction in pain intensity. Failure to detect change in absolute levels of pain at 12 and 60 months was also noted in a controlled study of a modified version of the ASMP delivered in Australia to groups of OA and RA patients (Lindroth *et al.*, 1995). Lindroth *et al.* suggest that the 'crude measure' typically used to assess pain (i.e. a visual analogue scale) reflects only one dimension of the pain experience, and this might account, in part, for the inconsistency among findings. Interventions that impact on all aspects of the pain experience (i.e. behaviour, severity, and psychological consequences) are rare. Furthermore, the ASMP emphasises enhancement of perceived ability to self-manage and reinterpretation of symptoms, rather than reduction of symptoms *per se*.

Many interventions have drawn on the lessons from the ASMP in the course of their development. One example is a mail-delivered programme (Self-Management Arthritis Relief Therapy; SMART), based on individualised, computer-generated advice, the ASMP, and the *Arthritis Helpbook*. A randomised, controlled trial produced similar improvements to the group programme among a mixed group of arthritis patients (Fries *et al.*, 1997). At six months, participants showed a decrease in pain, improved joint count, increased self-efficacy and increased use of exercise, and were making fewer visits to physicians. A further study compared SMART with usual care and with the classic, small-group

ASMP (K.R. Lorig *et al.*, 2004). Unlike previous studies of the ASMP in the US, participants were recruited through rheumatology clinics, and the sample comprised a much higher proportion of people with RA, a more severe disease. The length of time that people participated in SMART ranged from 12 to 18 months whereas the ASMP is conducted in six, weekly, 2.5-hour sessions with no reinforcement. Compared with patients receiving usual care, SMART participants had decreased disability, improved role function and increased self-efficacy at one-year follow-up. At two years, SMART participants had decreased global severity and doctor visits, and increased self-efficacy. There were no differences between the intervention and usual care group at three years. Comparisons with the ASMP showed that SMART was more effective at one year in terms of greater decreases in disability and increased self-efficacy. However, there were no differences between the groups at two years. At three-year follow-up, role function and doctor visits were improved in ASMP compared to SMART. The authors point out that both intervention groups showed moderate improvements compared to baseline. The improvements were equal or greater than the effects of non-steroidal anti-inflammatory drugs for pain, disability and global outcomes. Thus, optimal outcomes for participants may be achieved by using a combination of mail- and group-based programmes. The mailed programme is a useful alternative for those who dislike group interactions or who have difficulty attending an intervention location, because they are not able to travel or do not have time for instance.

A variation in delivery of self-management interventions was evaluated in a small randomised, controlled trial (Pariser, 2004). All 85 outpatient clinic participants received an information pack on self-management and developed an action plan and related goals over a six-week period. The intervention group (n = 40) also received a brief educational session based on the information pack and were called by telephone once a week for five weeks. Calls followed a script based on different sections of the information pack and were designed to be motivational and to provide instruction. Control group participants were contacted in week 6 only. Both groups showed significant increases in arthritis self-efficacy. Qualitative analysis revealed that the telephone support had assisted many participants in initiating exercise for the first time in their lives and that it was helpful in terms of facilitating medical care when needed (e.g. during arthritis exacerbation). Results illustrate the added value of telephone support during the intervention period. Whether exercise performance is maintained in the longer term after the end of the intervention remains to be examined.

Lindroth *et al.* held a workshop to develop an arthritis education programme for people with RA and OA. Doctors, nurses, physiotherapists, occupational therapists, social workers and patients attended the workshop and were presented with details of the ASMP and education programmes used by the rheumatology departments of Lund (Sweden) and Perth (Australia). The workshop participants went on to develop a new programme that covered the following topics: medical aspects of RA and OA, pain management, exercise, available treatment, stress management, self-awareness and communication skills, work simplification and joint protection, nutrition and leisure, and the availability of community resources. Health professionals delivered the programme to groups of 8 to 15 patients in multidisciplinary settings in six weekly sessions. Separate sessions were held for RA and OA. The evaluation compared an intervention group of 100 outpatients (55 per cent RA, 45 per cent OA) from one hospital in Sydney (Australia) with a non-random control group of 95 outpatients (80 per cent RA, 20 per cent OA) attending a different hospital in Sydney. Different hospitals were used in order to prevent contamination between the groups. The control group did not receive any form of education. Results showed that, at 12 months, the intervention group had improvements on knowledge and disability. In addition, those who increased their knowledge scores were also likely to increase their use of work simplification and reported a decreased number of problems. There were no differences in symptoms, adherence to therapy, pain or locus of control. Lack of change in pain following educational intervention is a common finding (see above) and general measures of health locus of control may not be sensitive to change among people with specific diseases. A five-year follow-up was conducted and managed to assess 53 of the intervention group and 39 of the control group. The only significant differences regarding arthritis knowledge were that the intervention group knew more about anatomy and therapies than the control group. The intervention group maintained similar levels of disability over time whereas the control group showed evidence of decline. Similarly, there was an increase in pain in both groups, but this was only significant for the control group. In conditions that are incurable and with typical worsening over time, maintenance or slowing down of both disability and pain are appropriate long-term aims. Interestingly, there was a difference in terms of internal health locus of control, with the intervention group showing an increase in internality at five years. Long-term studies of psycho-educational interventions are rare and attrition is an obvious problem. Responders in this study were those with more secondary education, who used more exercise and joint protection activities compared with non-responders.

Drawing on their earlier work in Sweden and Australia, Lindroth *et al.* (1997) developed and evaluated a Rheumatoid Arthritis School. Their Problem-Based Education Program was conducted for groups of five to seven RA patients over eight weekly sessions of 2.5 hours. Each week, group discussions were led by one of a team of health professionals (doctor, nurse, physiotherapist, occupational therapist, social worker and dietician). The first session focused on the main problems of the group members. These typically comprised physical problems (e.g. pain and immobility), emotional problems (e.g. fear of the future, depression and low self-esteem) and social problems (e.g. work disability, lack of social contact and inability to care for children). Fatigue was a major problem that patients classified as having physical, emotional and social impact. The remaining sessions focused on problem-solving for each group. For example, the nurse led discussions on medication, surgery and alternative treatments whilst the dietician focused on diet, fasting and basic nutrition. The patients were encouraged to bring a relative or friend to the final sessions.

Evaluation used a waiting-list control group design. At three months, compared with the control group, intervention group participants had greater knowledge, used exercise and joint protection more, and had less disability and pain. However, only the increase in knowledge and use of joint protection remained significantly improved at 12 months. The intervention group reported fewer problems concerning lack of disease information after the programme. There was no change on perceived helplessness throughout the study. The authors suggest that problems such as depressed mood, fear of the future and work disability are too profound to be significantly influenced by only 14 hours of education.

Personal Development Interventions

In the UK, Arthritis Care (www.arthritiscare.org.uk) successfully delivered personal development courses for younger people with arthritis for several years. Although these courses proved to be very popular, their effectiveness was not systematically investigated. However, anecdotal evidence suggests that younger people (under 40 years of age) became more aware of the social model of disability and often went on to become involved in campaigning for the rights of people with disability. The success of the personal development courses and delivery of the ASMP led to development of a community-empowerment initiative targeting older people with arthritis. Arthritis Care developed a three-phase programme comprising the ASMP (phase I), personal independence courses (phase II) and a conference (phase III). Thus, a group of older people (> 55 years of age) was able to attend the ASMP and progress to a two-day residential course focusing on personal independence. The latter was set within the theoretical framework of the social model of disability, whereby disability is conceived as a socially constructed phenomenon (Finkelstein & Stuart, 1996). This viewpoint contrasts with the biomedical model that construes disability as a consequence of disease pathology in the individual. The aim was to empower older people to understand, challenge and overcome disabling barriers inherent within society. Topics covered included concepts, aims and philosophy of personal independence, models of disability, applications to the world of medicine, transport and leisure, external barriers present in society and how to overcome them, making choices and risk-taking, and their role within organisations.

A process evaluation showed that participants expressed a strong preference for an individualised agenda specific to arthritis rather than a wider, social agenda (J. Barlow & Williams, 1999). Although maintaining the same overall objectives, subsequent delivery was adjusted to emphasise individual factors that may influence independence, such as expectations and fears, the meaning of independence, beliefs and attitudes, being in control, and the internal and external barriers to independence. Interestingly, despite the emphasis on 'disability', albeit from a social rather than an individual perspective, participants did not view themselves as disabled, before during or after the course at four-month follow-up. Indeed, they disliked the term and did not perceive themselves as part of a wider 'disabled' group. Indeed, use of the term 'disability' provoked negative emotions and feelings of stigmatisation. Nonetheless, after the course participants felt able to look beyond arthritis and to examine the wider societal implications of disability. They recognised the value of working together as a group to overcome barriers (e.g. access to buildings and transport) and some had become involved in community projects. Furthermore, several had contacted their local council to request adaptations to their homes making access easier and safer (e.g. a handrail, ramp). They felt more confident, were able to express their feelings and no longer felt constrained by arthritis, as is illustrated in the following quotes.

> My attitude to being a wheelchair has completely changed ... Being in a wheelchair is not the worst scenario, it can be a liberating experience. I felt freedom.

> Arthritis to me was a disease. But now arthritis is not a bad thing ... it is just a new way of life ... I now feel that I am not just a bit of left luggage.

Having tested the water by attending an ASMP, this older group of people was motivated to continue the learning process. Although the personal independence course was not what they expected, they realised that the ASMP focused on self-management at the individual level whereas personal independence explored how the individual can manage in society. They felt it was a 'bonus' to have attended both courses. The experiences of this group of older people are in keeping with a lifespan perspective on control. This suggests that, as people move through middle to old age, the probability of changing their external environment (primary control) gradually recedes and attention shifts to within the individual (Heckhausen & Schulz, 1995). Thus, although some participants went on to join in community projects, they were in the minority, and the campaigning stance adopted by younger adults who attend personal development courses was not adopted. Indeed, participants viewed tutors who promulgated 'campaigning' notions as having 'fixed' or 'rather blurred' visions of the needs of older people with arthritis. Unfortunately this innovative intervention has not been taken forward into service provision, but it does serve to indicate how attending the ASMP can consolidate the ability to self-manage and can reawaken the desire to take part in new learning experiences.

Interventions for Enhancing Employment Potential

Although work disability has emerged as a significant issue in arthritis (see Chapter 6) and return to work is a key outcome used in outpatient settings, there are few interventions targeting this topic. Exceptions are

Table 8.1. Structure and content of the Into Work Personal Development Programme (IWPD)

Structure	Five residential courses, lasting between two and five days delivered over a six-month period; mentor support; homework assignments
Content	
Stage 1	**Introduction to personal development**
	Social model of disability and comparisons with the medical model
Stage 2	**Achieving personal excellence**
	Recognising personal priorities and choices
	Problem-solving
	Interpersonal skills (e.g. listening)
Stage 3	**Goal-setting for personal excellence**
	Decision-making
Stage 4	**Development of personal action plans**
	Monitoring goal achievement
	Self-advocacy
Stage 5	**Getting into work: essential skills**
	CV writing
	Interview techniques
Training elements	Lectures, individual and group discussions, videos, individual and group activities, mentor support, homework assignments

the approaches developed and tested by Arthritis Care. The INTO Work Personal Development Programme (IWPD) aimed to address both the internal and external barriers faced by people with arthritis in seeking to fulfil their employment potential. The structure and content of the programme are summarised in Table 8.1.

A controlled study showed the programme to be effective in terms of improved psychological wellbeing (i.e. less anxiety, lower depression, more self-esteem, increased positive mood) and increased generalised self-efficacy to cope with the demands of life in general and job-seeking self-efficacy (e.g. producing a CV). Participants expressed greater satisfaction with their lives and accepted that arthritis was still a part of their life, but was not the dominant feature (J. Barlow, Wright & Kroll, 2001). They were more aware of the social model of disability and were able to identify strategies for overcoming perceived barriers to employment.

The improvement in mood among the intervention group was not mirrored by change in symptoms, increasing the likelihood that changes were due to the intervention. Moreover, quantitative findings were confirmed and extended by qualitative findings from focus groups and individual interviews. In accordance with many group intervention studies, the main benefit of course attendance to emerge from the qualitative data was the process of sharing with similar others who had arthritis. Participants believed this to be instrumental in facilitating personal change, and they reported a number of improved interpersonal skills including the ability to listen, greater respect for other people's views and greater openness. Interestingly, several participants had met with resistance and lack of understanding when trying to explain their changed outlook to their partners and other family members on returning home after the residential courses. This situation can create difficulties for intervention participants when they attempt to maintain their hard-earned changes in behaviours or emotional coping. After the IWPD programme, people with arthritis felt able to act autonomously, were able to self-regulate their behaviour and were psychologically empowered and self-realising. Not only were participants able to select personal goals that were salient to them, but they also possessed the knowledge and skills necessary to take steps towards achieving their goals in a structured manner. They possessed the characteristics of self-determined individuals, as exemplified in the quotes below.

> I've still got arthritis and other things wrong with me but it isn't ruling my life any more. It's taking second place because I'm getting to learn more about myself as a person.

> I was actually applying for office jobs. The reason I was applying for office jobs was because I had arthritis … I didn't actually sit down and think through what I really wanted to do … I will be doing some courses coming September … I realised I could do other things than just office work … I have always been interested in something in the arts … this course has given me an option …

> I feel more self-confident, value my life with other people, can cope better with disappointment and I am trying to live by my values.

> My partner and family have seen a great difference in me and they don't recognise me for the person that I was. There has been a lot of negative feelings … it's very difficult to understand why my personality has changed so much.

Change of any description and in any situation can be associated with difficulty, and this may help to explain why participants in many interventions that address emotional issues suggest that increased access to counsellors or mentors is warranted. Mentors were an integral aspect of the IWPD programme and played a key role in supporting participants. However, the time constraints, lack of face-to-face contact and the number of participants allocated to each mentor may have limited the amount of support that was actually available (Cullen & Barlow, 1998). Nonetheless, mentoring conducted by mentors who have similar conditions to mentees appears to be successful in providing much-needed emotional support for people with arthritis undergoing personal change. The advantage of using mentors with arthritis is that they possess a good understanding of mentees' experiences and can use their expert knowledge to good effect.

A subsequent intervention, developed by the same team as INTO Work, was called Working Horizons and aimed to facilitate job-seeking behaviour among people with arthritis currently not registered as 'available for work', and to provide assistance to those who wish to retain their current employment status. The programme offered participants one-to-one advice with an employment adviser, and work experience; a sub-group received personal development training and vocational training. The use of employment advisers and work experience placements were the main differences between Working Horizons and its predecessor INTO Work. Employment advisers who had arthritis themselves acted as peer mentors to participants, offering advice, support and guidance as required. A small controlled study showed that Working Horizons was effective in terms of increasing participants' job-seeking self-efficacy and satisfaction with life, and decreasing anxious mood (J. Barlow, Wright & Wright, 2000). Results of the qualitative analyses based on interviews and focus groups confirmed that participants felt more confident in relation to seeking employment, were more accepting of their condition, felt more positive and had a greater awareness of the social model of disability. Participants reported receiving valuable emotional and instrumental support from employment advisers. Both participants and employment advisers viewed the notion of 'feeling understood' as a vital aspect of Working Horizons and stressed the importance of having suitable role models with an inherent insight into the problems and issues encountered by people with a fluctuating condition. Working Horizons was perceived to fill a gap in that it helped prepare people to approach employment agencies or to register for appropriate training. It also provided much-needed experience of managing arthritis in the workplace.

Although Arthritis Care did not continue with these two work-focused interventions, they are currently offering 'Preparing for Work', an eight-week intervention that is similar to Challenging Arthritis but includes additional job-seeking skills such as knowing your limits, identifying transferable skills, completing an application form and preparing a CV, interview techniques and negotiation skills with employers.

Interventions in JIA

Evidence from the few published studies evaluating psychological interventions for children with JIA suggest this is a promising avenue worthy of greater attention in a field where treatment is ameliorative rather than curative, treatment adherence is poor and long-term adaptation is essential. Interventions for children include behavioural techniques, CBT, videos, computer programs, summer camps and family retreats.

The efficacy of a parent-managed behavioural (token) reinforcement programme designed to improve the medication compliance of a 14-year-old boy with JIA was examined in a withdrawal (single-subject) design (Rapoff *et al.*, 1988a) Results showed increased compliance, clinical improvements (assessed by a rheumatologist), and improvement on parental rating of symptoms. In an attempt to reduce the complexity and time-consuming nature of token reinforcement programmes, Rapoff *et al.* (1988b) used more simple behavioural strategies (e.g. self-monitoring and positive verbal feedback) combined with education among three female patients, aged 3, 10 and 13 years. Medication compliance increased for two patients but showed no change for the third patient. Moreover, for all three patients compliance had decreased at four-month follow-up, suggesting that long-term maintenance may require either continuous intervention or regular monitoring. It should be noted that the high level of compliance achieved by the youngest child might reflect more about the parents' attitudes to medication than the beliefs and behaviours of the child.

In the context of pain management, the effectiveness of CBT delivered in a series of individual sessions, was examined among 26 children (Walco *et al.*, 1992). Of the 13 children who completed the programme, pain ratings were improved in the short term and at six-month follow-up. Using similar methods, but with the addition of thermal biofeedback and autogenic exercises (e.g. positive self-statements and relaxing imagery), Lavigne *et al.* (1992) found improved pain ratings among four of the eight child participants post-intervention and at six-month follow-up. These findings were confirmed by maternal reports of children's pain and pain behaviour. Whilst indicating the potential of CBT for influencing pain management in children, generalisability is limited by the very small samples, high attrition rates and reliance on parametric statistical procedures in small data sets.

The impact of a very different intervention, a summer camp designed to foster independence and to promote disease self-management, was examined among children aged between 7 and 20 in an uncontrolled, pre-post test design (Stefl *et al.*, 1989). Given these aims, it is surprising to note that no measures of self-management were included in the assessment battery. Results showed that children's locus of control and self-esteem had significantly improved immediately following the one-week camp, but these changes were not maintained at six months. Acknowledging the fact that management of JIA occurs within a family context, Haggelund *et al.* (1996) examined the efficacy of a three-day family retreat held at a 'resort' hotel among 39 families. The retreat included formal educational and therapeutic sessions (e.g. coping with chronic illness, enhancing self-esteem) and family-oriented recreational activities. Caregivers reported that their children's internalising behaviour problems were significantly reduced six months after the retreat, and mothers reported reductions in strain on family leisure and occupational functioning. Mothers' psychological distress remained stable. A number of important methodological limitations were noted, such as the lack of a control group and the difficulty in controlling for intervening variables between initial and follow-up assessments.

One UK study evaluated the effects of two modes of disease education upon the knowledge, physical and psychosocial health of children with JIA (aged 7–17) and their parents (Southwood *et al.*, 2000). The interventions comprised a JIA-specific video, entitled *Kids Like Us* (Southwood, 1992), and an interactive multi-media computer program, developed by T. Southwood, S. Young and D. Cheseldine in 1998 whilst working at Birmingham Children's Hospital. Both the video and computer program were developed specifically to teach children with JIA about their disease and its treatment. Although designed for children, these videos and computer packages can also be used by other family members. Thus, parental outcomes were assessed in addition to those relating to children. A randomised, controlled study showed that there were no statistically, significant differences between the children in the computer (n = 62) and video (n = 66) groups on any of the study variables at the four-month follow-up. However, both groups of children showed evidence of an increase in arthritis-related knowledge and improvement in their sense of hope. Furthermore, children in the video group showed improvements in self-efficacy for managing symptoms, self-efficacy for managing activities, current stiffness, worst pain, and trait anxiety. There were no significant changes on parental measures of wellbeing. Interviews revealed that children had received little previous disease education and that the video and the computer program were welcome sources of information, with both being perceived as appropriate and user-friendly modes of disease education. The computer program was seen as a particularly enjoyable means of learning about JIA, and children appreciated its interactive nature (e.g. being able to take part in a quiz). Both children and parents indicated that the video and computer program might have different preferred uses. The video was seen as most useful for newly diagnosed families, providing general information at a basic level, whereas the computer program was viewed as a useful means of providing more specific and complex information to children throughout the course of their disease.

There have been a few interventions that specifically target other family members, usually parents. Ireys *et al.* (1996) evaluated a 15-month, family-to-family network, social support and mentoring intervention (Arthritis Parents: Learning, Understanding and Sharing, A-Plus). Mentors (mothers of young adults who had had JIA since childhood) were linked up with mothers of children with JIA aged between 2 and 11 years. The intervention aimed to enhance informational support (dealing with teachers), affirmational support (e.g. giving praise) and emotional support (e.g. feelings). Compared with the control group, the mentoring group showed improvements in maternal mental health and social support. A residential workshop and information pack for parents of adolescents with JIA (aged between 12 and 18) were evaluated in a controlled study (Turner & Barlow, 2001). The three-day workshop aimed to provide information, education, and social and emotional support. Content included discussion of the roles adopted by parents, parenting skills, social and medical models of disability, and presentations by a young adult with JIA focusing on coping and a research psychologist who presented the results of interviews with teenagers living with JIA. The information pack included a series of leaflets covering topics such as accessing resources, relationship issues, sexuality, education and employment. Twenty-three parents attended the workshop and 28 parents who had expressed an interest but were unable to attend formed the comparison group. At three-month follow-up, the workshop group reported fewer episodes of disease-related stress relating to their child and their own health. The study was somewhat underpowered to detect changes. Recruitment was outside of the control of the evaluators and the final sample was smaller than expected. However, there was a trend towards improvement on mental health among the workshop group. Interviews with workshop parents showed that almost half of them felt that they were communicating more effectively with their child, in terms of being able to raise issues (e.g. bullying) and in terms of listening more closely to their child's needs. Some parents felt more positive about their child's future and their own. One benefit that often derives from group interventions is that of the reduced isolation that results from meeting with similar others at the workshop. This point is particularly important where disease prevalence is relatively low such as in JIA. Parents also appeared to feel more assertive in accessing resources such as home tuition, information from health professionals and requesting special needs statements.

There are indications that psychological interventions may offer benefits to children and their families. However, a number of methodological issues remain to be addressed, such as the small sample sizes, lack of controlled studies, dearth of validated measuring instruments for children and scarcity of resources available for non-medical interventions. Furthermore, it has been argued that pain is not always viewed as a prominent issue in JIA (Lavigne *et al.*, 1992), which partly explain why pain management interventions are not used more frequently. Descriptive studies employing qualitative methodologies may offer greater insight into the experience of JIA from a child's perspective and would provide a useful framework for developing successful interventions in the future.

Effectiveness of Psycho-Educational Interventions

This section draws together findings from systematic reviews of psycho-educational interventions and considers some of the issues raised. It is important to note that the effectiveness of psycho-educational interventions is usually assessed over and above the effects of medical interventions. Contrary to the procedure in many drug trials, participants are not required to stop standard treatment for a wash-out period prior to entering the intervention. Wash-out periods serve to increase the probability of finding a significant effect in clinical trials, whilst maintenance of medication during an education intervention may limit the potential for improvement. One review of arthritis patient education studies (including psycho-educational interventions) suggests that clinical studies of the effects of medication alone demonstrate a 20 to 50 per cent improvement on health status, whereas educational interventions provide an additional 15 to 30 per cent improvement (Hirano *et al.*, 1994). A meta-analysis comparing the effects of educational interventions and NSAIDs on pain and functional disability in OA and RA concluded that, since most patients in education trials are in receipt of medications, the effect sizes of these trials represent additional, marginal effects of patient education beyond those achieved by medication alone (Superio-Cabuslay *et al.*, 1996). The weighted average effect sizes for pain, disability and tender joint count in educational interventions were 0.17, 0.03 and 0.34 respectively, compared with 0.66, 0.34 and 0.43 for NSAID trials. Among participants with OA, patient education was, on average, 20 per cent as efficacious as NSAID treatment in reducing pain (effect size .17) but had little effect on functional disability. One exception was the eight-week supervised walking programme developed by Allegrante *et al.* (1993), which showed an effect size of 1.11 on functional disability. Interestingly, there was evidence of a publication bias, with smaller NSAID trials reporting small or negative effects being under-represented in the meta-analysis. Hence, the averaged effect sizes for NSAID trials may be inflated. As may be expected, the effect on pain was greater for interventions incorporating cognitive-behavioural pain-management techniques. Also focusing on pain disability, a more recent meta-analysis of arthritis patient education by Warsi *et al.* (2003) reported effects sizes of 0.12 for pain and 0.07 for disability. Furthermore, there was no evidence of publication bias towards studies showing reductions in pain or disability.

A Cochrane Review of patient education for people with rheumatoid arthritis based on randomised, controlled trials found small but statistically significant effects for scores on disability, joint counts, patients' global assessment, psychological status and depression (Riemsma *et al.*, 2002) in the short term. Typical improvements found when comparing patient education to no education were in the order of a 12 per cent decrease on depression, a 4 per cent decrease on pain, and a 12 per cent improvement on impact. These findings were based on a range of patient education formats including information only (e.g. leaflets), counselling and support-style interventions, and more complex interventions including cognitive behavioural techniques. The findings should be viewed with caution since there is a sense in which comparing the effects of a leaflet with the effects of 12 hours of intensive interventions delivered by health professionals or trained tutors and including home work tasks cannot be considered fair and just. Indeed, many trials use a leaflet-only condition as the control group. In addition, including outcomes that are not of relevance to the content of the intervention seems rather odd. For example, few patient education interventions set out to reduce swollen joint counts or lower ESR (a blood test measuring disease activity). As noted by Edwards (2002), the core data set of clinical outcome measures in RA was established to determine the effects of anti-rheumatic drugs. Much of patient education aims to foster knowledge transfer and to empower patients in the management of their condition, enabling them to make informed decisions about their care. The emphasis is on reassurance rather than directly influencing clinical outcomes. The fact that Riemsma *et al.* found a reduction of 12 per cent on depression has been somewhat overlooked. We know that people with RA are vulnerable to depression; thus, any intervention that offers an effective means of reducing depression should be encouraged. Moreover, a large-scale WHO survey has shown that depression co-morbid with one or more chronic diseases such as arthritis results in the worst health scenario, thus emphasising the importance of addressing depression in the wider field of public health priority (Moussavi *et al.*, 2007) and not just within psychosocial rheumatology. Regarding the lack of longer-term effects, few studies are able to retain controlled conditions for more than six months. Funding and ethical issues act as constraining issues in this regard. For example, many evaluations use a randomised wait-list control design whereby the control group are offered the intervention after the follow-up assessments. Thus, most study participants will receive the intervention, and there is no longer a suitable control group.

One meta-analysis of 25 randomised, controlled trials of psychological interventions for RA set out to exclude from the review any interventions that simply provided information; the intervention had to include a psychological component such as biofeedback, cognitive behavioural therapy or relaxation (Astin *et al.*, 2002). Significant, pooled effect sizes were found post-intervention for pain (0.22), functional disability (0.27), psychological status (0.15), coping (0.46), and self-efficacy (0.35). At follow-up (average 8.5 months), there were significant pooled effect sizes for tender joints (0.33), psychological status (0.30), and coping (0.52). The authors rated the methodological quality of studies on a rating system. However, this system included ratings for 'blinding patients to treatment'. Clearly, this is not possible with a psychological intervention. The authors excluded any studies that failed to adequately describe the intervention, including one of our own studies (J.H. Barlow, Bishop & Pennington, 1996). Since this study was a trial of an information leaflet that was not intended to have a psychological component, it is not clear why we were singled out as an example of 'not describing the intervention clearly'. In fact, our study should have been excluded as one that provided information only. I have included this information here as such errors in reporting can raise doubts regarding the accuracy of other statements in the paper (at least it did for me!).

A later meta-analysis has focused on psychological interventions for managing pain and disability among a sample of RA, OA and mixed RA and OA samples (Dixon *et al.*, 2007). Interventions included were CBT, pain-coping skills, biofeedback, stress management, emotional disclosure, hypnosis and psychodynamic therapy. Twenty-seven studies were included in the final analysis, which covered 3409 participants with mean age 58.9 years, 69.5 per cent female, 81 per cent Caucasian. The mean number of sessions in each intervention was 8.5 (range 4–20), with the length of each session averaging 86 minutes. Effect sizes for the outcomes considered are summarised in Table 8.2 and range from 0.716 for active coping to 0.070 for fatigue. Overall, results show that psychological interventions are effective for people with RA or OA and lead to small improvements on pain, self-efficacy, and psychological wellbeing with a larger improvement on use of active coping strategies and little or no effect on fatigue.

Comparison across the various types of intervention was not possible since the majority of interventions included in the analysis were CBT (n = 23). It is worth noting that the majority of the study samples were female, Caucasian and middle-aged. Thus effectiveness for males, ethnic minority participants, the older elderly (aged 80+ years) and younger participants (aged <40 years) remains to be investigated.

Table 8.2. Summary of effect sizes of meta-analysis of psychological interventions reported by Dixon *et al.* (2007)

Outcome	Effect size	95% confidence intervals
Pain	0.177	0.259–0.094
Anxiety	0.282	0.455–0.110
Depression	0.208	0.363–0.052
Psychological disability	0.249	0.396–0.101
Pain self-efficacy	0.184	0.031–0.336
Active coping	0.716	0.490–0.941
Physical functioning	0.152	0.242–0.062
Swollen joints	0.349	0.593–0.105
Fatigue	0.070	0.261–0.121

Echoing early suggestions by Lindroth *et al.* (1995), Dixon *et al.* (2007) maintain that measuring pain by a visual analogue scale (VAS) may be more suited to patients with constant daily pain resulting from chronic, idiopathic pain conditions (e.g. low back pain). They suggest that the arthritis impact measurement scale (AIMS), which covers frequency of pain episodes, number of painful joints etc., may be more appropriate for assessing pain outcomes in psychological interventions. Furthermore, the meta-analysis illustrates quite clearly the impact of such interventions on active pain coping. Thus, targeting interventions at patients who show deficits in this area may be valuable, as would inclusion of pain coping as an outcome measure in relevant intervention studies. Finally, patients and healthcare providers need to be aware that the impact of psychological interventions is not just limited to pain or physical functioning but can be experienced as improvement in psychological wellbeing and overall quality of life.

Issues to be clarified

Although there is a growing body of evidence supporting the effectiveness of psycho-educational interventions, there are many questions that remain to be clarified. For example, little is known about the characteristics of people with arthritis who benefit most from psycho-educational interventions. Equally, little attempt has been made to understand the needs of under-served subgroups such as younger adults, people from ethnic minority groups, or those with learning disabilities. Strategies to maximise initial enrolment, to encourage attendance at all sessions, and to establish the optimal length or frequency of the intervention or the optimal timing of delivery are all areas that require attention. For example, many health professionals argue that education is needed early in the disease course but is less important as duration progresses. The reality is that people with arthritis may have different educational needs depending upon the degree of severity of their condition and the other psychosocial and environmental circumstances operating in their lives at any given point in time. For example, given the long-term nature of arthritis, an individual's needs at the age of 30 will differ from the same individual's needs at the age of 70. Finally, should partners be invited to attend the same intervention and will this enhance or detract from the session's effectiveness for people with arthritis? One of the few studies in this area focused on people with OA and spousal caregivers (Martire *et al.*, 2003). The intervention comprised what the authors describe as 'standard patient education' supplemented by specific information related to managing arthritis as a couple. Participants with OA were randomly assigned to attend the standard patient education or the 'couples' format. Both interventions were favourably evaluated, although the 'couples' format had better attendance rates and a greater increase in arthritis self-efficacy.

One area that has been subjected to investigation concerns the length of an intervention. The comparative effectiveness of the ASMP (six weekly sessions) and a shorter, three-week version was investigated in an uncontrolled design (Lorig *et al.*, 1998). The shortened ASMP excluded sessions on nutrition, medications and making judgements about non-traditional treatments, there were fewer sessions on cognitive pain management, problem-solving, and contracting (goal-setting) and less emphasis was placed on exercise. Results showed the traditional six-week ASMP was more effective at four-month follow-up; participants in the shortened version had significantly fewer improvements on key outcomes, such as pain and use of self-management techniques. Three sessions may be insufficient for behaviour change to become embedded in the routine of participants and severely limits the opportunities for sharing with similar others and receiving feedback and encouragement about one's achievements.

The other area that has received some attention is motivation to change behaviour and was based on the Transtheoretical Model of

Table 8.3. Stages of change based on Prochaska *et al.* (1994)

Stage	Action
Pre-contemplation	Do not intend to change
Contemplation	Intending to change but not decided when to take action
Preparation	Decided to change and completed plans/some small behaviours
Action	Overt changes in behaviour
Maintenance	Sustaining change and resisting temptation to relapse

Change. This model has been used most extensively in the field of health promotion and was developed in the area of smoking cessation. It suggests that individuals are at different stages of change in relation to adopting and maintaining health behaviours. Thus, interventions should be tailored to meet the needs of people within each stage, encouraging them to move towards action and maintenance. The Transtheoretical Model has been shown to be relevant across 12 different behaviours (Prochaska *et al.*, 1994), some of which are salient to people with arthritis (e.g. weight loss and exercise). Motivation to initiate and sustain change is represented as a series of stages that people move through (see Table 8.3).

Keefe *et al.* (2000) conducted separate cluster analyses of people with OA (n = 74) and people with RA (n = 103), to determine whether homogeneous groups of patients within each condition could be identified in terms of stages of change for adoption of self-management behaviours. Participants with a confirmed diagnosis were recruited through rheumatology clinics, public posters and newspaper adverts. As in previous studies of self-management usage, results for OA paralleled those for RA; therefore both groups were merged in presentation of results. Five homogeneous subgroups were identified.

The largest subgroup (44 per cent) was in pre-contemplation, and not only lacked the motivation to take action but also used few coping strategies. This lack of action may have been associated with lower levels of pain, physical disability and psychological disability. Keefe *et al.* (2000) suggest that pre-contemplaters may benefit from interventions that raise their awareness about the benefits of adopting self-management behaviours. In addition, there is a need for a support-ive relationship with a friend, a peer with arthritis, or a health profes-sional who can act as a source of feedback or reflection on their behaviours. This finding supports anecdotal evidence concerning the difficulties of recruiting people with OA onto educational interventions despite the use of personalised letters and home visits from a rheuma-tology nurse practitioner (D. Doyle, personal communication, 1999).

The second subgroup (11 per cent) was in the contemplation stage. Keefe *et al.* suggest interventions aiming to develop self-monitoring skills, and a re-evaluation of the pros and cons of self-management may encourage movement into the action stage.

The third subgroup (22 per cent) was in preparation, and it is sug-gested that setting a date to commence self-management, taking small steps towards action, and making an open commitment to family, friends and colleagues may help to move people forwards (Prochaska *et al.*, 1994).

A small subgroup (6 per cent) was labelled as in 'unprepared action'; that is they were taking action but had not contemplated or prepared for their actions. They were characterised as adequately managing pain, physical disability and psychological disability and had high arthritis self-efficacy.

The final subgroup (17 per cent) was coping with the most pain, physical disability and psychological distress. It is important to note that none of the patients in this study had attended a self-management intervention and that subgroup membership was independent of dis-ease duration. Although the sample size was relatively small, the results are interesting and indicate the need to consider a wide variety of routes to psycho-educational and self-management outcomes whilst acknowl-edging that individuals vary in their starting positions.

Few studies of psycho-educational interventions find differences between responders and non-responders in psychosocial rheumatol-ogy. Thus the factors contributing to attrition from interventions and their evaluation remain largely unknown. For example, a series of studies by Barlow *et al.* evaluating the ASMP did not find any statisti-cally significant differences between responders and non-responders on any study variables (e.g. physical, psychological or social health status, health behaviours or beliefs). Failure to complete the interven-tion was attributed to transport difficulties, disease flares and illness (not arthritis) of self or family member. Insight into the problem of attrition from psycho-educational evaluations is provided by Shaw *et al.* (1994), in a randomised, controlled study. Participants, aged over 60 (mean 70, SD 6.7) with symptoms of OA (130 male and 234 female), were recruited from a health maintenance organisation in the US, and were randomly assigned to one of three experimental groups (education, social support or a combination) or a control group. The content of the interventions is described in more detail earlier in this chapter (see Cronan *et al.*, 1998). The response rate was lower for the control group but similar across the three intervention groups. Responders were those who completed all three assessments (i.e. baseline, three-month and six-month follow-up). Non-responders in the intervention groups had higher levels of depression, as indicated by the depressed affect sub-scale of the CES-D. Non-responders in the control group had extreme scores on social activity (high or low) and more informational social support. A good attender was defined by the authors as one who 'attended at least four out of ten weekly meetings'. This seems a very liberal definition of a good attender and needs to be borne in mind when considering the findings. The most robust predictor of attrition was either a very high or a very low score on depression. It is noteworthy that dealing with depression was not covered in the content of the intervention. Hence participants scoring high on depression may have found that their main concern was not being addressed and thus ceased attending. Alternatively, people with high levels of depression may find it difficult to cope with the social interactions inherent in group situations and to concentrate on learning new skills. Attrition of high- and low-scoring respondents means that those who remain form a more homogeneous group. Thus, in social comparison terms, attendees who perceive their fellow group members as similar to themselves may be more willing to persist, whilst those who feel they have less in common may decide to quit. Better attendance in the social support group was predicted by less social isolation and a smaller informational social support network. This contrasts with previous research among older adults suggesting a weak social support network is predictive of attrition (e.g. Powell *et al.*, 1990). However, it may be that attending the social support group met the social network needs of participants. Indeed, interviews with participants attending a range of group interventions in the UK revealed that reduced isolation, finding a peer group and sharing with similar others are valued components of the group educational experience.

Chapter Summary

A wide range of psycho-educational interventions has been developed for people with arthritis. Examples of interventions have been presented under the broad headings of cognitive behavioural interventions, multi-component interventions focused primarily on exercise, multi-component self-management interventions, emotional disclosure, personal development, social support interventions, interventions for enhancing employment potential and interventions in JIA.

Cognitive behavioural therapy offers an effective means of changing behaviour and mood, although published studies of interventions have tended to focus on RA, and thus less is known about effectiveness for people with other forms of arthritis. Furthermore, in some countries such as the UK there is a shortage of professionals trained to deliver CBT, so the number of people with arthritis who are able to receive CBT intervention is likely to be relatively low. However, changing behaviour is a key theme of many psycho-educational interventions for people with arthritis, and many interventions draw on the principles of CBT or include a CBT component.

Multi-component interventions focusing on exercise, such as walking in OA or specific stretching exercises in AS, have been shown to be effective in the short term, although few longer-term changes are reported. Such interventions are often sited away from traditional healthcare settings, taking education into the community locations (e.g. a sports centre) and the home environment.

Multi-component self-management interventions typically draw on a range of methods to assist change in behaviour, cognitions, and emotions. One such intervention that is widely used is the Arthritis Self-Management Program that was developed for people at the mild to moderate end of the disease spectrum (Lorig & Gonzalez, 1992) and is delivered by pairs of lay tutors in community settings. The ASMP aims to enhance arthritis self-efficacy, defined as perceived ability to control or manage various aspects of arthritis such as pain, fatigue or depressed mood. Results of randomised, controlled trials suggest the ASMP has some success in meeting these aims, particularly in terms of increasing arthritis self-efficacy, decreasing pain, and reducing depressed mood. Studies conducted in the US tend to report a reduction in use of healthcare resources, whereas UK studies report little or no change in this respect. In addition, some UK studies have included assessment of positive affect and find improvements on this dimension. Qualitative findings suggest that further exploration of positive parameters, such as purpose in life, may be a fruitful area of enquiry. The ASMP is important as it has influenced development of many other psycho-educational interventions, including culturally adapted programmes, and mailed or internet-delivered programmes.

Interventions focused on social support have been developed and tested, although results are somewhat disappointing with few effects for provision of social support as the sole component. Online support groups are on the increase and have the advantage of being accessible 24/7 and not limited by geographical barriers, and they allow participants to remain anonymous until they feel comfortable with the group and its norms.

Interventions based on emotional disclosure are beginning to appear and have an impact on disease activity in RA and physical functioning in AS, at least in the short term. However, recruitment to such interventions can be difficult – this is an issue shared by many psycho-educational interventions.

Given the prevalence of work disability among people with arthritis, interventions designed to enhance employment potential and assist people who wish to remain in employment are needed. A couple of examples of interventions based around the social model of disability, personal development and job-seeking tasks were presented. Interestingly, in accordance with many group intervention studies, the main benefit of course attendance was reported to be the process of sharing with similar others, which participants believed to be instrumental in facilitating personal change (e.g. increased job-seeking self-efficacy, improved satisfaction with life, and decreased mood disturbance). Interventions for children with JIA, parents and siblings were relatively scarce but included behavioural techniques, CBT, videos, computer programs, summer camps and family retreats. Group-based interventions, the video and computer programs are popular and perceived to be of value among children and parents.

In sum, the main benefits of psycho-educational interventions appear to centre on promoting use of health behaviours, enhancing positive mood, fostering confidence in self-management (i.e. self-efficacy) and reducing psychological distress. Systematic reviews have focused mainly on RA although a few have included both RA and OA. Such reviews report statistically significant effects of patient education on disability, joint counts (in RA), pain, psychological status, coping and self-efficacy although the absolute level of effects tends to be small or moderate at best. In this respect, it is important that an element of reality is retained in relation to what is expected from psycho-educational interventions. Taking the widely used ASMP as an example, the intervention takes place over a period of six weeks in sessions of 2.5 hours led by lay tutors. There is no booster session or contact with health professionals. Nonetheless, both short-term (up to 12 months) and longer-term change in participants' attitudes to their condition and related self-management have been reported. During interviews many ASMP participants report that arthritis is no longer the dominant feature in their lives and that they have been reconnected with hope for the future. The typical outcome measures used in effectiveness studies may not tap into these reported changes. Thus future studies may benefit from including a wider range of measures, including positive parameters, and also cost-effectiveness data. Other issues that remain to be clarified include identifying the characteristics of those who benefit most from psycho-educational interventions, the needs of underserved subgroups such as children and younger adults, people from ethnic minority groups, or those with learning disabilities, recruitment, the optimal length or frequency of the intervention and optimal timing of attendance in the context of the individual's arthritis journey.

The relative merits of various types of intervention remain largely unknown since patient education is usually compared to standard care. Indeed, the variety and range of intervention predicates against comparative studies and combining studies in meta-analyses. For example, comparison of the effects of written materials with a cognitive-behavioural intervention using performance of healthcare behaviours as the outcome measure is likely to be loaded in favour of the latter. However, in terms of the number of people who receive the intervention and cost, written materials probably have the advantage. Nonetheless, among healthcare professionals and providers comparisons across different styles of intervention remain of great interest and may be driven by the need to manage scarce resources.

Overall, psycho-educational interventions have an important role to play in the lives of many people with arthritis.

9

Agenda for the Future

I have worked as a researcher since the early 1990s, and thus my perspective has a research bias. In this final chapter, I propose to present my personal view about where psychological research and psychologists could usefully focus their attention in the future based on the issues that have been raised throughout the book – basically, it's a 'research wish list'.

Under-Researched Groups

I chose to cover four main types of arthritis in this book: RA, OA, AS and JIA. One reason for choosing this approach was that research in psychosocial rheumatology has tended to focus on people with RA. Thus, we know a great deal about a very narrow band of the very diverse population with arthritis. One way of illustrating the comparative number of research studies conducted on the various types of arthritis is via a literature search. Using search engines (e.g. BioMed Central Journals, CINAHL, MEDLINE, and PsycINFO), a search conducted for psychological studies published between 2000 and 28 May 2008 revealed that there were 417 records for RA, 336 records for OA, but only 190 records for AS. Searching on 'JIA 'resulted in 344 records; searching on 'children and arthritis' resulted in 233 records, suggesting that research activity in psychosocial domains among children with JIA/arthritis is on the increase.

By including different types of arthritis I hoped to cover a range of perspectives and issues which would not have been possible by focusing on one condition alone. Many types of arthritis are more prevalent among women; both RA and OA fall into this category. Hence the inclusion of research findings from studies of AS, which is one of the few types of arthritis to exhibit a male predominance, enables another perspective to be considered. Furthermore, AS typically affects the spine whereas RA and OA tend to have more impact on hands, feet, hips and knees. Disease management and managing the consequences of any physical impairment may differ according to part of the body affected. By including JIA and OA, I hoped to cover the age span (i.e. from young children to the older elderly). I have found parents of children with JIA to be one of the most distressed groups that I have worked with, and make no apology for devoting space to their perspectives as well as those of children and young people.

In the context of children with JIA, their parents and siblings, there is a need to extend the evidence base for psychosocial wellbeing. Children with JIA appear to be at slightly elevated risk of psychological distress, although the number of those who fall within clinical parameters is relatively small. Paralleling published literature on adults, this finding does contrast with qualitative accounts of life with JIA, where children and young people describe themselves as 'being' and 'feeling' different and withdrawing from physical activities. Encouragingly, a few studies reporting aspects of positive psychological wellbeing are beginning to appear in the literature and point the way for further exploration. Little is known about the psychological wellbeing of siblings or parents of children with JIA. The few studies that have focused on parental functioning suggest an increased risk of psychosocial symptomatology among mothers that is consistent with the wider literature on chronic conditions of childhood (e.g. Eiser, 1993; Singer, 2006). Gaining a more informed understanding of the psychosocial needs of the child with JIA and the impact on their families will help in the development and targeting of interventions that are timely and effective, thus improving the quality of care. Thus, I view parents of children with JIA as comprising an under-researched group deserving more attention.

Other under-researched groups include the children of parents who have arthritis, some of whom take on the role of carer at a relatively early age, the older elderly and people from ethnic minority backgrounds. Regarding the latter, there are moves in the UK to set up a special interest group focusing on the needs of people from ethnic minorities and there are a few exploratory studies commencing in this topic area. For example, Alison Hipwell is currently examining the self-management needs of South Asians living in the Midlands region of the UK as part of her doctoral research at Coventry University.

At the top of my research wish list is the hope that researchers will not only continue to include people with RA but will also consider the situation of people with other types of arthritis, including OA, AS, JIA and some of the less prevalent conditions such as systemic lupus erythematosus, Scleroderma, Sjogren's syndrome, psoriatic arthritis and gout. Although there are a number of commonalities across conditions from a psychological perspective (e.g. vulnerability to depression), there are likely to be challenges associated with the nature of each condition and its resultant impact. Psychologists have a role to play in helping people to meet these challenges and to secure a satisfactory, purposeful quality of life filled with hope.

Under-Researched Psychosocial Domains

My research 'wish list' contains a range of topic areas that I feel require increased attention. Pain already receives a great deal of attention in outpatient settings and is used by patients as a touchstone for determining the degree of severity of their condition (J.H. Barlow, 1998). However, pain management using psychologically based techniques in place of, or in addition to, medication may be worthy of greater exploration and implementation in rheumatology, especially as many patients express concern about the toxic side effects of the drugs used to treat their condition. Equally, fatigue tends to receive less attention than pain in clinical settings but clearly is salient for patients' satisfaction with life and ability to function. The precise mechanism leading to fatigue in arthritis remains to be clarified. It is known that there can be a tendency towards anaemia in some patients, and also the extra effort required to accomplish simple tasks can serve to place further strain on scarce resources (i.e. patients' energy reserves). Thus, after ruling out biological causes of fatigue (e.g. anaemia), instruction in techniques such as pacing and other self-management strategies may help patients to cope better with this symptom in the home environment.

The impact of arthritis on the important social role of parenting has received relatively little attention despite being such a crucial aspect of the life course. Thus parenting is one psychosocial domain that warrants increased attention. I have found that working with an occupational therapist to be of great value in this context, resulting in production of the *Handbook for Parents and Grandparents with Arthritis* (Grant & Barlow, 2008), which is full of tips and ideas for coping according to the age of the child. Referral to occupational therapy does not seem to be high in some conditions and yet this discipline has lots to offer.

Arthritis can interfere with the ability to obtain employment, with maintenance of employment and with long-term plans for retirement – a situation referred to as work disability. However, it is important to note that not all changes in working life or pattern as a consequence of arthritis are negative. Reduced working hours can leave more time to spend on valued activities with partners, family and friends. Despite the fact that some people find that positive features emerge from changes to working life imposed by arthritis, there does appear to be a general lack of assistance available, or it could be that the appropriate source of support or assistance is not clearly signposted. Equally, individuals seeking work or workplace adjustment need to feel confident in their ability to negotiate for their arthritis-related needs. It is important that employers understand the needs of people with arthritis in the work environment, where even relatively simple adjustments can make life much easier for the individual concerned. This point was confirmed in a qualitative study that included the views of eight National Health Service managers who were interviewed about their role in supporting people with long-term conditions (J.H. Barlow & Ellard, 2007). Managers cited the need for a pool of readily available information about long-term conditions, signposts to the appropriate methods of providing support and adequate resources.

Given the established links between stressful events and symptom severity, training in stress-management strategies may be helpful for some people with arthritis. In relation to stress, the indications that traumatic experiences, including sexual abuse, in childhood (Kopec & Sayre, 2004) and sexual assault in adults (Stein & Barrett-Connor, 2000) are worthy of further investigation both in terms of possible mechanisms of action in later development of arthritis and also to identify those in need of appropriate psychological intervention. One other area that can lead to unresolved stress and anger is that of diagnostic delay (i.e. delay between onset of symptoms and diagnosis). This has been reported by people with AS and also some parents of children with JIA. Indeed, internalisation of anger and fear, irrespective of the cause, could manifest as pain, stiffness and restricted movement and would be an indicator of need for psychological intervention and support.

One issue likely to become more salient in the field of arthritis concerns the implications of genetic screening. As more genetic indicators become identified, so will the likelihood that individuals with those genetic markers may be faced with issues connected with telling their children that they are at risk or taking the decision not to have children.

Expand Research on Positive Dimensions

There is a need to understand more about how to promote positive psychological wellbeing as well as to identify what helps to alleviate psychological distress such as depression. The picture painted by qualitative accounts of living with arthritis and the results of quantitative investigation using standard measures is one that is in stark contrast to notions of 'health'. Blaxter (1983) conceptualised health as encompassing fitness (e.g. energy, strength and an efficient body), ability to perform various roles normally, and psychological health (e.g. being unstressed, able to cope, and happy). Life with arthritis is characterised by pain, fatigue, lack of vitality, and adverse bodily changes leading to limited physical functioning and, in some cases, visible deformity. Performance of normal roles, such as parenting, work, housework, gardening and leisure pursuits can be adversely affected. The good news is that the majority of people with arthritis appear able to gradually adapt to their condition and its consequences over time, experiencing a satisfactory quality of life. Indeed, some people positively thrive in the face of apparent adversity despite the loss of valued activities. However, some appear to struggle at various points in the disease course and a minority continue to experience persistent psychological distress described qualitatively in terms of anger, frustration, uncertainty, depression, anxiety about the future, isolation and loss of control. Findings about the nature of the distress experienced are consistent regardless of type of arthritis, gender and age. Given this scenario, people who manage to live happily with their condition are to be applauded on their substantial achievement. Researchers and health professionals can learn much from such experts, and could better utilise this knowledge to assist those who find life with arthritis to be a continual struggle. For example, there are indications that a minority of people with RA become psychologically distressed early in the disease course and that raised levels of anxiety and depression remain fairly stable throughout their arthritis journey. We need to know whether this finding generalises to people with other types of arthritis and to find ways to identify those at increased risk in order to target treatment effectively. More extensive research aimed at enhancing our understanding about how people with various types of arthritis achieve adaptation is called for and would serve as a useful guide for developing interventions.

Although there is little evidence of an association between personality traits and arthritis, there are indications that traits such as optimism may be linked to more positive psychosocial adjustment. This suggests that exploration of the coping strategies used by individuals with arthritis who are highly optimistic may offer valuable insight. In addition, people who are pessimistic may need assistance in adapting to their condition through training in greater use of positive strategies such as benefit-finding or the three blessings exercise (Emmons & McCullough, 2003). Being able to express emotions such as anger may assist wellbeing, although finding 'safe' ways to express powerful emotions can be difficult. Increased use of emotional disclosure as an intervention in its own right or as a component in an intervention may assist in this regard.

Evaluation of psycho-educational interventions has tended to focus on a core set of outcomes revolving around health status, health behaviours and healthcare utilisation. However, there is increasing evidence that the impact of such interventions resides in the psychosocial domain. When psychological measures are included in intervention studies there is a tendency to focus on psychological pathology, particularly depression. Whilst understanding that the impact of the psycho-educational interventions on depression is important, it is not the whole story. Qualitative studies of lay-led, arthritis self-management interventions have revealed that participants report a much wider range of positive outcomes, including renewed hope and a sense of purpose (J.H. Barlow, Williams & Wright, 1999; Turner *et al.*, 2002). Furthermore, interviews with lay tutors have revealed additional benefits, such as feeling a useful member of society, altruism and increased self-worth (Hainsworth & Barlow, 2003). How such outcomes are related to health status in the short and longer term and also the potential impact on future healthcare utilisation remain to be investigated. In addition, some tutors begin to transfer their newly acquired skills to other areas such as advocacy groups or other community support networks. Such social outcomes have received little research attention.

Health Care and Interventions

We have seen in previous chapters that there are few studies of inpatient care from either patient or provider perspectives, and few studies of the experience of care provision in primary care. However, there are examples of innovative studies that include a range of perspectives, such as the investigation of quality of life among parents compared with paediatricians by Janse *et al.* (2005). Inclusion of a range of perspectives is welcomed as a means to understand where 'mis'understandings occur and where clarity and further support are needed.

The impact of the rapid growth of e-Health technologies needs to be carefully examined in order to ensure that the quality of provision does not suffer at the expense of technological advances. Developments, such as remote monitoring by handheld devices that enable ratings of pain, for example, to be uploaded and sent to a remote monitor, need testing among people with arthritis. Internet provision of written information has the advantage of being available 24/7, although the quality of internet sites is not always assured since at present there are few controls over the quality and reliability of internet-based arthritis information.

There are indications that depression among people with RA is unrecognised and under-treated (Dickens & Creed, 2001). Whilst this may be understandable give the overlap of symptoms of arthritis and depression, ways to help people with arthritis receive interventions for depression are clearly needed. In the UK, the National Institute for Clinical Excellence (NICE) guidelines for treating the most common episodes of mental health problems (e.g. mild anxiety and depression) recommend that patients should not be prescribed medication 'because the risk-benefit ratio is poor'. Rather, psychological therapies (e.g. self-help/self-management, cognitive behavioural therapy) with an established evidence base should be the first treatment option. However, few patients are routinely offered these therapies due to a shortage of trained therapists. Effective psycho-educational interventions have an important role to play in this regard. A stepped approach could be used, whereby people with arthritis presenting with mild depression could be referred to a lay-led self-management course or recommended to try an internet- or manual-based intervention. If no improvement occurs, then referral options could be reconsidered.

Lifestyle issues, such as exercise, following a healthy diet and improved management of daily stress, are areas where psychologists could have useful input. Among people with arthritis commencing and maintaining exercise can be hindered by levels of pain and fatigue, which are both commonly experienced symptoms. Some intriguing findings are emerging, such as the failure of people with OA to experience a post-exercise improvement in mood, and these warrant further investigation.

Given that a relatively large proportion of people with arthritis use complementary or alternative medicine at some point during their disease journey, further systematic evaluation of CAM therapies that may help to provide relaxation (e.g. meditation, yoga), and stress reduction would be a useful avenue of investigation in psychosocial rheumatology. For example, the effects of mindfulness-based meditation and a four-month programme of continued reinforcement as a means of reducing stress among people with RA (Pradhan *et al.*, 2007) found significant reduction of psychological distress and improvements in well-being.

Patient education has become an integral aspect of disease management for people with arthritis, and is an area where psychologists can have a useful input. Educational strategies may be most effective if tailored to match the needs of the target population, although the optimal time for presenting patients with disease-related information (i.e. at diagnosis, after several years, or at repeated intervals throughout the disease course) has yet to be identified. It is important that people with arthritis are provided with updates of the latest developments and therapeutic strategies. Thus, education at one point in time (e.g. at diagnosis) is not sufficient.

Whilst it is important that we continue to amass a robust evidence base regarding the effectiveness of psycho-educational interventions through high-quality randomised controlled trials, it is equally important that we establish how many interventions delivered as part of a research study actually make it through to implementation as a service. This point echoes Nicassio's (2008) concern that research findings on depression 'may not be penetrating clinical practice'. Equally, we need to understand more about the impact of such interventions when they move away from rigidly controlled research settings to implementation. Randomised controlled trials with strict inclusion and exclusion criteria yield homogeneous research samples but may not represent the wide range of potential participants when the intervention is delivered in a real-life setting as a service. In this respect, implementation studies can be extremely useful but are rarely conducted. Indeed, widespread adoption of evidence-based, health-related education interventions can be problematic and can result in poor implementation, with interventions failing to reach their target populations (King *et al.*, 1998; Prochaska *et al.*, 2000). Adoption can be enhanced if interventions are shown to be feasible and effective in real life in a range of locations (De Jong *et al.*, 2004). Implementation studies are more flexible than randomised, controlled trials, where adjustment of recruitment procedures or intervention delivery violates a trial protocol thus rendering data unusable. In an implementation study, the intervention can be adjusted to match available resources and circumstances. Furthermore, implementation studies can be used to examine who chooses to enrol on an intervention and why, who benefits most and who benefits least, and to examine what factors predict positive health change. One example of the last of these in the field of psychosocial rheumatology is a study by R.H. Osborne *et al.* (2007) based on 452 participants of the ASMP delivered in Australia. Assessments were conducted at six months and two years post-course attendance. Approximately half the sample had a positive change on self-efficacy, and this predicted improvement in health status.

Implementation studies rarely have a control or comparison group and acknowledge that participants cannot be blinded to the intervention. This is particularly relevant when studying psycho-educational interventions, which require participants to be actively involved in terms of time, effort, commitment and motivation. However, it is worth noting that these inherent participant 'costs' of intervention attendance rarely feature in cost-effectiveness analysis. On that note, inclusion of cost-effectiveness data is relatively rare but is an issue that is becoming more pertinent given increasingly scarce resources.

The most widely examined mechanism of action for psycho-educational interventions in rheumatology is that of self-efficacy. Whilst the value of self-efficacy is largely supported, it is unlikely to be the sole mediator of change following intervention. Interview-based studies shed some light on this issue, suggesting that disclosure of emotions in a safe environment to others similar to oneself may be one means through which change in psychosocial wellbeing occurs (Turner *et al.*, 2002). One other mechanism of action may be linked to the enhanced level of social support inherent in group interventions. Many participants feel that they have benefited from being with similar others and sharing common experiences to such an extent that they plan to maintain contact with fellow participants after the intervention.

Finally, there is a need to be realistic about the changes that can result from attending psycho-educational interventions. For example, the ASMP is a lay-led, group-based intervention delivered in the community by pairs of lay tutors in six, weekly sessions (i.e. approximately 15 hours in total) with no follow-up or booster sessions. As noted by Osborne *et al.* (2007), absolute changes in health status tend to be small. However, low-cost, community-based interventions have the potential to reach a wide audience and thus could have 'substantial public health impact'. Moreover, interventions such as the ASMP are open to anyone with arthritis and therefore can be accessed by people with milder disease who may not have the opportunity to attend hospital-based educational interventions. Implementation or transition studies have an important role to play in furthering knowledge about the impact of the ASMP and similar programmes. One important point to note, though, is that the Arthritis Foundation in the US reports that the ASMP has reached less than 1 per cent of the US population with arthritis (Arthritis Foundation, 1999). Recruitment to studies and similar courses in the UK has been similarly low, and it is hard to achieve targets for studies. Other issues that remain to be examined include methods for enabling health professionals to better support patients who embark on the self-management journey, ways to encourage greater participation, including those referred to as 'hard to reach' (e.g. young adults, males) and how greater attendance at ASMP sessions can be encouraged in order to maximise outcomes.

The topic of prevention deserves a mention as an important public health issue. Nothing can be done about certain risk factors for OA such as age, female gender or genetic predisposition. However, prevention of other risk factors such as obesity, repetitive use and excessive mechanical loading of joints, along with maintaining physical fitness, could help to prevent onset of OA and may assist in the management of the condition after onset. Greater input from weight-management specialists, occupational therapists and sports therapists working alongside psychologists trained in promotion of physical activity would be helpful.

Longitudinal Studies

Longitudinal studies documenting the pattern of change on psychological dimensions through the life course are sorely needed. This is much more difficult to do when samples are recruited through the community compared to samples recruited via outpatient clinics. Few randomised, controlled trials have a follow-up period longer than 12 months, hence little is known about the longer-term impact of attending psycho-educational interventions, or even about the pattern of change (or not) on psychological variables. For example, it is quite likely that people with arthritis who feel confident that they can deal with the anxious and depressed moods that can occur as a consequence of arthritis may be less likely to require prescription medication for these conditions. Thus, in the longer term there may be cost savings on medication.

Chapter Summary

My research wish list covers the following:

- Expand the research remit to include a wider range of types of arthritis and under-researched groups, including children with JIA, their parents and siblings, children of parents with arthritis, the older elderly and ethnic minorities.
- Increase research on a number of psychosocial domains, including parenting, work disability, the effects of traumatic experience and sexual abuse in children and adults, diagnostic delay and genetic screening.
- Expand research on positive dimensions and interventions.
- Increase research attention on the healthcare experience from a range of perspectives (both provider and patient), and for inpatients and primary care patients. In addition, further attention is needed regarding e-Health developments to make sure they are of high quality and meet the needs of the target population. Lifestyle interventions, psycho-educational interventions and interventions targeting depression are needed, along with implementation studies of how interventions work in service mode.
- Longitudinal studies documenting the pattern of psychological wellbeing from diagnosis onwards are sorely needed, as well as longer-term follow-ups of intervention studies.

Appendix

Malcolm Macdonald's Arthritis Journey

Adapted from an interview conducted by Dr A. Turner

The following case study has been selected to provide insight into one man's arthritis journey from development of symptoms, to attaining a diagnosis, through to current self-management. Malcolm's story is based on an interview and the words used in the narrative are those used by Malcolm to describe his life with OA. Direct quotes appear in quotation marks.

Malcolm was aged 51 years at the time of the interview. He was divorced and an ex-professional footballer who represented England during his playing career. He was known as 'Supermac, the scoring ace of the seventies'. He now works as a football commentator and lives in the north of England. Both of Malcolm's knees are affected by OA, and he has had one knee replaced. In addition, Malcolm has another long-term health condition, asthma.

Diagnosis, Disease Course and Treatment

Malcolm does not recall being given a diagnosis until several years after the onset of symptoms. He felt that doctors were reluctant to discuss his knee problems. He remembers talking about the pain and discomfort in his knees with doctors but felt that 'they only talk about the weather' and would not discuss his condition. He was relieved when finally 'doctors had the courage to tell me something I'd known all along': his GP told him that he had OA.

His surgeon first used the word 'trauma' in 1977 during an explanation of the effects that trauma can have on a joint. Malcolm recalls being told that the body can accept and recover from one trauma; it may even get away with two traumas, but in Malcolm's case a third trauma was too much and resulted in more lasting damage. Malcolm well remembers the day he saw the surgeon who did a great deal of work for the Football Association. The surgeon took one look at Malcolm's X-rays and said that an operation was called for immediately. Malcolm felt that, at last, someone accepted his condition and did not accuse him of 'being a baby'.

Eventually, he had his left cartilage removed. Since this time he has not been able to straighten his leg. A further operation was followed by an arthrogram, which showed a 'little speck of damage that sort of concertinaed its way throughout the joint'. Malcolm believes that the rubbing of bone on bone in the knee joint, led to the bones 'flaking away'. Malcolm was still playing professional football at this time. He had a further operation to remove the 'growth'. Malcolm reports that the surgeon 'left the attachment' in his knee in the belief that it would encourage new cartilage to grow. The reality was that a pencil-like piece of gristle grew in an uncontrolled way. Malcolm believes that this was not put in his medical records. After this operation, Malcolm managed to play one game but felt 'it was no good': he could not cope with demands of playing professional football and was forced to retire.

The pain and discomfort became so bad at one stage that painkillers had no effect, Malcolm felt that doctors would not discuss his condition and would not prescribe any different medication to help him to cope. At this time, Malcolm began to resort to drinking scotch 'as the one thing that would guarantee him a night's sleep'. By now, Malcolm was no longer part of a football team and was receiving health care via a GP. He found this to be a totally different experience compared with the approach adopted by the medical teams working with football clubs. He feels that the aim of football medical teams was to get players 'fit for Saturday' regardless of any long-term consequences and regardless of the cost of medication. When he became part of 'Joe Public', Malcolm believed the approach to his condition became very different and he reiterated that doctors did not want to discuss his condition with him or to prescribe 'expensive' medication. He felt he had to find ' his own way to survive, to get through the ordinary day'.

Malcolm spent eight years getting about one hour of sleep per night, but he feels that the problem is much deeper, and is not just about getting a good night's sleep. He feels strongly that arthritis affects 'you mentally.

Your eyes sting because all you really want to do is sleep', but you become a television addict just to while away the long hours of the night.

He had a knee replacement three to four years ago. Malcolm is currently not on any prescribed medication because 'nobody will give me anything'. He is trying herbal supplements to see if these improve his condition.

Attributed Cause

Malcolm attributes OA to playing football with injuries and to being a sprinter, which meant that his joints received an 'absolute pounding'. Unlike many other players, Malcolm refused cortisone injections whilst playing because he knew that being able to get back on the field of play quicker may 'not be the long-term answer'. However, he recalls observing other players disappear five minutes before football games started and again at half time, and presumes these players were given injections to help keep them playing.

Malcolm feels that his body shape did not help his risk of injury or recovery. He claims to be hollow-backed, narrow-waisted (compared with his chest and hips), and also to be bow-legged. He feels these factors placed 'a different kind of stress' on his knees and ankles. In addition he was a sprinter, a skill that Malcolm believes places even more stress on joints from the hip downwards. He likens his body to a machine that 'sooner or later' will give out 'under that constant pounding'.

Getting on with Life

After retiring from professional football, Malcolm has worked as a sports commentator. This has proven to be difficult because of the physical effects of OA. Press boxes in football grounds tend to be down lots of stairs and are very confined in terms of space. Both of these facts cause problems for Malcolm. Even when he can get down to the press box, he sometimes is not able to sit comfortably and spends the whole time commentating through gritted teeth whilst trying to bear the pain.

When Malcolm meets up with 'old playing colleagues', they discuss 'how to cope with life'. Thus, Malcolm knows that he is not alone in suffering from arthritis-related injuries sustained whilst playing professional football. For example, one old playing colleague (in his early fifties) has not been able to work for the past 10 years because of OA in his back. This man's children have now left home but he is still struggling financially and is not able to just enjoy his 'later years'.

Although Malcolm and his colleagues succeed in attending reunions and other events, there is a lack of spontaneity about their lives in that all activities must be planned for and may have an adverse effect on their wellbeing. If Malcolm plans to attend an event, he has to leave the four days before the event clear so that he can prepare himself physically.

Malcolm uses a 'mind over matter 'approach in trying to cope with his symptoms, detaching from his body, away from the part with the problem. He believes this approach works to some degree, but when 'you find yourself doing this all of the time, 24 hours a day, that is when you need help and there is likely to be breakdown'. Malcolm can now only sleep on his front with his foot (same side as knee replacement) over the edge of the bed. He feels that his right knee is like ' a 36 hour warning of bad weather'.

Malcolm's main fears regarding his OA are that the functional limitations and pain will worsen and he will not be able to walk to his car or drive it, and thus his freedom would be severely curtailed. Regarding the latter, Malcolm feels that this would impact on the 'normal, social things of a family'. He finds lack of mobility to be very frightening and attributes his second divorce to this. He feels that arthritis becomes the focal point of one's life, 'the centre of your universe', and that it is very difficult for partners and family to understand, especially where the condition is not visible:

> It becomes very difficult for other people to live according to it [arthritis]. They can't see it, they can't feel it, and it's completely intangible. You can have all the plans in the world but if you wake up one morning and one of your legs just doesn't want to work … everything has to be changed.

The only 'visible' sign of OA that Malcolm mentions is the creak his knee gives when he moves, and yet if he has difficulty walking this must be obvious to those around him. He attributes the 'creak' to a piece of bone that is floating' in his knee joint. Malcolm has linked the 'creak' to being able to move easily the following day; thus when he does not hear it, he expects moving to be difficult.

Malcolm feels that the general public is 'naive' about arthritis and its effects. He has difficulty keeping up with friends and acquaintances, even if the activity is simply standing in a bar. He no longer offers an explanation as to why he cannot join in such activities. Instead, he prefers to spend time at home where he can 'do funny movements' if needed. In addition, he can sit with his feet up and find a comfortable position without causing disruption to other people. He admits that arthritis has caused him to become somewhat of a 'recluse'.

Despite the obvious costs of being injured whilst playing professional football, Malcolm would not change any of his life.

> In spite of the pain, I got to the top in football, I had the most wonderful few years. It still brings me work to this day. If I had been warned as a 14 or 16 year old kid – this is going to be your future after football, I would have still done it.

He believes that 'the warning' should go to those 'in control of players, to have respect for their future'. He cites medical teams, coaches, managers and boards of directors as those whose duty it is to become as 'informed as possible medically' and then to inform the players.

> When you're in your peak fitness in your 20s, you think you're going to be like that forever. But middle age, it seems a million miles away. You feel as if you can carry 2 or 3 injuries, get away with it, but it takes its toll.

Commentary

Malcolm's story illustrates the risks faced by professional footballers, for whom performance 'on the day' is the overriding goal. He appears to have had a confusing time in terms of contact with the medical profession in the early years following disease onset. He felt that his reports of pain and discomfort were not taken seriously to begin with. It is acknowledged that Malcolm experienced problems in other areas of his life (e.g. business) after retiring from professional football. Nonetheless, the pain and discomfort that he suffered were very real and led to dependence on alcohol as a means of coping. Malcolm recognises that the effects of OA are not limited to the physical body but can adversely influence psychological wellbeing, social relationships, working life and leisure pursuits. Interestingly, and despite a lack of formal psycho-educational intervention, Malcolm uses distraction as part of his self-management repertoire. Also evident in Malcolm's story are the lack of spontaneity, the need to plan for events and activities and the determination to resist disruption to one's life, even at the cost of increased discomfort and pain. The unique aspect of Malcolm's story is that he does not regret his playing career despite attributing playing whilst injured as a contributory factor in the development of OA. This situation accords with the results of studies by Turner *et al.* (2000, 2002) referred to in Chapter 2.

References

Abbott, C.A., Helliwell, P.S. & Chamberlain, M.A. (1994). Functional assessment in ankylosing spondylitis: Evaluation of a new self-administered questionnaire and correlation with anthropometric variables. *British Journal of Rheumatology*, 33(11), 1060–1066.

Abdel-Nasser, A.M., Abd El-Azim, S., Taal, E., El-Badawy, S.A., Rasker, J.J. & Valkenburg, H.A. (1998). Depression and depressive symptoms in rheumatoid arthritis patients: An analysis of their occurrence and determinants. *British Journal of Rheumatology*, 37(4), 391–397.

Achenbach, T.M. & Edelbrock, C.S. (1983). *Manual for the child behavior checklist and revised profile*. Burlington: University of Vermont.

Adab, P., Rankin, E.C., Witney, A.G., Miles, K.A., Bowman, S., Kitas, G.D. et al. (2004). Use of a corporate needs assessment to define the information requirements of an arthritis resource centre in Birmingham: Comparison of patients' and professionals' views. *Rheumatology (Oxford)*, 43(12), 1513–1518.

Adam, V., St-Pierre, Y., Fautrel, B., Clarke, A.E., Duffy, C.M. & Penrod, J.R. (2005). What is the impact of adolescent arthritis and rheumatism? Evidence from a national sample of Canadians. *Journal of Rheumatology*, 32(2), 354–361.

Affleck, G. & Tennen, H. (1991). Social comparison and coping with major medical problems. In J. Suls & T.A. Wills (Eds.) *Social comparison: Contemporary theory and research*. Hillsdale, NJ: Erlbaum.

Affleck, G., Tennen, H. & Apter, A. (2001). Optimism, pessimism and daily life with chronic illness. In E.C. Chang (Ed.) *Optimism and pessimism: Implications for theory research and practice*, (pp.145–168). Washington, DC: American Psychological Association.

Affleck, G., Tennen, H., Pfeiffer, C. & Fifield, J. (1987). Appraisals of control and predictability in adapting to a chronic disease. *Journal of Personality and Social Psychology*, 53(2), 273–279.

Affleck, G., Tennen, H., Pfeiffer, C. & Fifield, J. (1998). Social support and psycho-social adjustment to rheumatoid arthritis. *Arthritis Care and Research*, 1, 71–77.

Affleck, G., Tennen, H., Urrows, S. & Higgins, P. (1994). Person and contextual features of daily stress reactivity: Individual differences in relations of undesirable daily events with mood disturbance and chronic pain intensity. *Journal of Personality and Social Psychology, 66*(2), 329–340.

Affleck, G., Urrows, S., Tennen, H. & Higgins, P. (1992). Daily coping with pain from rheumatoid arthritis: Patterns and correlates. *Pain, 51*(2), 221–229.

Akikusa, J.D. & Allen, R.C. (2002). Reducing the impact of rheumatic diseases in childhood. *Best Practice & Research Clinical Rheumatology, 16*(3), 333–345.

Al-Allaf, A.W., Sanders, P.A., Ogston, S.A. & Marks, J.S. (2001). A case-control study examining the role of physical trauma in the onset of rheumatoid arthritis. *Rheumatology (Oxford), 40*(3), 262–266.

Albers, J.M., Kuper, H.H., van Riel, P.L., Prevoo, M.L., van 't Hof, M.A., van Gestel, A.M. *et al.* (1999). Socio-economic consequences of rheumatoid arthritis in the first years of the disease. *Rheumatology (Oxford), 38*(5), 423–430.

Allaire, S., Wolfe, F., Niu, J., Lavalley, M. & Michaud, K. (2005). Work disability and its economic effect on 55–64-year-old adults with rheumatoid arthritis. *Arthritis & Rheumatism, 53*(4), 603–608.

Allaire, S.H. (1996). Work disability. In S.T. Wegener, B.A. Belza & E.P. Gall (Eds.) *Clinical care in the rheumatic diseases.* Atlanta, GA: ACR.

Allegrante, J.P., Kovar, P.A., MacKenzie, C.R., Peterson, M.G. & Gutin, B. (1993). A walking education program for patients with osteoarthritis of the knee: Theory and intervention strategies. *Health Education Quarterly, 20*(1), 63–81.

Anderson, K.O., Bradley, L.A., Young, L.D., McDaniel, L.K. & Wise, C.M. (1985). Rheumatoid arthritis: Review of psychological factors related to etiology, effects, and treatment. *Psychological Bulletin, 98*(2), 358–387.

Andersson, S., Nilsson, B., Hessel, T., Saraste, M., Noren, A., Stevens-Andersson, A. *et al.* (1989). Degenerative joint disease in ballet dancers. *Clinical Orthopaedics and Related Research, 238,* 233–236.

Ang, D.C., Choi, H., Kroenke, K. & Wolfe, F. (2005). Comorbid depression is an independent risk factor for mortality in patients with rheumatoid arthritis. *Journal of Rheumatology, 32*(6), 1013–1019.

Ansani, N.T., Fedutes-Henderson, B., Weber, R., Smith, R., Dean, J., Vogt, M. *et al.* (2006). The Drug Information Center Arthritis Project: Providing patients with interactive and reliable arthritis internet education. *Drug Information Journal, 40*(1), 39–49.

Ansani, N.T., Vogt, M., Henderson, B.A., McKaveney, T.P., Weber, R.J., Smith, R.B. *et al.* (2005). Quality of arthritis information on the internet. *American Journal of Health System Pharmacy, 62*(11), 1184–1189.

Applebaum, K.A., Blanchar, E.B., Hickling, E.J. & Alfonso, M. (1988). Cognitive behavioral treatment of a veteran population with moderate to severe rheumatoid arthritis. *Behavior Therapy, 19,* 489–502.

April, K.T., Feldman, D.E., Platt, R.W. & Duffy, C.M. (2006). Comparison between children with Juvenile Idiopathic Arthritis (JIA) and their parents concerning perceived quality of life. *Quality of Life Research, 15*(4), 655–661.

Arnett, F.C. (1989). A new look at ankylosing spondylitis. *Patient Care, 23*(19), 82–101.

Arthritis Foundation, A.o.S.a.T.H.O., Centers for Disease Control and Prevention. (1999). *National arthritis action plan: A public health strategy.* Atlanta, GA.

Astin, J.A., Beckner, W., Soeken, K., Hochberg, M.C. & Berman, B. (2002). Psychological interventions for rheumatoid arthritis: A meta-analysis of randomized controlled trials. *Arthritis & Rheumatism, 47*(3), 291–302.

Backman, C.L., Kennedy, S.M., Chalmers, A. & Singer, J. (2004). Participation in paid and unpaid work by adults with rheumatoid arthritis. *Journal of Rheumatology, 31*(1), 47–56.

Badley, E.M. & Tennant, A. (1993). Disablement associated with rheumatic disorders in a British population: Problems with activities of daily living and level of support. *British Journal of Rheumatology, 32*(7), 601–608.

Badley, E.M. & Wood, P.H. (1979). Attitudes of the public to arthritis. *Annals of the Rheumatic Diseases, 38*(2), 97–100.

Bandura, A. (1977). Self-efficacy: Toward a unifying theory of behavioral change. *Psychology Review, 84*(2), 191–215.

Bandura, A. (1982). Self-efficacy mechanism in human agency. *American Psychologist, 37*(2), 122–147.

Bandura, A. (1997). *Self-efficacy: The exercise of control.* New York: W.H. Freeman.

Barlow, J. (1997). Living with arthritis: Pain management in the homecare setting. *Home Healthcare Consultant, 4,* 23–40.

Barlow, J. (1998a). Arthritis. In A. S. Bellack & M. Hersen (Eds.) *Comprehensive clinical psychology* (pp. 427–443). Oxford: Pergamon.

Barlow, J. (1998b). Setting a research agenda for psychosocial rheumatology. *Journal of Psychosomatic Research, 44*(6), 619–623.

Barlow, J., Cullen, L.A., Davis, S. & Williams, R.B. (1997). The power of sharing common experiences: The 'hidden' benefit of group education for people with arthritis. *British Journal of Therapy and Rehabilitation, 4*(1), 38–41.

Barlow, J., Cullen, L.A. & Rowe, I.F. (2001). Educational preferences, psychological wellbeing and self-efficacy among people with rheumatoid arthritis. *Patient Education and Counseling, 46*(1), 11–19.

Barlow, J. & Hainsworth, J. (2001). Volunteerism among older people with arthritis. *Ageing and Society, 21,* 203–217.

Barlow, J. & Harrison, K. (1996). Focusing on empowerment: Facilitating self-help in young people with arthritis through a disability organisation. *Disability & Society, 11*(4), 539–551.

Barlow, J., Harrison, K. & Shaw, K. (1998). The experience of parenting in juvenile chronic arthritis. *Clinical Child Psychology and Psychiatry, 3*(3), 445–463.

Barlow, J. & Lorig, K. (2003). Patient education, In M. Doherty *et al.* (Eds.) *Osteoarthritis* (pp. 321–326). Oxford: Oxford University Press.

Barlow, J., Macey, S.J., Pugh, M. & Struthers, G. (1994). Perceptions of control in rheumatoid arthritis. *British Journal of Rheumatology, 33*(S2), 23.

Barlow, J., Macey, S.J. & Struthers, G. (1993). Control-related cognitions, chronic disease and gender, In H. Schroeder, K. Reshke, M. Johnston & S. Maes (Eds.) *Health psychology: Potential in diversity* (pp.272–278). Regensburg: Roderer.

Barlow, J. & Pennington, D.C. (1996). *Evaluation of patient education materials.* Arthritis and Rheumatism Council for Research, Scientific Reports 1995. Chesterfield, UK.

Barlow, J., Pennington, D.C. & Bishop, P.E. (1997). Patient education leaflets for people with rheumatoid arthritis: A controlled study. *Psychology, Health & Medicine, 2*(3), 221–235.

Barlow, J., Shaw, K.L. & Southwood, T.R. (1998). Do psychosocial interventions have a role to play in paediatric rheumatology? *British Journal of Rheumatology, 37*(5), 573–578.

Barlow, J., Turner, A. & Wright, C. (1998a). A longer term follow up of an arthritis self-management programme. *British Journal of Rheumatology, 37*(12), 1315–1319.

Barlow, J., Turner, A. & Wright, C. (1998b). Sharing, caring and learning to take control: Self-management training for people with arthritis. *Psychology, Health & Medicine, 3*(4), 387–393.

Barlow, J. & Williams, B. (1999). 'I now feel that I'm not just a bit of left luggage': The experiences of older women with arthritis attending a personal independence course. *Disability & Society, 14*(1), 53–64.

Barlow, J., Williams, R.B. & Wright, C. (1997a). Improving arthritis self-management among older adults: 'Just what the doctor didn't order'. *British Journal of Health Psychology, 2,* 175–186.

Barlow, J., Williams, R.B. & Wright, C. (1997b). The Arthritis Self-Efficacy Scale in a UK context. *Psychology, Health & Medicine, 2*(1), 5–19.

Barlow, J., Wright, C., Carr, A., Hughes, R., Sheasby, J.E. & Stowers, K. (2001). *Final report: Incorporating patients' priorities and objectives in the management of chronic disease.* Submitted to the Department of Health Physical & Complex Disabilities Programme.

Barlow, J., Wright, C. & Krol, T. (2001). Overcoming perceived barriers to employment among people with arthritis. *Journal of Health Psychology, 6*(2), 205–216.

Barlow, J., Wright, C., Shaw, K., Luqmani, R. & Wyness, I.J. (2002). Maternal stressors, maternal wellbeing and children's wellbeing in the context of juvenile idiopathic arthritis. *Early Child Development and Care, 172*(1), 89–98.

Barlow, J., Wright, S. & Wright, C. (2000). *Evaluation of working horizons: Final report*. London: Arthritis Care.

Barlow, J.H. (1998). Understanding exercise in the context of chronic disease: An exploratory investigation of self-efficacy. *Perceptual and Motor Skills, 87*(2), 439–446.

Barlow, J.H. (2001). How to use education as an intervention in osteoarthritis. In M. Docherty & M. Dougados (Eds.) *Osteoarthritis: Balliere's best practice and research*. London: Harcourt (*Clinical Rheumatology, 15*(4), 545–558).

Barlow, J.H. & Barefoot, J. (1996). Group education for people with arthritis. *Patient Education & Counseling, 27*(3), 257–267.

Barlow, J.H., Bishop, P.E. & Pennington, D.C. (1996). How are printed patient educational materials used in out-patient clinics? Insight from rheumatology. *Health Education, 55*, 275–284.

Barlow, J.H. & Cullen L. (1996). Parenting and ankylosing spondylitis: 'I can't see where my baby is feeding'. *Disability, Pregnancy and Parenthood International, 16*, 4–5.

Barlow, J.H., Cullen, L.A., Foster, N.E., Harrison, K. & Wade, M. (1999). Does arthritis influence perceived ability to fulfill a parenting role? Perceptions of mothers, fathers and grandparents. *Patient Education & Counseling, 37*(2), 141–151.

Barlow, J.H., Cullen, L.A. & Rowe, I.F. (1999). Comparison of knowledge and psychological well-being between patients with a short disease duration (< or = 1 year) and patients with more established rheumatoid arthritis (> or = 10 years duration). *Patient Education & Counseling, 38*(3), 195–203.

Barlow, J.H. & Ellard, D.R. (2006). The psychosocial well-being of children with chronic disease, their parents and siblings: An overview of the research evidence base. *Child Care Health Development, 32*(1), 19–31.

Barlow J.H. & Ellard D.R. (2007) Implementation of a self-management programme for people with long-term medical conditions in a workplace setting. *Journal of Applied Rehabilitation Counselling, 38*(2), 24–34.

Barlow, J.H., Macey, S.J. & Struthers, G. (1992). Psychosocial factors and self-help in ankylosing spondylitis patients. *Clinical Rheumatology, 11*(2), 220–225.

Barlow, J.H., Macey, S.J. & Struthers, G.R. (1993a). Gender, depression, and ankylosing spondylitis. *Arthritis Care and Research, 6*(1), 45–51.

Barlow, J.H., Macey, S.J. & Struthers, G.R. (1993b). Health locus of control, self-help and treatment adherence in relation to ankylosing spondylitis patients. *Patient Education & Counseling, 20*(2/3), 153–166.

Barlow, J.H., Shaw, K.L. & Harrison, K.(1999). Consulting the 'experts': Children's and parents' perceptions of psycho-educational interventions in the context of juvenile chronic arthritis. *Health Education Research, 14*(5), 597–610.

Barlow, J.H., Shaw, K.L. & Wright, C.C. (2000). Development and preliminary validation of a self-efficacy measure for use among parents of children with juvenile idiopathic arthritis. *Arthritis Care and Research, 13*(4), 227–236.

Barlow, J.H., Shaw, K.L. & Wright, C.C. (2001). Development and preliminary validation of a children's arthritis self-efficacy scale. *Arthritis & Rheumatism, 45*(2), 159–166.

Barlow, J.H., Turner, A.P. & Wright, C.C. (1998). Comparison of clinical and self-reported diagnoses for participants on a community-based arthritis self-management programme. *British Journal of Rheumatology, 37*(9), 985–987.

Barlow, J.H., Turner, A.P. & Wright, C.C. (2000). A randomized controlled study of the Arthritis Self-Management Programme in the UK. *Health Education Research, 15*(6), 665–680.

Barlow, J.H., Williams, B. & Wright, C. (1996). The Generalized Self-Efficacy Scale in people with arthritis. *Arthritis Care and Research, 9*(3), 189–196.

Barlow, J.H., Williams, B. & Wright, C.C. (1999). 'Instilling the strength to fight the pain and get on with life': Learning to become an arthritis self-manager through an adult education programme. *Health Education Research, 14*(4), 533–544.

Barlow, J.H., Williams, B. & Wright, C.C. (2001). Patient education for people with arthritis in rural communities: The UK experience. *Patient Education & Counseling, 44*(3), 205–214.

Barlow, J.H. & Wright, C.C. (1998a). Dimensions of the Center of Epidemiological Studies-Depression Scale for people with arthritis from the UK. *Psychological Reports, 83*(3/1), 915–919.

Barlow, J.H. & Wright, C.C. (1998b). Knowledge in patients with rheumatoid arthritis: A longer term follow-up of a randomized controlled study of patient education leaflets. *British Journal of Rheumatology, 37*(4), 373–376.

Barlow, J.H., Wright, C.C. & Lorig, K. (2001). The perils and pitfalls of comparing UK and US samples of people enrolled in an arthritis self-management program: The case of the Center for Epidemiological Studies-Depression (CES-D) Scale. *Arthritis & Rheumatism, 45*(1), 77–80.

Barlow, J.H., Wright, C.C., Williams, B. & Keat, A. (2001). Work disability among people with ankylosing spondylitis. *Arthritis & Rheumatism, 45*(5), 424–429.

Baron, R.M. & Kenny, D.A. (1986). The moderator-mediator variable distinction in social psychological research: Conceptual, strategic, and statistical considerations. *Journal of Personality and Social Psychology, 51*(6), 1173–1182.

Barrett, E.M., Scott, D.G., Wiles, N.J. & Symmons, D.P. (2000). The impact of rheumatoid arthritis on employment status in the early years of disease: A UK community-based study. *Rheumatology (Oxford), 39*(12), 1403–1409.

Basler, H.D. (1993). Group treatment for pain and discomfort. *Patient Education & Counseling, 20*(2–3), 167–175.

Beales, J.G., Holt, P.J., Keen, J.H. & Mellor, V.P. (1983). Children with juvenile chronic arthritis: Their beliefs about their illness and therapy. *Annals of the Rheumatic Diseases, 42*(5), 481–486.

Beaton, D.E., Tarasuk, V., Katz, J.N., Wright, J.G. & Bombardier, C. (2001). 'Are you better?' A qualitative study of the meaning of recovery. *Arthritis & Rheumatism, 45*(3), 270–279.

Beckham, J.C., Burker, E.J., Rice, J.R. & Talton, S.L. (1995). Patient predictors of caregiver burden, optimism, and pessimism in rheumatoid arthritis. *Behavioural Medicine, 20*(4), 171–178.

Beckham, J.C., Rice, J.R., Talton, S.L. & Helms, M.J. (1994). Relationship of cognitive constructs to adjustment in rheumatoid arthritis patients. *Cognitive Theory and Research, 18*(5), 479–497.

Bediako, S.M. & Friend, R. (2004). Illness-specific and general perceptions of social relationships in adjustment to rheumatoid arthritis: The role of interpersonal expectations. *Annals of Behavioural Medicine, 28*(3), 203–210.

Belot, H. (1999). *The language of the body*. Australia: Sekhem Association.

Belza, B.L., Henke, C.J., Yelin, E.H., Epstein, W.V. & Gilliss, C.L. (1993). Correlates of fatigue in older adults with rheumatoid arthritis. *Nursing Research, 42*(2), 93–99.

Benjamin, C.M. (1990). Review of UK data on the rheumatic diseases – 1. Juvenile chronic arthritis. *British Journal of Rheumatology, 29*(3), 231–233.

Beresford, B. (1995). Expert opinions: A national survey of parents caring for a severely disabled child. Bristol: Policy Press.

Berkanovic, E., Oster, P. & Wong, W.K. (1996). The relationship between socioeconomic status and recently diagnosed rheumatoid arthritis. *Arthritis Care and Research, 9*, 257–262.

Bermas, B.L., Tucker, J.S., Winkelman, D.K. & Katz, J.N. (2000). Marital satisfaction in couples with rheumatoid arthritis. *Arthritis Care and Research, 13*(3), 149–155.

Billings, A.G., Moos, R.H., Miller, J.J. & Gottlieb, J. (1987). Psychological adaptation in juvenile rheumatic disease: A controlled evaluation. *Health Psychology, 6*, 343–359.

Blalock, S.J., deVellis, B.M. & deVellis, R.F. (1989). Social comparisons among individuals with rheumatoid arthritis. *Journal of Applied Social Psychology, 19*(8), 665–680.

Blalock, S.J., deVellis, B.M., deVellis, R.F. & Sauter, S.H. (1988). Self-evaluation processes and adjustment to rheumatoid arthritis. *Arthritis & Rheumatism, 31*(10), 1245–1251.

Blalock, S.J., deVellis, B.M., Holt, K. & Hahn, P.M. (1993). Coping with rheumatoid arthritis: Is one problem the same as another? *Health Education Quarterly, 20*(1), 119–132.

Blalock, S.J., deVellis, R.F., Brown, G.K. & Wallston, K.A. (1989). Validity of the Center for Epidemiological Studies Depression Scale in arthritis populations. *Arthritis & Rheumatism, 32*(8), 991–997.

Blaxter, M. (1983). The causes of disease: Women talking. *Social Science and Medicine, 17*(2), 59–69.

Boonen, A. (2002). Socioeconomic consequences of ankylosing spondylitis. *Clinical and Experimental Rheumatology, 20*(6, suppl. 28), S23–26.

Boonen, A., Chorus, A., Miedema, H., van der Heijde, D., van der Tempel, H. & van der Linden, S. (2001). Employment, work disability, and work days lost in patients with ankylosing spondylitis: A cross sectional study of Dutch patients. *Annals of the Rheumatic Diseases, 60*(4), 353–358.

Booth, G.C. (1937). Personality and chronic arthritis. *Journal of Nervous Mental Disorders, 85*, 637–662.

Bradford, R. (1994). Children with liver disease: Maternal reports of their adjustment and the influence of disease severity on outcomes. *Child Care Health Development, 20*(6), 393–407.

Bradley, L.A. (1989). Adherence with treatment regimens among adult rheumatoid arthritis patients: Current status and future directions. *Arthritis Care and Research, 2*(3), S33–39.

Bradley, L.A. (1996). Pain management, In S.T. Wegener, B.L. Belza & E.P. Gall (Eds.) *Clinical care in the rheumatic diseases* (pp.59–64). Atlanta, GA: ACR.

Bradley, L.A., Young, L.D., Anderson, K.O., Turner, R.A., Agudelo, C.A., McDaniel, L.K. *et al.* (1987). Effects of psychological therapy on pain behavior of rheumatoid arthritis patients. Treatment outcome and six-month followup. *Arthritis & Rheumatism, 30*(10), 1105–1114.

Bradley, L.A., Young, L.D., Anderson, K.O., Turner, R.A., Agudelo, C.A., McDaniel, L.K. *et al.* (1988). Effects of cognitive behavioral therapy on rheumatoid arthritis pain behavior: One-year follow-up, In R. Dubner, G. Gebhardt & M. Bond (Eds.) *Pain research and clinical management, 3*, proceedings of the fifth World Congress on Pain (pp.310–314). Amsterdam: Elsevier.

Brekke, M., Hjortdahl, P. & Kvien, T.K. (2001a). Involvement and satisfaction: A Norwegian study of health care among 1024 patients with rheumatoid arthritis and 1509 patients with chronic noninflammatory musculoskeletal pain. *Arthritis Care and Research, 45*, 8–15.

Brekke, M., Hjortdahl, P. & Kvien, T.K. (2001b). Self-efficacy and health status in rheumatoid arthritis: A two-year longitudinal observational study. *Rheumatology (Oxford), 40*(4), 387–392.

Brekke, M., Hjortdahl, P., Thelle, D.S. & Kvien, T.K. (1999). Disease activity and severity in patients with rheumatoid arthritis: Relations to socioeconomic inequality. *Social Science and Medicine, 48*(12), 1743–1750.

Brenner, G.F., Melamed, B.G. & Panush, R.S. (1994). Optimism and coping determinants of psychological adjustment to rheumatoid arthritis. *Journal of Clinical Psychology in Medical Settings*, 1(2), 115–134.

Breuer, G.S., Orbach, H., Elkayam, O., Berkun, Y., Paran, D., Mates, M. *et al.* (2005). Perceived efficacy among patients of various methods of complementary alternative medicine for rheumatologic diseases. *Clinical and Experimental Rheumatology*, 23(5), 693–696.

Breuer, G.S., Orbach, H., Elkayam, O., Berkun, Y., Paran, D., Mates, M. *et al.* (2006). Use of complementary and alternative medicine among patients attending rheumatology clinics in Israel. *Israel Medical Association Journal*, 8(3), 184–187.

Brewerton, D.A., Hart, F.D., Nicholls, A., Caffrey, M., James, D.C. & Sturrock, R.D. (1973). Ankylosing spondylitis and HL-A 27. *Lancet*, 1(7809), 904–907.

Britton, C. (2000). *Families' experiences of the management of Juvenile Idiopathic Arthritis: Views from the inside*. Bristol: University of Bristol.

Britton, C. & Moore, A. (2002a). Views from the inside, part 1: Routes to diagnosis – families' experience of living with a child with arthritis. *British Journal of Occupational Therapy*, 65(8), 374–380.

Britton, C. & Moore, A. (2002b). Views from the inside, part 2: What the children with arthritis said, and the experiences of siblings, mothers, fathers and grandparents. *British Journal of Occupational Therapy*, 65(9), 413–419.

Brown, G.K. (1990). A causal analysis of chronic pain and depression. *Journal of Abnormal Psychology*, 99(2), 127–137.

Brown, G.K., Wallston, K.A. & Nicassio, P.M. (1989). Social support and depression in rheumatoid arthritis: A one-year prospective study. *Journal of Applied Social Psychology*, 19, 1164–1181.

Brus, H., van de Laar, M., Taal, E., Rasker, J. & Wiegman, O. (1999). Determinants of compliance with medication in patients with rheumatoid arthritis: The importance of self-efficacy expectations. *Patient Education & Counseling*, 36(1), 57–64.

Buckelew, S.P., Shutty, M.S., Jr., Hewett, J., Landon, T., Morrow, K. & Frank, R.G. (1990). Health locus of control, gender differences and adjustment to persistent pain. *Pain*, 42(3), 287–294.

Bulstrode, S.J., Barefoot, J., Harrison, R.A. & Clarke, A.K. (1987). The role of passive stretching in the treatment of ankylosing spondylitis. *British Journal of Rheumatology*, 26(1), 40–42.

Burckhardt, C.S. (1985). The impact of arthritis on quality of life. *Nursing Research*, 34(1), 11–16.

Burckhardt, C.S., Lorig, K., Moncur, C., Melvin, J., Beardmore, T., Boyd, M. *et al.* (1994). Arthritis and musculoskeletal patient education standards. Arthritis Foundation. *Arthritis Care and Research*, 7(1), 1–4.

Burton, W., Morrison, A., Maclean, R. & Ruderman, E. (2006). Systematic review of studies of productivity loss due to rheumatoid arthritis. *Occupational Medicine, 56*(1), 18–27.

Bury, M. (1991). The sociology of chronic illness: A review of research and prospects. *Sociology of Health & Illness, 13*, 451–468.

Buszewicz, M., Rait, G., Griffin, M., Nazareth, I., Patel, A., Atkinson, A. *et al.* (2006). Self-management of arthritis in primary care: Randomised controlled trial. *British Medical Journal, 333*(7574), 879.

Buunk B.P. (1995). Comparison direction and comparison dimension among disabled individuals: Towards a refined conceptualization of social comparison under stress. *Journal of Personality and Social Psychology, 59*, 1238–1249.

Callahan, L. & Pincus, T. (1988). Formal education level as a significant marker of clinical status in rheumatoid arthritis. *Arthritis and Rheumatism, 31*, 1346–1347.

Callahan, L.F., Bloch, D.A. & Pincus, T. (1992). Identification of work disability in rheumatoid arthritis: Physical, radiographic and laboratory variables do not add explanatory power to demographic and functional variables. *Journal of Clinical Epidemiology, 45*(2), 127–138.

Callahan, L.F., Kaplan, M.R. & Pincus, T. (1991). The Beck Depression Inventory, Center for Epidemiological Studies Depression Scale (CES-D), and General Well-Being Schedule Depression Subscale in rheumatoid arthritis: Criterion contamination of responses. *Arthritis Care and Research, 4*(1), 3–11.

Caracciolo, B. & Giaquinto, S. (2005). Self-perceived distress and self-perceived functional recovery after recent total hip and knee arthroplasty. *Archives of Gerontology and Geriatrics – Elsevier, 41*(2), 177–181.

Carette, S., Graham, D., Little, H., Rubenstein, J. & Rosen, P. (1983). The natural disease course of ankylosing spondylitis. *Arthritis & Rheumatism, 26*(2), 186–190.

Carlisle, A.C., John, A.M., Fife-Schaw, C. & Lloyd, M. (2005). The self-regulatory model in women with rheumatoid arthritis: Relationships between illness representations, coping strategies, and illness outcome. *British Journal of Health Psychology, 10*(4), 571–587.

Carter, M.A. (2004). Review: Group interventions may improve coping, quality of life, and social support in patients with arthritic conditions, but more research is needed. *Evidence Based Nursing, 7*(2), 51.

Cassidy, J. & Petty, R. (1990). *Textbook of pediatric rheumatology* (2nd edn.). New York: Churchill Livingstone.

Cassileth, B.R., Lusk, E. J., Strouse, T.B., Miller, D.S., Brown, L.L., Cross, P.A. *et al.* (1984). Psychosocial status in chronic illness: A comparative analysis of six diagnostic groups. *New England Journal of Medicine, 311*(8), 506–511.

Castenada, D., Bigatti, S. & Cronan, T.A. (1998). Gender and exercise behaviour among women and men with osteoarthritis. *Women and Health, 27*(4), 33–53.

Chandrashekara, S., Anilkumar, T. & Jamuna, S. (2002). Complementary and alternative drug therapy in arthritis. *Journal of Associations of Physicians of India, 50,* 225–227.

Chaney, J.M., Uretsky, D., Mullins, L., Doppler, M., Palmer, W., Wees, S. *et al.* (1996). Differential effects of age and illness duration on pain-depression and disability-depression relationships in rheumatois arthritis. *International Journal of Rehabilitation and Health, 2,* 101–112.

Charles, C., Whelan, T. & Gafni, A. (1999). What do we mean by partnership in making decisions about treatment? *British Medical Journal, 319,* 780–782.

Chehata, J.C., Hassell, A.B., Clarke, S.A., Mattey, D.L., Jones, M.A., Jones, P.W. *et al.* (2001). Mortality in rheumatoid arthritis: Relationship to single and composite measures of disease activity. *Rheumatology (Oxford), 40*(4), 447–452.

Chipperfield, J. & Greenslade, L. (1999). Perceived control as a buffer in the use of health care services. *Journals of Gerontology, Series B: Psychological Siences and Social Services, 54*(3), 146–154.

Chorus, A.M., Miedema, H.S., Boonen, A. & van der Linden, S. (2003). Quality of life and work in patients with rheumatoid arthritis and ankylosing spondylitis of working age. *Annals of the Rheumatic Diseases, 62*(12), 1178–1184.

Clark, N., Becker, M., Janz, N. & Lorig, K. (1991). Self-management of chronic disease by older adults: A review and questions for research. *Journal of Ageing and Health, 3,* 3–27.

Claudpierre, P. (2005). Spa therapy for ankylosing spondylitis: Still useful? *Joint Bone Spine, 72,* 283–285.

Cohen, J.L., Sauter, S.V., deVellis, R.F. & deVellis, B.M. (1986). Evaluation of arthritis self-management courses led by laypersons and by professionals. *Arthritis & Rheumatism, 29*(3), 388–393.

Conrad, P. (1990). Qualitative research on chronic illness: A commentary on method and conceptual development. *Social Science and Medicine, 30*(11), 1257–1263.

Cornel, U., Schiaffino, K.M. & Ilowite, N. (2001). Predictors of sibling relationship characteristics in youths with juvenile chronic arthritis. *Children's Health Care, 30*(1), 67–77.

Crawford, J.R., Henry, J.D., Crombie, C. & Taylor, E.P. (2001). Brief report: Normative data for the HADS from a large non-clinical sample. *British Journal of Clinical Psychology, 40,* 429–434.

Creamer, P. & Hochberg, M.C. (1997). Osteoarthritis. *Lancet, 350*(9076), 503–508.

Creed, F. & Ash, G. (1992). Depression in rheumatoid arthritis: Aetiology and treatment. *International Review of Psychiatry, 4,* 23–34.

Croft, P., Cooper, C., Wickham, C. & Coggon, D. (1992). Osteoarthritis of the hip and occupational activity. *Scandinavian Journal of Work, Environment and Health, 18*(1), 59–63.

Cronan, T.A., Hay, M., Groessl, E., Bigatti, S., Gallagher, R. & Tomita, M. (1998). The effects of social support and education on health care costs after three years. *Arthritis Care and Research, 11*(5), 326–334.

Cullen, L.A. & Barlow, J.H. (1998). Mentoring in the context of a training programme for young unemployed adults with physical disability. *International Journal of Rehabilitation Research, 21*(4), 389–391.

Curtis, R., Groarke, A., Coughlan, R. & Gsel, A. (2005). Psychological stress as a predictor of psychological adjustment and health status in patients with rheumatoid arthritis. *Patient Education & Counseling, 59*(2), 192–198.

Dagfinrud, H., Kjeken, I., Mowinckel, P., Hagen, K.B. & Kvien, T.K. (2005). Impact of functional impairment in ankylosing spondylitis: Impairment, activity limitation, and participation restrictions. *Journal of Rheumatology, 32*(3), 516–523.

Daltroy, L.H., Eaton, L., Hashimoto, H. & Liang, M.H. (1995). Rheumatoid arthritis patients' expectations for treatment outcomes. *Arthritis and Rheumatism, 38*(9), 945.

Daltroy, L. H., Larson, M.G., Eaton, H.M., Partridge, A.J., Pless, I.B., Rogers, M.P. *et al.* (1992). Psychosocial adjustment in juvenile arthritis. *Journal of Pediatric Psychology, 17*(3), 277–289.

Damush, T.M., Perkins, S.M., Mikesky, A.E., Roberts, M. & O'Dea, J. (2005). Motivational factors influencing older adults diagnosed with knee osteoarthritis to join and maintain an exercise program. *Journal of Aging & Physical Activity, 13*(1), 45–60.

Danoff-Burg, S., Agee, J.D., Romanoff, N.R., Kremer, J.M. & Strosberg, J.M. (2006). Benefit finding and expressive writing in adults with lupus or rheumatoid arthritis. *Psychology and Health, 21*, 651–665.

Danoff-Burg, S., Ayala, J. & Revenson, T.A. (2000). Researcher knows best? Toward a closer match between the concept and measurement of coping. *Journal of Health Psychology, 5*(2), 183–194.

Danoff-Burg, S. & Revenson, T.A. (2005). Benefit-finding among patients with rheumatoid arthritis: Positive effects on interpersonal relationships. *Journal of Behavioural Medicine, 28*(1), 91–103.

Danoff-Burg, S., Revenson, T.A., Trudeau, K.J. & Paget, S.A. (2004). Unmitigated communion, social constraints, and psychological distress among women with rheumatoid arthritis. *Journal of Personality, 72*(1), 29–46.

De Jong, O., Hopman-Rock, M., Tak, E. & Klazinga, N. (2004). An implementation study of two evidence-based exercise and health education programmes for older with osteoarthritis of the knee and hip. *Health Education Research, 19*(3), 316–325.

De Roos, A.J. & Callahan, L.F. (1999). Differences by sex in correlates of work status in rheumatoid arthritis patients. *Arthritis Care and Research, 12*(6), 381–391.

Dekker, J., Boot, B., van der Woude, L.H. & Bijlsma, J.W. (1992). Pain and disability in osteoarthritis: A review of biobehavioral mechanisms. *Journal of Behavioural Medicine, 15*(2), 189–214.

Dekker, J., Tola, P., Aufdemkampe, G. & Winckers, M. (1993). Negative affect, pain and disability in osteoarthritis patients: The mediating role of muscle weakness. *Behaviour Research & Therapy, 31*(2), 203–206.

Dekker-Saeys, A.J. (1976). *Spondylitis ankylopetica syndroom.* Amsterdam: Academic Press.

Dekkers, J.C., Geenen, R., Evers, A.W., Kraaimaat, F.W., Bijlsma, J.W. & Godaert, G.L. (2001). Biopsychosocial mediators and moderators of stress-health relationships in patients with recently diagnosed rheumatoid arthritis. *Arthritis & Rheumatism, 45*(4), 307–316.

DeLongis, A. & Holtzman, S. (2005). Coping in context: The role of stress, social support, and personality in coping. *Journal of Personality, 73*(6), 1633–1656.

Demange, V., Guillemin, F., Baumann, M., Suurmeijer, T.P., Moum, T., Doeglas, D. et al. (2004). Are there more than cross-sectional relationships of social support and support networks with functional limitations and psychological distress in early rheumatoid arthritis? The European Research on Incapacitating Diseases and Social Support Longitudinal Study. *Arthritis & Rheumatism, 51*(5), 782–791.

Dexter, P. & Brandt, K. (1994). Distribution and predictors of depressive symptoms in osteoarthritis. *Journal of Rheumatology, 21*(2), 279–286.

Deyo, R.A. (1982). Compliance with therapeutic regimens in arthritis: Issues, current status, and a future agenda. *Seminars in Arthritis and Rheumatism, 12*(2), 233–244.

Dickens, C. & Creed, F. (2001). The burden of depression in patients with rheumatoid arthritis. *Rheumatology (Oxford), 40*(12), 1327–1330.

Dickens, C., McGowan, L., Clark-Carter, D. & Creed, F. (2002). Depression in rheumatoid arthritis: A systematic review of the literature with meta-analysis. *Psychosomatic Medicine, 64*(1), 52–60.

Diehl, S.F., Moffitt, K.A. & Wade, S.M. (1991). Focus group interview with parents of children with medically complex needs: An intimate look at their perceptions and feelings. *Child Health Care, 20*(3), 170–178.

Dildy, S.M.P. (1992). A naturalistic study of the nature, meaning and impact of suffering in people with rheumatoid arthritis. Doctoral dissertation, University of Texas at Austin.

DiMatteo, M., Lepper, H. & Croghan, T. (2000). Depression is a risk factor for non-compliance with medical treatment: Meta-analysis of the effects of anxiety and depression on patient adherence. *Archives of Internal Medicine, 160*, 2101–2107.

Dishman, R.K. (1982). Compliance/adherence in health-related exercise. *Health Psychology, 1*(3), 237–267.

Dixon, K.E., Keefe, F.J., Scipio, C.D., Perri, L.M. & Abernethy, A.P. (2007). Psychological interventions for arthritis pain management in adults: A meta-analysis. *Health Psychology, 26*(3), 241–250.

Doeglas, D., Suurmeijer, T., Krol, B., Sanderman, R., van Rijswijk, M. & van Leeuwen, M. (1994). Social support, social disability and psychological well-being in rheumatoid arthritis. *Arthritis Care & Research, 7*, 10–15.

Doeglas, D., Suurmeijer, T., Krol, B., Sanderman, R., van Leeuwen, M. & van Rijswijk, M. (1995). Work disability in early rheumatoid arthritis. *Annals of Rheumatic Disease, 54*(6), 455–460.

Doeglas, D.M., Suurmeijer, T.P., van den Heuvel, W.J., Krol, B., van Rijswijk, M.H., van Leeuwen, M.A. *et al.* (2004). Functional ability, social support, and depression in rheumatoid arthritis. *Quality of Life Research, 13*(6), 1053–1065.

Donovan, J.L. & Blake, D.R. (1992). Patient non-compliance: Deviance or reasoned decision-making? *Social Science and Medicine, 34*(5), 507–513.

Donovan, J.L., Blake, D.R. & Fleming, W.G. (1989). The patient is not a blank sheet: Lay beliefs and their relevance to patient education. *British Journal of Rheumatology, 28*(1), 58–61.

Dowdy, S.W., Dwyer, K.A., Smith, C.A. & Wallston, K.A. (1996). Gender and psychological well-being of persons with rheumatoid arthritis. *Arthritis Care and Research, 9*(6), 449–456.

Duff, I.F., Carpenter, J.O. & Neukom, J.E. (1974). Comprehensive management of patients with rheumatoid arthritis. Some results of the regional Arthritis Control Program in Michigan. *Arthritis & Rheumatism, 17*(5), 635–645.

Duffy, C.M. (2005). Measurement of health status, functional status, and quality of life in children with juvenile idiopathic arthritis: Clinical science for the pediatrician. *Paediatric Clinics of North America, 52*(2), 359–372, v.

Dwyer, K.A. (1997). Psychosocial factors and health status in women with rheumatoid arthritis: Predictive models. *American Journal of Preventative Medicine, 13*(1), 66–72.

Eberhardt, K., Larsson, B.M. & Nived, K. (1993). Psychological reactions in patients with early rheumatoid arthritis. *Patient Education & Counseling, 20*(2–3), 93–100.

Ebringer, R.W., Cawdell, D.R., Cowling, P. & Ebringer, A. (1978). Sequential studies in ankylosing spondylitis: Association of klebsiella pneumoniae with active disease. *Annals of the Rheumatic Diseases, 37*(2), 146–151.

Edwards, J., Mulherin, D., Ryan, S. & Jester, R. (2001). The experience of patients with rheumatoid arthritis admitted to hospital. *Arthritis & Rheumatism, 45*(1), 1–7.

Edwards, S. (2002). Patient education programmes for adults with rheumatoid arthritis. Electronic letter. *British Medical Journal.*

Eiser, C. (1993) *Growing up with chronic illness: The impact on children and their families.* London: Jessica Kingsley.

Elder, R.G. (1973). Social class and lay explanations of the etiology of arthritis. *Journal of Health and Social Behaviour, 14*(1), 28–38.

Elfant, E., Gali, E. & Perlmuter, L. (1999). Learned illness behaviour and adjustment to arthritis. *Arthritis Care and Research, 12*(6), 411–416.

Emmons R.A. & McCullough M.E. (2003) Counting blesings versus burdens: An experimental investigation of gratitude and subjective well-being in daily life. *Journal of Personality and Social Psychology.* 84, (2), 377–389.

Ennett, S.T., DeVellis, B.M., Earp, J.A., Kredich, D., Warren, R.W. & Wilhelm, C.L. (1991). Disease experience and psychosocial adjustment in children with juvenile rheumatoid arthritis: Children's versus mothers' reports. *Journal of Pediatric Psychology, 16*(5), 557–568.

Eskanazi, D. (1998). Factors that shape alternative medicine. *Journal of the American Medical Association, 280*(18), 1621–1623.

Evers, A.W., Kraaimaat, F.W., Geenen, R. & Bijlsma, J.W. (1997). Determinants of psychological distress and its course in the first year after diagnosis in rheumatoid arthritis patients. *Journal of Behavioural Medicine, 20*(5), 489–504.

Evers, A.W., Kraaimaat, F.W., Geenen, R., Jacobs, J.W. & Bijlsma, J.W. (2002). Long term predictors of anxiety and depressed mood in early rheumatoid arthritis: A 3- and 5-year follow-up. *Journal of Rheumatology, 29*(11), 2327–2336.

Evers, A.W., Kraaimaat, F.W., Geenen, R., Jacobs, J.W. & Bijlsma, J.W. (2003). Stress-vulnerability factors as long-term predictors of disease activity in early rheumatoid arthritis. *Journal of Psychosomatic Research, 55*(4), 293–302.

Falkenbach, A. (2003). Disability motivates patients with ankylosing spondylitis for more frequent physical exercise. *Archives of Physical Medicine & Rehabilitation, 84*(3), 382–383.

Faucett, J. & Levine, J. (1991). The contribution of interpersonal conflict to chronic pain in the presence or absence of organic pathology. *Pain, 44,* 35–43.

Fautrel, B., Adam, V., St-Pierre, Y., Joseph, L., Clarke, A.E. & Penrod, J.R. (2002). Use of complementary and alternative therapies by patients self-reporting arthritis or rheumatism: Results from a nationwide Canadian survey. *Journal of Rheumatology, 29*(11), 2435–2441.

Feifel, H., Strack, S. & Nagy, V.T. (1987). Degree of life-threat and differential use of coping modes. *Journal of Psychosomatic Research, 31*(1), 91–99.

Feldman, D.E., Duffy, C., De Civita, M., Malleson, P., Philibert, L., Gibbon, M. *et al.* (2004). Factors associated with the use of complementary and alternative medicine in juvenile idiopathic arthritis. *Arthritis & Rheumatism, 51*(4), 527–532.

Felson, D. (1994). Do occupation-related physical factors contribute to arthritis? *Baillieres Best Practice & Research Clinical Medicine, 8*(1), 63–77.

Felson, D.T., Anderson, J.J., Lange, M.L., Wells, G. & LaValley, M.P. (1998). Should improvement in rheumatoid arthritis clinical trials be defined as fifty percent or seventy percent improvement in core set measures, rather than twenty percent? *Arthritis & Rheumatism, 41*(9), 1564–1570.

Felson, D., Anderson, J.J., Naimark, A., Hannan, M., Kannel, W. & Meenan, R.F. (1989). Does smoking protect against osteoarthritis? *Arthritis and Rheumatism, 32,* 166–172.

Felson, D.T., Zhang, Y., Anthony, J.M., Naimark, A. & Anderson, J.J. (1992). Weight loss reduces the risk for symptomatic knee osteoarthritis in women. The Framingham Study. *Annals of Internal Medicine, 116*(7), 535–539.

Felton, B.J. & Revenson, T.A. (1984). Coping with chronic illness: A study of illness controllability and the influence of coping strategies on psychological adjustment. *Journal of Consulting & Clinical Psychology, 52*(3), 343–353.

Felton, B.J., Revenson, T.A. & Hinrichsen, G.A. (1984). Stress and coping in the explanation of psychological adjustment among chronically ill adults. *Social Science and Medicine, 18*(10), 889–898.

Fifield, J., McQuillan, J., Armeli, S., Tennen, H., Reisine, S. & Affleck, G. (2004). Chronic strain, daily work stress and pain among workers with rheumatoid arthritis: Does job stress make a bad day worse? [peer reviewed]. *Work & Stress, 18*(4), 275.

Fifield, J., Reisine, S.T. & Grady, K. (1991). Work disability and the experience of pain and depression in rheumatoid arthritis. *Social Science and Medicine, 33*(5), 579–585.

Finkelstein, V. & Stuart, O. (1996). Developing new services. In G. Hales (Ed.) *Beyond Disability: Towards an enabling society.* London: Sage Publications.

Fischer, D., Stewart, A.L., Bloch, D.A., Lorig, K., Laurent, D. & Holman, H. (1999). Capturing the patient's view of change as a clinical outcome measure. *Journal of the American Medical Association, 282*(12), 1157–1162.

Fisher, P. & Ward, A. (1994). Complementary medicine in Europe. *British Medical Journal, 309*(6947), 107–111.

Fitzpatrick, R., Newman, S., Archer, R. & Shipley, M. (1991). Social support, disability and depression: A longitudinal study of rheumatoid arthritis. *Social Science and Medicine, 33*(5), 605–611.

Fitzpatrick, R., Newman, S., Lamb, R. & Shipley, M. (1988). Social relationships and psychological well-being in rheumatoid arthritis. *Social Science and Medicine, 27*(4), 399–403.

Flor, H., Haag, G. & Turk, D.C. (1986). Long-term efficacy of EMG biofeedback for chronic rheumatic back pain. *Pain, 27*(2), 195–202.

Focht, B.C., Gauvin, L. & Rejeski, W.J. (2004). The contribution of daily experiences and acute exercise to fluctuations in daily feeling states among older, obese adults with knee osteoarthritis. *Journal of Behavioural Medicine, 27*(2), 101–121.

Foster, H.E., Eltringham, M.S., Kay, L.J., Friswell, M., Abinun, M. & Myers, A. (2007). Delay in access to appropriate care for children presenting with musculoskeletal symptoms and ultimately diagnosed with juvenile idiopathic arthritis. *Arthritis & Rheumatism, 57*(6), 921–927.

Foster, H.E., Marshall, N., Myers, A., Dunkley, P. & Griffiths, I.D. (2003). Outcome in adults with juvenile idiopathic arthritis: A quality of life study. *Arthritis & Rheumatism, 48*(3), 767–775.

Fraenkel, L., Bogardus, S., Concato, J. & Felson, D. (2001). Preference for disclosure of information among patients with rheumatoid arthritis. *Arthritis & Rheumatism, 45*(2), 136–139.

Fries, J.F., Carey, C. & McShane, D.J. (1997). Patient education in arthritis: Randomized controlled trial of a mail-delivered program. *Journal of Rheumatology, 24*(7), 1378–1383.

Fries, J.F., Spitz, P., Kraines, R.G. & Holman, H.R. (1980). Measurement of patient outcome in arthritis. *Arthritis & Rheumatism, 23*(2), 137–145.

Fries, J.F., Williams, C.A., Morfeld, D., Singh, G. & Sibley, J. (1996). Reduction in long-term disability in patients with rheumatoid arthritis by disease-modifying antirheumatic drug-based treatment strategies. *Arthritis & Rheumatism, 39*(4), 616–622.

Fyrand, L., Moum, T., Finset, A. & Glennas, A. (2002). The impact of disability and disease duration on social support of women with rheumatoid arthritis. *Journal of Behavioural Medicine, 25*(3), 251–268.

Gamsa, A., Braha, R. & Catchlove, R. (1985). The use of structured group therapy sessions in the treatment of chronic pain patients. *Pain, 22*, 91–96.

Geenen, R., Van Middendorp, H. & Bijlsma, J.W. (2006). The impact of stressors on health status and hypothalamic-pituitary-adrenal axis and autonomic nervous system responsiveness in rheumatoid arthritis. *Annals of the New York Academy of Sciences, 1069*, 77–97.

Geirdal, O. (1990). Supportive groupwork with young arthritic mothers. *Groupwork, 2*, 220–236.

Gerhardt, U. (1989). Ideas about illness: An intellectual and political history of medical sociology. London: Macmillan.

Gignac, M.A. (2003). Leisure time physical activity and well-being: Learning from people living with arthritis. *Journal of Rheumatology, 30*(11), 2299–2301.

Gignac, M.A., Badley, E.M., Lacaille, D., Cott, C.C., Adam, P. & Anis, A.H. (2004). Managing arthritis and employment: Making arthritis-related work changes as a means of adaptation. *Arthritis & Rheumatism, 51*(6), 909–916.

Gignac, M.A., Cott, C. & Badley, E.M. (2000). Adaptation to chronic illness and disability and its relationship to perceptions of independence and dependence. *Journals of Gerontology Series B: Psychological Sciences and Social Sciences, 55*(6), P362–372.

Gignac, M.A., Sutton, D. & Badley, E.M. (2006). Reexamining the arthritis-employment interface: Perceptions of arthritis-work spillover among employed adults. *Arthritis & Rheumatism, 55*(2), 233–240.

Glazier, R.H., Badley, E.M., Lineker, S.C., Wilkins, A.L. & Bell, M.J. (2005). Getting a grip on arthritis: An educational intervention for the diagnosis and treatment of arthritis in primary care. *Journal of Rheumatology, 32*(1), 137–142.

Goemaere, S., Ackerman, C., Goethals, K., De Keyser, F., Van der Straeten, C., Verbruggen, G. *et al.* (1990). Onset of symptoms of rheumatoid arthritis in relation to age, sex and menopausal transition. *Journal of Rheumatology, 17*(12), 1620–1622.

Goeppinger, J., Armstrong, B., Schwartz, T., Ensley, D. & Brady, T.J. (2007). Self-management education for persons with arthritis: Managing comorbidity and eliminating health disparities. *Arthritis & Rheumatism, 57*(6), 1081–1088.

Gonzalez, A., Maradit Kremers, H., Crowson, C.S., Nicola, P.J., Davis, J.M. III, Therneau, T.M. *et al.* (2007). The widening mortality gap between rheumatoid arthritis patients and the general population. *Arthritis & Rheumatism, 56*(11), 3583–3587.

Gonzalez, V.M., Goeppinger, J. & Lorig, K. (1990). Four psychosocial theories and their application to patient education and clinical practice. *Arthritis Care and Research, 3*, 132–143.

Gorter, S., van der Linden, S. & Brauer, J. (2001). Rheumatologists' performance in daily practice. *Arthritis Care and Research, 45*(1), 16–28.

Gran, J.T. & Husby, G. (1990). Ankylosing spondylitis in women. *Seminars in Arthritis and Rheumatism, 19*(5), 303–312.

Gran, J.T. & Husby, G. (2003). Epidemiology of ankylosing spondylitis. In M.C. Hochberg, A.S. Silman, J.S. Smolen, M.E. Weinblatt & E. Weisman (Eds.) *Rheumatology*, 3rd edn. (pp.1153–1159). London: Mosby.

Grant, M. & Barlow, J. (2000). *A handbook for parents and grandparents with arthritis*. Coventry: Coventry University.

Griffin, K.W., Friend, R., Kaell, A.T. & Bennett, R.S. (2001). Distress and disease status among patients with rheumatoid arthritis: Roles of coping styles and perceived responses from support providers. *Annals of Behavioural Medicine, 23*(2), 133–138.

Groessl, E.J. & Cronan, T.A. (2000). A cost analysis of self-management programs for people with chronic illness. *American Journal of Community Psychology, 28*(4), 455–480.

Groessl, E.J., Kaplan, R.M. & Cronan, T.A. (2003). Quality of well-being in older people with osteoarthritis. *Arthritis & Rheumatism, 49*(1), 23–28.

Hackett, J. (2003). Perceptions of play and leisure in junior school aged children with juvenile idiopathic arthritis: What are the implications for occupational therapy? *British Journal of Occupational Therapy, 66*(7), 303–310.

Hafstrom, I., Ringertz, B., Spangberg, A., von Zweigbergk, L., Brannemark, S., Nylander, I. *et al.* (2001). A vegan diet free of gluten improves the signs and symptoms of rheumatoid arthritis: The effects on arthritis correlate with a reduction in antibodies to food antigens. *Rheumatology (Oxford), 40*(10), 1175–1179.

Hagen, L.E., Schneider, R., Stephens, D., Modrusan, D. & Feldman, B.M. (2003). Use of complementary and alternative medicine by pediatric rheumatology patients. *Arthritis & Rheumatism, 49*(1), 3–6.

Haggelund, K.J., Doyle, N.M., Clay, D.L., Frank, R.G., Johnson, J.C. & Pressly, T.A. (1996). A family retreat as a comprehensive intervention for children with arthritis and their families. *Arthritis Care and Research, 9*(1), 35–41.

Hainsworth, J. & Barlow, J. (2003). The experience of older volunteers training to become self-management tutors. *Health Education Journal, 62*(3), 266–277.

Hakkinen, A., Kautiainen, H., Hannonen, P., Ylinen, J., Makinen, H. & Sokka, T. (2006). Muscle strength, pain, and disease activity explain individual sub-dimensions of the health assessment questionnaire disability index, especially in women with rheumatoid arthritis. *Annals of the Rheumatic Diseases, 65*(1), 30–34.

Hall, J.A., Milburn, M.A., Roter, D.L. & Daltroy, L.H. (1998). Why are sicker patients less satisfied with their medical care? Tests of two explanatory models. *Health Psychology, 17*(1), 70–75.

Hamilton-West, K.E. & Quine, L. (2007). Effects of written emotional disclosure on health outcomes in patients with ankylosing spondylitis. *Psychology and Health, 22*(6), 637–657.

Hampson, S.E., Glasgow, R.E. & Zeiss, A.M. (1994). Personal models of osteoarthritis and their relation to self-management activities and quality of life. *Journal of Behavioural Medicine, 17*(2), 143–158.

Harris, J.A., Newcomb, A.F. & Gewanter, H.L. (1991). Psychosocial effects of juvenile rheumatic disease: The family and peer systems as a context for coping. *Arthritis Care and Research, 4*(3), 123–130.

Harrison, H. & Barlow, J. (1996). Focus group technique: A consumer perspective on outpatient therapeutic services. *British Journal of Therapy and Rehabilitation., 2*, 323–327.

Harrison, M.J. (2003). Young women with chronic disease: A female perspective on the impact and management of rheumatoid arthritis. *Arthritis & Rheumatism, 49*(6), 846–852.

Hartman, C.A., Manos, T.M., Winter, C., Hartman, D.M., Li, B. & Smith, J.C. (2000). Effects of T'ai Chi training on function and quality of life indicators in older adults with osteoarthritis. *Journal of the American Geriatrics Association, 48*(12), 1553–1559.

Haugli, L., Strand, E. & Finset, A. (2004). How do patients with rheumatic disease experience their relationship with their doctors? A qualitative study of experiences of stress and support in the doctor-patient relationship. *Patient Education & Counseling, 52*(2), 169–174.

Hawley, D.J. & Wolfe, F. (1991). Pain, disability, and pain/disability relationships in seven rheumatic disorders: A study of 1,522 patients. *Journal of Rheumatology, 18*(10), 1552–1557.

Hawley, D.J. & Wolfe, F. (1993). Depression is not more common in rheumatoid arthritis: A 10-year longitudinal study of 6,153 patients with rheumatic disease. *Journal of Rheumatology, 20*(12), 2025–2031.

Hay, L. (1984). *You can heal your life*. Santa Monica, CA: Hay House.

Haynes, R.B., Taylor, W.D. & Sackett, D.L. (Eds.) (1979). *Compliance in health care*. Baltimore: John Hopkins University Press.

Hazes, J.M. & Silman, A.J. (1990). Review of UK data on the rheumatic diseases, 2: Rheumatoid arthritis. *British Journal of Rheumatology, 29*(4), 310–312.

Headland, M. (2006). Using a website containing patient narratives to understand people's experiences of living with arthritis. *Journal of Orthopaedic Nursing, 10*(2), 106–112.

Heckhausen, J., Schulz, R. (1995). A life-span theory of control. *Psychological Review, 102*(2), 284–304.

Heiberg, T. & Kvien, T.K. (2002). Preferences for improved health examined in 1,024 patients with rheumatoid arthritis: Pain has highest priority. *Arthritis & Rheumatism, 47*(4), 391–397.

Helmick, C.G., Lawrence, R.C., Pollard, R.A., Lloyd, E. & Heyse, S.P. (1995). Arthritis and other rheumatic conditions: Who is affected now, who will be affected later? National Arthritis Data Workgroup. *Arthritis Care and Research, 8*(4), 203–211.

Hendry, M., Williams, N.H., Markland, D., Wilkinson, C. & Maddison, P. (2006). Why should we exercise when our knees hurt? A qualitative study of primary care patients with osteoarthritis of the knee. *Journal of Family Practice, 23*(5), 558–567.

Herman, C.J., Allen, P., Hunt, W.C., Prasad, A. & Brady, T.J. (2004). Use of complementary therapies among primary care clinic patients with arthritis. *Preventing Chronic Disease, 1*(4), A12.

Hidding, A., van der Linden, S., Boers, M., Gielen, X., de Witte, L., Kester, A. et al. (1993). Is group physical therapy superior to individualized therapy in ankylosing spondylitis? A randomized controlled trial. *Arthritis Care and Research, 6*(3), 117–125.

Hidding, A., van der Linden, S., Boers, M., Gielen, X., Kester, A. & Vlaeyen, J. (1992). Fake good test taking attitude in ankylosing spondylitis patients. *Arthritis and Rheumatism, 35,* 5244.

Hill, J. (1992). A nurse practitioner rheumatology clinic. *Nursing Standard, 7*(11), 35–37.

Hill, J. (1997). Patient satisfaction in a nurse-led rheumatology clinic. *Journal of Advanced Nursing, 25*(2), 347–354.

Hill, J., Bird, H.A., Hopkins, R., Lawton, C. & Wright, V. (1991). The development and use of patient knowledge questionnaire in rheumatoid arthritis. *British Journal of Rheumatology, 30*(1), 45–49.

Hirano, P.C., Laurent, D.D. & Lorig, K. (1994). Arthritis patient education studies, 1987–1991: A review of the literature. *Patient Education & Counseling, 24*(1), 9–54.

Hirsch, B.J., Moos, R.H. & Reischl, T.M. (1985). Psychosocial adjustment of adolescent children of a depressed, arthritic, or normal parent. *Journal of Abnormal Psychology, 94*(2), 154–164.

Hirst, M. & Baldwin, S. (1994). *Unequal opportunities: Growing up disabled.* London: Social Policy Research Unit.

Hollander, J. & Comroe, B. (1949). *Arthritis and allied conditions* (4th edn.). Philadelphia: Lea & Febiger.

Holman, H. & Lorig, K. (1992). Perceived self-efficacy in self-management of chronic disease. In Ralf Schwarzer (Ed.) *Self-efficacy: Thought control of action* (pp.305–324). Bristol, PA: Taylor & Francis.

Hommel, K.A., Wagner, J.L., Chaney, J.M., White, M.M. & Mullins, L.L. (2004). Perceived importance of activities of daily living and arthritis helplessness in rheumatoid arthritis; a prospective investigation. *Journal of Psychosomatic Research, 57*(2), 159–164.

Hughes, S.L., Dunlop, D., Edelman, P., Chang, R.W. & Singer, R.H. (1994). Impact of joint impairment on longitudinal disability in elderly persons. *Journals of Gerontology, 49*(6), S291–300.

Hutton, C.W. (1995). Osteoarthritis: Clinical features and management. In R.C. Butler and I.V. Jayson (Eds.) *Collected reports on the rheumatic diseases* (pp.35–38). Chesterfield: Arthritis and Rheumatism Council.

Huygen, A.C., Kuis, W. & Sinnema, G. (2000). Psychological, behavioural, and social adjustment in children and adolescents with juvenile chronic arthritis. *Annals of the Rheumatic Diseases, 59*(4), 276–282.

Huyser, B.A., Parker, J.C., Thoreson, R., Smarr, K.L., Johnson, J.C. & Hoffman, R. (1998). Predictors of subjective fatigue among individuals with rheumatoid arthritis. *Arthritis & Rheumatism, 41*(12), 2230–2237.

Ireys, H.T., Sills, E.M., Kolodner, K.B. & Walsh, B.B. (1996). A social support intervention for parents of children with juvenile rheumatoid arthritis: Results of a randomized trial. *Journal of Pediatric Psychology, 21*(5), 633–641.

Ishii, H., Nagashima, M., Tanno, M., Nakajima, A. & Yoshino, S. (2003). Does being easily moved to tears as a response to psychological stress reflect response to treatment and the general prognosis in patients with rheumatoid arthritis? *Clinical and Experimental Rheumatology, 21*(5), 611–616.

Iverson, M.D., Fossel, A.H. & Daltroy, L.H. (1999). Rheumatologist-patient communication about exercise and physical therapy in the management of rheumatoid arthritis. *Arthritis Care and Research, 12*(3), 180–192.

Jackson, S.W. (1994). Catharsis and abreaction in the history of psychological healing. *Psychiatric Clinic North America, 17*(3), 471–491.

Jacobi, C.E., Rupp, I., Boshuizen, H.C., Triemstra, M., Dinant, H.J. & van den Bos, G.A. (2004). Unmet demands for health care among patients with rheumatoid arthritis: Indications for underuse? *Arthritis & Rheumatism, 51*(3), 440–446.

Jacoby, R.K., Newell, R.L. & Hickling, P. (1985). Ankylosing spondylitis and trauma, the medicolegal implications: A comparative study of patients with non-specific back pain. *Annals of the Rheumatic Diseases, 44*(5), 307–311.

Jahn, L. (1997). *Women who have survived childhood sexual abuse: Do their coping strategies vary by personality type as measured by the Myers-Briggs Type Indicator?* Dissertation. University of North Texas.

James, N.T., Miller, C.W., Brown, K.C. & Weaver, M. (2005). Pain disability among older adults with arthritis. *Journal of Aging and Health, 17*(1), 56–69.

Janse, A.J., Sinnema, G., Uiterwaal, C.S., Kimpen, J.L. & Gemke, R.J. (2005). Quality of life in chronic illness: Perceptions of parents and paediatricians. *Archives of Disease in Childhood, 90*(5), 486–491.

Jenkinson, C., Wright, L. & Coulter, A. (1993). *Quality of life measurement in health care: A review of measures and population norms for the UK SF–36.* Oxford: Health Services Research Unit.

Jones, R.L. (1909). Arthritis deformans. *New York: William Wood Pub. and Research, 9*(4), 273–278.

Jordan, J.M., Luta, G., Renner, J.B., Linder, G.F., Dragomir, A., Hochberg, M.C. *et al.* (1996). Self-reported functional status in osteoarthritis of the knee in a rural southern community: The role of sociodemographic factors, obesity, and knee pain. *Arthritis Care and Research, 9*(4), 273–278.

Julious, S.A. (2005). Sample size of 12 per group rule of thumb for a pilot study. *Pharmaceutical Statistics, 4*, 287–291.

Kaarela, K., Lehtinen, K. & Luukkainen, R. (1987). Work capacity of patients with inflammatory joint diseases: An eight-year follow-up study. *Scandinavian Journal of Rheumatology, 16*(6), 403–406.

Kaboli, P.J., Doebbeling, B.N., Saag, K.G. & Rosenthal, G.E. (2001). Use of complementary and alternative medicine by older patients with arthritis: A population-based study. *Arthritis & Rheumatism, 45*(4), 398–403.

Kahn, A.N. & van der Linden, S. (1990). Ankylosing spondylitis and other spondylarthropathies. *Rheumatic Disease Clinics of North America, 16*(30), 551–579.

Katz, P.P. (2005). Use of self-management behaviors to cope with rheumatoid arthritis stressors. *Arthritis & Rheumatism, 53*(6), 939–949.

Katz, P.P. & Alfieri, W.S. (1997). Satisfaction with abilities and well-being: Development and validation of a questionnaire for use among persons with rheumatoid arthritis. *Arthritis Care and Research, 10*(2), 89–98.

Katz, P.P. & Neugebauer, A. (2001). Does satisfaction with abilities mediate the relationship between the impact of rheumatoid arthritis on valued activities and depressive symptoms? *Arthritis & Rheumatism, 45*(3), 263–269.

Katz, P.P., Pasch, L.A. & Wong, B. (2003). Development of an instrument to measure disability in parenting activity among women with rheumatoid arthritis. *Arthritis & Rheumatism, 48*(4), 935–943.

Katz, P.P. & Yelin, E.H. (1993). Prevalence and correlates of depressive symptoms among persons with rheumatoid arthritis. *Journal of Rheumatology, 20*(5), 790–796.

Katz, P.P. & Yelin, E.H. (1994). Life activities of persons with rheumatoid arthritis with and without depressive symptoms. *Arthritis Care and Research, 7*(2), 69–77.

Katz, P.P. & Yelin, E.H. (1995). The development of depressive symptoms among women with rheumatoid arthritis. The role of function. *Arthritis & Rheumatism, 38*(1), 49–56.

Kavale, S. (1996). *Interviews: An introduction to qualitative research interviewing.* London: Sage Publications.

Kay, E.A. & Punchak, S.S. (1988). Patient understanding of the causes and medical treatment of rheumatoid arthritis. *British Journal of Rheumatology, 27*(5), 396–398.

Kazis, L.E., Anderson, J.J. & Meenan, R.F. (1989). Effect sizes for interpreting changes in health status. *Medical Care, 27*(3, suppl.), S178–189.

Kean, W.F., Hart, L. & Buchanan, W.W. (1997). Disease-modifying drugs: Auranofin. *British Journal of Rheumatology, 36*, 560–572.

Kee, C.C. (2003). Older adults with osteoarthritis. Psychological status and physical function. *Journals of Gerontology Nursing, 29*(12), 26–34.

Keefe, F.J., Affleck, G., Lefebvre, J., Underwood, L., Caldwell, D.S., Drew, J. *et al.* (2001). Living with rheumatoid arthritis: The role of daily spirituality and daily religious and spiritual coping. *Journal of Pain, 2*(2), 101–110.

Keefe, F.J. & Caldwell, D.S. (1996). Cognitive behavioural interventions for arthritis pain management. In S.T. Wegener, B.A. Belza & E.P. Gall (Eds.) *Clinical care in the rheumatic diseases* (pp.221–226). Atlanta, GA: ACR.

Keefe, F.J., Caldwell, D.S., Martinez, S., Nunley, J., Beckham, J. & Williams, D.A. (1991). Analyzing pain in rheumatoid arthritis patients: Pain coping strategies in patients who have had knee replacement surgery. *Pain, 46*(2), 153–160.

Keefe, F.J., Caldwell, D.S., Queen, K.T., Gil, K.M., Martinez, S., Crisson, J.E. *et al.* (1987). Pain coping strategies in osteoarthritis patients. *Journal of Consulting & Clinical Psychology, 55*(2), 208–212.

Keefe, F.J., Caldwell, D.S., Williams, D.A., Gil, K.M., Mitchell, D.M. *et al.* (1990). Pain coping and training in the management of osteoarthritic knee pain: A comparative study. *Behavior Therapy, 21*, 49–62.

Keefe, F.J., Lefebvre, J.C., Egert, J.R., Affleck, G., Sullivan, M.J. & Caldwell, D.S. (2000). The relationship of gender to pain, pain behavior, and disability in osteoarthritis patients: The role of catastrophizing. *Pain, 87*(3), 325–334.

Keefe, F.J., Lefebvre, J.C., Kerns, R.D., Rosenberg, R., Beaupre, P., Prochaska, J. *et al.* (2000). Understanding the adoption of arthritis self-management: Stages of change profiles among arthritis patients. *Pain, 87*(3), 303–313.

Keefe, F.J., Lefebvre, J.C., Maixner, W., Salley, A.N., Jr. & Caldwell, D.S. (1997). Self-efficacy for arthritis pain: Relationship to perception of thermal laboratory pain stimuli. *Arthritis Care and Research, 10*(3), 177–184.

Keefe, F.J., Smith, S.J., Buffington, A.L., Gibson, J., Studts, J.L. & Caldwell, D.S. (2002). Recent advances and future directions in the biopsychosocial assessment and treatment of arthritis. *Journal of Consulting & Clinical Psychology, 70*(3), 640–655.

Kelley, J.E., Lumley, M.A. & Leisen, J.C. (1997). Health effects of emotional disclosure in rheumatoid arthritis patients. *Health Psychology, 16*(4), 331–340.

Kessler, R.C., Berglund, P., Demler, O., Jin, R., Koretz, D., Merikangas, K.R. *et al.* (2003). The epidemiology of major depressive disorder: Results from the National Comorbidity Survey Replication (NCS-R). *Journal of the American Medical Association, 289*(23), 3095–3105.

Kim, H.A., Bae, Y.D. & Seo, Y.I. (2004). Arthritis information on the Web and its influence on patients and physicians: A Korean study. *Clinical and Experimental Rheumatology, 22*(1), 49–54.

Kim, S., Drabinski, A., Williams, G. & Formica, C. (2001). The impact of early rheumatoid arthritis on productivity. [peer reviewed]. *Value in Health, 4*(5), 69.

King, L., Hawe, P. & Wise, M. (1998). Making dissemination a two-way process. *Health Promotion International, 3*, 237–244.

Kitzinger, J. (1995). Qualitative research. Introducing focus groups. *British Medical Journal, 311*(7000), 299–302.

Kocher, M. (1994). Mother with disabilities. *Sexuality Disability, 12*(2), 127–133.

Konkol, L., Lineberry, J., Gottlieb, J., Shelby, P.E., Miller, J.J. III & Lorig, K. (1989). Impact of juvenile arthritis on families: An educational assessment. *Arthritis Care and Research, 2*(2), 40–48.

Kopec, J.A. & Sayre, E.C. (2004). Traumatic experiences in childhood and the risk of arthritis: A prospective cohort study. *Canadian Journal of Public Health, 95*(5), 361–365.

Kovar, P.A., Allegrante, J.P., MacKenzie, C.R., Peterson, M.G., Gutin, B. & Charlson, M.E. (1992). Supervised fitness walking in patients with osteoarthritis of the knee: A randomized, controlled trial. *Annals of Internal Medicine, 116*(7), 529–534.

Kraag, G.R., Gordon, D.A., Menard, H.A., Russell, A.S. & Kalish, G.H. (1994). Patient compliance with tenoxicam in family practice. *Clinical Therapeutics, 16*(3), 581–593.

Kraimaat, F.W., van Dam-Baggen, C.M.J. & Bijlsma, J.W. (1995). Depression, anxiety and social support in rheumatoid arthritic women without and with a spouse. *Psychology and Health, 10*, 387–396.

Kralik, D., Koch, T., Price, K. & Howard, N. (2004). Chronic illness self-management: Taking action to create order. *Journal of Clinical Nursing, 13*(2), 259–267.

Krol, B., Sanderman, R., Suurmeijer, T.P., Doeglas, D., van Sonderen, E., Rijswijk *et al.* (1998). Early rheumatoid arthritis, personality and psychological status: A follow-up study. *Psychology and Health, 13*, 35–48.

Krol, T., Barlow, J.H. & Shaw, K. (1999). Treatment adherence in juvenile rheumatoid arthritis: A review. *Scandinavian Journal of Rheumatology, 28*(1), 10–18.

Krol, T. & Peake, S. (1996). *Employment situation of young adults in Scandinavia: Research report.* Oslo: Norwegian Arthritis Organisation (NRF).

Kruger, J.M., Helmick, C.G., Callahan, L.F. & Haddix, A.C. (1998). Cost-effectiveness of the arthritis self-help course. *Archives of Internal Medicine, 158*(11), 1245–1249.

Kujala, U.M., Kettunen, J., Paananen, H., Aalto, T., Battie, M.C., Impivaara, O. *et al.* (1995). Knee osteoarthritis in former runners, soccer players, weight lifters, and shooters. *Arthritis & Rheumatism, 38*(4), 539–546.

Kyngas, H. (2004). Support network of adolescents with chronic disease: Adolescents' perspective. *Nursing and Health Sciences, 6*(4), 287–293.

Kyngas, H., Kukkurainen, M. & Makelainen, P. (2004). Patients' education from the perspective of patients with arthritis [Finnish]. *Hoitotiede, 16*(5), 225–234.

La Montagna, G., Tirri, G., Cacace, E., Perpignano, G., Covelli, M., Pipitone, V. *et al.* (1998). Quality of life assessment during six months of NSAID treatment [Gonarthrosis and quality of life (GOAL) study]. *Clinical and Experimental Rheumatology, 16*(1), 49–54.

La Plante, M.P. (1988). *Data on disability from the National Health Interview Survey: An info. use report (1983–1985).* Washington, DC: National Institute on Disability and Rehabilitation.

Labyak, S.E., Bourguignon, C. & Docherty, S. (2003). Sleep quality in children with juvenile rheumatoid arthritis. *Holistic Nursing Practice, 17*(4), 193–200.

Lacaille, D., Sheps, S., Spinelli, J.J., Chalmers, A. & Esdaile, J.M. (2004). Identification of modifiable work-related factors that influence the risk of work disability in rheumatoid arthritis. *Arthritis & Rheumatism, 51*(5), 843–852.

Lacaille, D., White, M.A., Backman, C.L. & Gignac, M.A. (2007). Problems faced at work due to inflammatory arthritis: New insights gained from understanding patients' perspective. *Arthritis & Rheumatism, 57*(7), 1269–1279.

Latman, N.S. & Walls, R. (1996). Personality and stress: An exploratory comparison of rheumatoid arthritis and osteoarthritis. *Archives of Physical Medicine & Rehabilitation, 77*(8), 796–800.

Lavigne, J.V., Ross, C.K., Berry, S.L., Hayford, J.R. & Pachman, L.M. (1992). Evaluation of a psychological treatment package for treating pain in juvenile rheumatoid arthritis. *Arthritis Care and Research, 5*(2), 101–110.

Lawrence, J.S., Bremner, J.M. & Bier, F. (1966). Osteo-arthrosis. Prevalence in the population and relationship between symptoms and X-ray changes. *Annals of the Rheumatic Diseases, 25*(1), 1–24.

Lazarus, R.S. & Folkman, S. (1984). Coping with adaptation. In W.D. Gentry (Ed.) *Handbook of behavioural medicine* (pp.282–325) New York: Guilford Press.

LeBovidge, J.S., Lavigne, J.V., Donenberg, G.R. & Miller, M.L. (2003). Psychological adjustment of children and adolescents with chronic arthritis: A meta-analytic review. *Journal of Pediatric Psychology, 28*(1), 29–39.

LeBovidge, J.S., Lavigne, J.V. & Miller, M.L. (2005). Adjustment to chronic arthritis of childhood: The roles of illness-related stress and attitude toward illness. *Journal of Pediatric Psychology, 30*(3), 273–286.

Lehtinen, K. (1981). Working ability of 76 patients with ankylosing spondylitis. *Scandinavian Journal of Rheumatology, 10*(4), 263–265.

Lempp, H., Scott, D.L. & Kingsley, G.H. (2006). Patients' views on the quality of health care for rheumatoid arthritis. *Rheumatology (Oxford), 45*(12), 1522–1528.

Lenker, S.L., Lorig, K. & Gallagher, D. (1984). Reasons for the lack of association between changes in health behavior and improved health status: An exploratory study. *Patient Education & Counseling, 6*(2), 69–72.

Lerman, C.E. (1987). Rheumatoid arthritis: Psychosocial factors in etiology, course and treatment. *Clinical Psychology Review, 7*, 413–425.

Leventhal, H., Meyer, D. & Nerenz, D. (1980). The common sense model of illness danger. In S. Rachman (Ed.) *Medical psychology* (vol.2, pp.7–30). New York: Pergamon Press.

Li, J., Schiottz-Christensen, B. & Olsen, J. (2005). Psychological stress and rheumatoid arthritis in parents after death of a child: A national follow-up study. *Scandinavian Journal of Rheumatology, 34*(6), 448–450.

Lichtenberg, P.A., Skehan, M.W. & Swensen, C.H. (1984). The role of personality, recent life stress and arthritic severity in predicting pain. *Journal of Psychosomatic Research, 28*(3), 231–236.

Lim, H.J., Lee, M.S. & Lim, H.S. (2005). Exercise, pain, perceived family support, and quality of life in Korean patients with ankylosing spondylitis. *Psychological Reports, 96*(1), 3–8.

Lin, E.H., Katon, W., Von Korff, M., Tang, L., Williams, J.W., Jr., Kroenke, K. *et al.* (2003). Effect of improving depression care on pain and functional outcomes among older adults with arthritis: A randomized controlled trial. *Journal of the American Medical Association, 290*(18), 2428–2429.

Lindroth, Y., Bauman, A., Barnes, C., McCredie, M. & Brooks, P.M. (1989). A controlled evaluation of arthritis education. *British Journal of Rheumatology, 28*(1), 7–12.

Lindroth, Y., Bauman, A., Brooks, P.M. & Priestley, D. (1995). A 5-year follow-up of a controlled trial of an arthritis education programme. *British Journal of Rheumatology, 34*(7), 647–652.

Lindroth, Y., Brattström, M., Bellman, I., Ekestaf, G., Olofsson, Y., Strömbeck, B., Stenshed, B., Wikström, I., Nilsson, J.A., Wollheim, F.A. (1997). A problem-based education program for patients with rheumatoid arthritis: Evaluation after three and twelve months. *Arthritis Care & Research, 10*(5), 325–332.

Lineker, S.C., Hughes, A. & Badley, E.M. (1995). *Educational needs of clients with rheumatoid arthritis: A focus group experience.* Working Paper 95-1. Wellesley, Canada: ACREU, Wellesley Hospital Research Institute.

Locker, D. (1983). *Disability and disadvantage: The consequences of chronic illness* (pp.14–42). London: Tavistock Publications.

Loffer, S.L. (2000). *Returning to ourselves: Women thriving with chronic illness.* Dissertation. Institute of Transpersonal Psychology, USA.

Lorig, K. (1998). Personal communication. Palo Alto, CA: Stanford University, Patient Education Research Center.

Lorig, K., Chastain, R.L., Ung, E., Shoor, S. & Holman, H.R. (1989). Development and evaluation of a scale to measure perceived self-efficacy in people with arthritis. *Arthritis & Rheumatism, 32*(1), 37–44.

Lorig, K., Feigenbaum, P., Regan, C., Ung, E., Chastain, R.L. & Holman, H.R. (1986). A comparison of lay-taught and professional-taught arthritis self-management courses. *Journal of Rheumatology, 13*(4), 763–767.

Lorig, K. & Fries, J.F. (1990). *The arthritis helpbook: A tested self-management program for coping with arthritis and fibromyalgia.* New York: Addison-Wesley.

Lorig, K. & Gonzalez, V. (1992). The integration of theory with practice: A 12-year case study. *Health Education Quarterly, 19*(3), 355–368.

Lorig, K., Gonzalez, V.M., Laurent, D.D., Morgan, L. & Laris, B.A. (1998). Arthritis self-management program variations: Three studies. *Arthritis Care and Research, 11*(6), 448–454.

Lorig, K. & Holman, H.R. (1989). Long-term outcomes of an arthritis self-management study: Effects of reinforcement efforts. *Social Science and Medicine, 29*(2), 221–224.

Lorig, K. & Holman, H.R. (1993). Arthritis self-management studies: A twelve-year review. *Health Education Quarterly, 20*(1), 17–28.

Lorig, K., Ritter, P.L. & Plant, K. (2005). A disease-specific self-help program compared with a generalized chronic disease self-help program for arthritis patients. *Arthritis & Rheumatism, 53*(6), 950–957.

Lorig, K., Seleznick, M., Lubeck, D., Ung, E., Chastain, R.L. & Holman, H.R. (1989). The beneficial outcomes of the arthritis self-management course are not adequately explained by behavior change. *Arthritis & Rheumatism, 32*(1), 91–95.

Lorig, K., Sobel, D., Stewart, A., Brown, B., Bandura, A., Ritter, P., Gonzalez, V., Laurent, D. & Holman, H. (1999). Evidence suggesting that a chronic disease self-management program can improve health status while reducing hospitalization: A randomized trial, *Medical Care, 37,* 1, 5–14.

Lorig, K.R., Mazonson, P.D. & Holman, H.R. (1993). Evidence suggesting that health education for self-management in patients with chronic arthritis has sustained health benefits while reducing health care costs. *Arthritis & Rheumatism, 36*(4), 439–446.

Lorig, K.R., Ritter, P.L., Laurent, D.D. & Fries, J.F. (2004). Long-term randomized controlled trials of tailored-print and small-group arthritis self-management interventions. *Medical Care, 42*(4), 346–354

Lovell, D.J., Athreya, B., Emery, H.M., Gibbas, D.L., Levinson, J.E., Lindsley, C.B., Spencer, C.H. & White, P.H. (1990). School attendance and patterns, special services and special needs in pediatric patients with rheumatic diseases. *Arthritis Care and Research, 3,* 196-203.

Lowe, R., Cockshott, Z., Greenwood, R., Kirwan, J.R., Almeida, C., Richards, P. *et al.* (2008). Self-efficacy as an appraisal that moderates the coping-emotion relationship: Associations among people with rheumatoid arthritis. *Psychology and Health, 23*(2), 155–174.

Lubeck, D.P. (1995). The economic impact of arthritis. *Arthritis Care and Research, 8*(4), 304–310.

Lustig, J.L., Ireys, H.T., Sills, E.M. & Walsh, B.B. (1996). Mental health of mothers of children with juvenile rheumatoid arthritis: Appraisal as a mediator. *Journal of Pediatric Psychology, 21*(5), 719–733.

MacKinnon, J.R., Avison, W.R. & McCain, G.A. (1994). Pain and functional limitations in individuals with rheumatoid arthritis. *International Journal of Rehabilitation Research, 17*(1), 49–59.

Maggs, F.M., Jubb, R.W. & Kemm, J.R. (1996). Single-blind randomized controlled trial of an educational booklet for patients with chronic arthritis. *British Journal of Rheumatology, 35*(8), 775–777.

Mancuso, C.A., Rincon, M., Sayles, W. & Paget, S.A. (2006). Psychosocial variables and fatigue: A longitudinal study comparing individuals with rheumatoid arthritis and healthy controls. *Journal of Rheumatology, 33*(8), 1496–1502.

Manne, S.L. & Zautra, A.J. (1989). Spouse criticism and support: Their association with coping and psychological adjustment among women with rheumatoid arthritis. *Journal of Personality and Social Psychology, 56*(4), 608–617.

Manne, S.L. & Zautra, A.J. (1990). Couples coping with chronic illness: Women with rheumatoid arthritis and their healthy husbands. *Journal of Behavioural Medicine, 13*(4), 327–342.

Manninen, P., Riihimaki, H., Heliovaara, M. & Suomalainen, O. (2001). Physical exercise and risk of severe knee osteoarthritis requiring arthroplasty. *Rheumatology (Oxford), 40*(4), 432–437.

Manuel, J.C. (2001). Risk and resistance factors in the adaptation in mothers of children with juvenile rheumatoid arthritis. *Journal of Pediatric Psychology, 26*(4), 237–246.

March, L.M. & Bachmeier, C.J. (1997). Economics of osteoarthritis: A global perspective. *Baillieres Clinical Rheumatology, 11*(4), 817–834.

Marinker, M., Blenkinsopp, A., Bond, C. *et al.* (1997). *From compliance to concordance: Achieving shared goals in medicine taking.* London: Royal Pharmaceutical Society of Great Britain. Available at: http://www.medicines-partnership. org/about-us/history-context. Accessed 15 Feb. 2008.

Marks, R. & Allegrante, J.P. (2005). Chronic osteoarthritis and adherence to exercise: A review of the literature. *Journal of Aging & Physical Activity, 13*(4), 434–460.

Martin, J., Meltzer, H. & Elliott, D. (1988). *The prevalence of disability among adults.* OPCS Surveys of Disability in Great Britain. London: HMSO.

Martire, L.M., Keefe, F.J., Schulz, R., Ready, R., Beach, S.R., Rudy, T.E. *et al.* (2006). Older spouses' perceptions of partners' chronic arthritis pain: Implications for spousal responses, support provision, and caregiving experiences. *Psychology and Aging, 21*(2), 222–230.

Martire, L.M., Schulz, R., Keefe, F.J., Starz, T.W., Osial, T.A., Jr., Dew, M.A. *et al.* (2003). Feasibility of a dyadic intervention for management of osteoarthritis: A pilot study with older patients and their spousal caregivers. *Aging & Mental Health, 7*(1), 53–60.

Masdottir, B., Jonsson, T., Manfredsdottir, V., Vikingsson, A., Brekkan, A. & Valdimarsson, H. (2000). Smoking, rheumatoid factor isotypes and severity of rheumatoid arthritis. *Rheumatology (Oxford), 39*(11), 1202–1205.

Mau, W., Bornmann, M., Weber, H., Weidemann, H.F., Hecker, H. & Raspe, H.H. (1996). Prediction of permanent work disability in a follow-up study of early rheumatoid arthritis: Results of a tree structured analysis using RECPAM. *British Journal of Rheumatology, 35*(7), 652–659.

Mazzuca, S.A., Brandt, K.D., Katz, B.P., Chambers, M., Byrd, D. & Hanna, M. (1997). Effects of self-care education on the health status of inner-city patients with osteoarthritis of the knee. *Arthritis & Rheumatism, 40*(8), 1466–1474.

Mazzuca, S.A., Brandt, K.D., Katz, B.P., Hanna, M.P. & Melfi, C.A. (1999). Reduced utilization and cost of primary care clinic visits resulting from self-care education for patients with osteoarthritis of the knee. *Arthritis & Rheumatism, 42*(6), 1267–1273.

McAnarney, E.R., Pless, I.B., Satterwhite, B. & Friedman, S.B. (1974). Psychological problems of children with chronic juvenile arthritis. *Pediatrics, 53*(4), 523–528.

McAuley, E. (1992). The role of efficacy cognitions in the prediction of exercise behavior in middle-aged adults. *Journal of Behavioural Medicine, 15*(1), 65–88.

McCauley, J., Tarpley, M.J., Haaz, S. & Bartlett, S.J. (2008). Daily spiritual experiences of older adults with and without arthritis and the relationship to health outcomes. *Arthritis & Rheumatism, 59*(1), 122–128.

McDougall, J., Bruce, B., Spiller, G., Westerdahl, J. & McDougall, M. (2002). Effects of a very low-fat, vegan diet in subjects with rheumatoid arthritis. *Journal of Alternative & Complementary Medicine, 8*(1), 71–75.

MacFarland, L. (2007) Emotional disclosure associated with attendance on the chronic disease self-management course. Ph.D. thesis, Coventry University.

McFarlane, A.C. & Brooks, P.M. (1988). Determinants of disability in rheumatoid arthritis. *British Journal of Rheumatology, 27*(1), 7–14.

McGuigan, L.E., Hart, H.H., Gow, P.J., Kidd, B.L., Grigor, R.R. & Moore, T.E. (1984). Employment in ankylosing spondylitis. *Annals of the Rheumatic Diseases, 43*(4), 604–606.

McIntosh, E. (1996). The cost of rheumatoid arthritis. *British Journal of Rheumatology, 35*(8), 781–790.

McMurray, R., Heaton, J., Sloper, P. & Nettleton, S. (1999). Measurement of patient perceptions of pain and disability in relation to total hip replacement: The place of the Oxford hip score in mixed methods. *Quality in Health Care, 8*(4), 228–233.

McPherson, K.M., Brander, P., Taylor, W.J. & McNaughton, H.K. (2001). Living with arthritis: What is important? *Disability & Rehabilitation, 23*(16), 706–721.

McVeigh, C.M. & Cairns, A.P. (2006). Diagnosis and management of ankylosing spondylitis. *British Medical Journal, 333*(7568), 581–585.

Meenan, R.F., Callahan, L.F. & Helmick, C.G. (1999). The National Arthritis Action Plan: A public health strategy for a looming epidemic. *Arthritis Care and Research, 12*(2), 79–81.

Meenan, R.F., Kazis, L.E., Anthony, J.M. & Wallin, B.A. (1991). The clinical and health status of patients with recent-onset rheumatoid arthritis. *Arthritis & Rheumatism, 34*(6), 761–765.

Meenan, R.F., Mason, J.H., Anderson, J.J., Guccione, A.A. & Kazis, L.E. (1992). AIMS2. The content and properties of a revised and expanded arthritis impact measurement scales health status questionnaire. *Arthritis & Rheumatism, 35*(1), 1–10.

Melanson, P.M. & Downe-Wamboldt, B. (2003). Confronting life with rheumatoid arthritis. *Journal of Advanced Nursing, 42*(2), 125–133.

Middence, K. (1994). The effects of chronic illness on children and their families: An overview. *Genetic, Social and General Psychological Monographs, 20,* 309–329.

Miller, J.J. (1993). Psychological factors related to rheumatic disease in childhood. *Journal of Rheumatolgy, 20*(S38), 1–11.

Miller, J.J. III, Spitz, P.W., Simpson, U. & Williams, G.F. (1982). The social function of young adults who had arthritis in childhood. *Journal of Pediatrics, 100*(3), 378–382.

Mindham, R.H., Bagshaw, A., James, S.A. & Swannell, A.J. (1981). Factors associated with the appearance of psychiatric symptoms in rheumatoid arthritis. *Journal of Psychosomatic Research, 25*(5), 429–435.

Minnock, P., Fitzgerald, O. & Bresnihan, B. (2003). Quality of life, social support, and knowledge of disease in women with rheumatoid arthritis. *Arthritis & Rheumatism, 49*(2), 221–227.

Minor, M.A., Hewett, J.E., Webel, R.R., Anderson, S.K. & Kay, D.R. (1989). Efficacy of physical conditioning exercise in patients with rheumatoid arthritis and osteoarthritis. *Arthritis & Rheumatism, 32*(11), 1396–1405.

Moll, J.M. (1986). Doctor-patient communication in rheumatology: Studies of visual and verbal perception using educational booklets and other graphic material. *Annals of the Rheumatic Diseases, 45*(3), 198–209.

Moos, R.H. (1964). Personality factors associated with rheumatoid arthritis: A review. *Journal of Chronic Diseases, 17,* 41–55.

Morgan, M. (1989). Social ties, support and well-being. In. D.L. Patrick & H. Peach (Eds.) *Disablement in the community.* Oxford: Oxford University Press.

Morrill, J.A. (2004). Demographic, illness-related, social, and psychological correlates and predictors of happiness and anxiety in children and adolescents with juvenile rheumatoid arthritis. *Dissertation Abstracts International: Section B: The Sciences and Engineering, 64*(7-B), 3535.

Moussavi, S., Chatterji, S., Verdes, E., Tandon, A., Patel, V. & Ustun, B. (2007). Depression, chronic diseases, and decrements in health: Results from the World Health Surveys. *Lancet, 370*(9590), 851–858.

Muller-Godeffroy, E., Lehmann, H., Kuster, R.M. & Thyen, U. (2005). Quality of life and psychosocial adaptation in children and adolescents with juvenile idiopathic arthritis and reactive arthritis. *Journal of Rheumatology, 64*(3), 177–187.

Mullick, M.S., Nahar, J.S. & Haq, S.A. (2005). Psychiatric morbidity, stressors, impact, and burden in juvenile idiopathic arthritis. *Journal of Health Population Nutrition, 23*(2), 142–149.

Mulligan, K., Newman, S.P., Taal, E., Hazes, M. & Rasker, J.J. (2005). The design and evaluation of psychoeducational/self-management interventions. *Journal of Rheumatology, 32*(12), 2470–2474.

Multon, K.D., Parker, J.C., Smarr, K.L., Stucky, R.C., Petroski, G., Hewett, J.E. *et al.* (2001). Effects of stress management on pain behavior in rheumatoid arthritis. *Arthritis & Rheumatism, 45*(2), 122–128.

Munthe, E. (1990). The care of the rheumatic child. *EULAR Bulletin, Basle,* 47–50.

Murphy, H., Dickens, C., Creed, F. & Bernstein, R. (1999). Depression, illness perception and coping in rheumatoid arthritis. *Journal of Psychosomatic Research, 46*(2), 155–164.

Nagyova, I., Stewart, R.E., Macejova, Z., van Dijk, J.P. & van den Heuvel, W.J. (2005). The impact of pain on psychological well-being in rheumatoid arthritis: The mediating effects of self-esteem and adjustment to disease. *Patient Education & Counseling, 58*(1), 55–62.

Naidoo, P. & Pretorius, T.B. (2006). The moderating role of helplessness in rheumatoid arthritis, a chronic disease. [peer reviewed]. *Social Behavior & Personality: An International Journal, 34*(2), 103.

Nasser-Abdel, A. (1996). *Egyptian and Dutch rheumatoid arthritis patients: A biopsychsocial analysis.* Dissertation: University Twente, Enschede.

Neame, R. & Hammond, A. (2005). Beliefs about medications: A questionnaire survey of people with rheumatoid arthritis. *Rheumatology (Oxford), 44*(6), 762–767.

Neugebauer, A. & Katz, P.P. (2004). Impact of social support on valued activity disability and depressive symptoms in patients with rheumatoid arthritis. *Arthritis & Rheumatism, 51*(4), 586–592.

Neugebauer, A., Katz, P.P. & Pasch, L.A. (2003). Effect of valued activity disability, social comparisons, and satisfaction with ability on depressive symptoms in rheumatoid arthritis. *Health Psychology, 22*(3), 253–262.

Neville, C., Fortin, P.R., Fitzcharles, M.A., Baron, M., Abrahamowitz, M., Du Berger, R. *et al.* (1999). The needs of patients with arthritis: The patient's perspective. *Arthritis Care and Research, 12*(2), 85–95.

Newman, S. & Mulligan, K. (2000). The psychology of rheumatic diseases. *Baillieres Best Practice & Research Clinical Medicine, 14*(4), 773–786.

Newman, S.P., Fitzpatrick, R., Lamb, R. & Shipley, M. (1989). The origins of depressed mood in rheumatoid arthritis. *Journal of Rheumatology, 16*(6), 740–744.

Newman, S.P., Fitzpatrick, R., Lamb, R. & Shipley, M. (1990). Patterns of coping in rheumatoid arthritis. *Psychology and Health, 4,* 187–200.

Newth, S. & Delongis, A. (2004). Individual differences, mood, and coping with chronic pain in rheumatoid arthritis: A daily process analysis. [peer reviewed]. *Psychology and Health, 19*(3), 283.

258   *References*

Nicassio, P.M. (2008). The problem of detecting and managing depression in the rheumatology clinic. *Arthritis & Rheumatism, 59*(2), 155–158.

Nicassio, P.M. & Wallston, K.A. (1992). Longitudinal relationships among pain, sleep problems, and depression in rheumatoid arthritis. *Journal of Abnormal Psychology, 101*(3), 514–520.

O'Leary, A., Shoor, S., Lorig, K. & Holman, H.R. (1988). A cognitive-behavioral treatment for rheumatoid arthritis. *Health Psychology, 7*(6), 527–544.

Oliver, M. (1992). Changing the social relations of research production. *Disability, Handicap and Society, 7*, 101–115.

Oliveria, S.A., Felson, D.T., Cirillo, P.A., Reed, J.I. & Walker, A.M. (1999). Body weight, body mass index, and incident symptomatic osteoarthritis of the hand, hip, and knee. *Epidemiology, 10*(2), 161–166.

Ong, L.M., de Haes, J.C., Hoos, A.M. & Lammes, F.B. (1995). Doctor-patient communication: A review of the literature. *Social Science and Medicine, 40*(7), 903–918.

Orbell, S., Espley, A., Johnston, M. & Rowley, D. (1998). Health benefits of joint replacement surgery for patients with osteoarthritis: Prospective evaluation using independent assessments in Scotland. *Journal of Epidemiology & Community Health, 52*(9), 564–570.

Orbell, S., Johnston, M., Rowley, D., Davey, P. & Espley, A. (1998). Self-efficacy and goal importance in the prediction of physical disability in people following hospitalisation: A prospective study. *British Journal of Health Psychology, 6*, 25–40.

Orbell, S., Johnston, M., Rowley, D., Davey, P. & Espley, A. (2001). Self-efficacy and goal importance in the prediction of physical disability in people following hospitalization: A prospective study. *British Journal of Health Psychology, 6*(Pt 1), 25–40.

O'Reilly, S.C., Muir, K.R. & Doherty, M. (1999). Effectiveness of home exercise on pain and disability from osteoarthritis of the knee: A randomised controlled trial. *Annals of the Rheumatic Diseases, 58*(1), 15–19.

Osborn, C.E. (2001). *Complementary and alternative medicine and the treatment of rheumatic diseases: Focusing on aromatherapy.* Coventry: Coventry University.

Osborn, C.E., Barlas, P., Baxter, G.D. & Barlow, J.H. (2001). Aromatherapy: A survey of current practice in the management of rheumatic disease symptoms. *Complementary Therapies in Medicine, 9*(2), 62–67.

Osborne, R.H., Wilson, T., Lorig, K.R. & McColl, G.J. (2007). Does self-management lead to sustainable health benefits in people with arthritis? A 2-year transition study of 452 Australians. *Journal of Rheumatology, 34*(5), 1112–1117.

Packham, J.C. & Hall, M.A. (2002). Long-term follow-up of 246 adults with juvenile idiopathic arthritis: Functional outcome. *Rheumatology (Oxford), 41*(12), 1428–1435.

Palermo, T.M. & Kiska, R. (2005). Subjective sleep disturbances in adolescents with chronic pain: Relationship to daily functioning and quality of life. *Journal of Pain, 6*(3), 201–207.

Palermo, T.M., Zebracki, K., Cox, S., Newman, A.J. & Singer, N.G. (2004). Juvenile idiopathic arthritis: Parent-child discrepancy on reports of pain and disability. *Journal of Rheumatology, 31*(9), 1840–1846.

Pariser, D.A. (2004). *The effects of telephone intervention on arthritis self-efficacy, depression, pain, and fatigue in older adults with arthritis.* New Orleans: University of New Orleans.

Parker, J.C., Buckelew, S.P., Smarr, K.L., Buescher, K.L., Beck, N.C., Frank, R.G. *et al.* (1990). Psychological screening in rheumatoid arthritis. *Journal of Rheumatology, 17*(8), 1016–1021.

Parker, J.C., Frank, R.G., Beck, N.C., Smarr, K.L., Buescher, K.L., Phillips, L.R. *et al.* (1988). Pain management in rheumatoid arthritis patients. A cognitive-behavioral approach. *Arthritis & Rheumatism, 31*(5), 593–601.

Parker, J.C., Smarr, K.L., Angelone, E.O., Mothersead, P.K., Lee, B.S., Walker, S.E. *et al.* (1992). Psychological factors, immunologic activation, and disease activity in rheumatoid arthritis. *Arthritis Care and Research, 5*(4), 196–201.

Parker, J.C., Smarr, K.L., Slaughter, J.R., Johnston, S.K., Priesmeyer, M.L., Hanson, K.D. *et al.* (2003). Management of depression in rheumatoid arthritis: A combined pharmacologic and cognitive-behavioral approach. *Arthritis & Rheumatism, 49*(6), 766–777.

Parker, J.C. & Wright, G.E. (1995). The implications of depression for pain and disability in rheumatoid arthritis. *Arthritis Care and Research, 8*(4), 279–283.

Pashler H.E. (2002) *Steven's Handbook of Experimental Psychology, vol. 2: Memory and Cognitive Processes.* New York: John Wiley.

Perrin, J.M., MacLean, W.E. & Perrin, E.C. (1989). Parental perceptions of health status and psychologic adjustment of children with asthma. *Pediatrics, 83*(1), 26–30.

Persson, L.O., Larsson, B.M., Nived, K. & Eberhardt, K. (2005). The development of emotional distress in 158 patients with recently diagnosed rheumatoid arthritis: A prospective 5-year follow-up study. *Scandinavian Journal of Rheumatology, 34*(3), 191–197.

Persson, L.O. & Sahlberg, D. (2002). The influence of negative illness cognitions and neuroticism on subjective symptoms and mood in rheumatoid arthritis. *Annals of the Rheumatic Diseases, 61*(11), 1000–1006.

Peterson, M.G., Kovar-Toledano, P.A., Otis, J.C., Allegrante, J.P., Mackenzie, C.R., Gutin, B. *et al.* (1993). Effect of a walking program on gait characteristics in patients with osteoarthritis. *Arthritis Care and Research, 6*(1), 11–16.

Pincus, T. & Callahan, L.F. (1986). Taking mortality in rheumatoid arthritis seriously: Predictive markers, socioeconomic status and comorbidity. *Journal of Rheumatology, 13*(5), 841–845.

Pincus, T. & Callahan, L.F. (1993). What is the natural history of rheumatoid arthritis? *Rheumatic Disease Clinics of North America, 19*(1), 123–151.

Pincus, T., Griffith, J., Pearce, S. & Isenberg, D. (1996). Prevalence of self-reported depression in patients with rheumatoid arthritis. *British Journal of Rheumatology, 35*(9), 879–883.

Pincus, T., Swearingen, C., Cummins, P. & Callahan, L.F. (2000). Preference for nonsteroidal anti-inflammatory drugs versus acetaminophen and concomitant use of both types of drugs in patients with osteoarthritis. *Journal of Rheumatology, 27*(4), 1020–1027.

Pisters, M.F., Veenhof, C., van Meeteren, N.L., Ostelo, R.W., de Bakker, D.H., Schellevis, F.G. *et al.* (2007). Long-term effectiveness of exercise therapy in patients with osteoarthritis of the hip or knee: A systematic review. *Arthritis & Rheumatism, 57*(7), 1245–1253.

Plach, S.K., Heidrich, S.M. & Waite, R.M. (2003). Relationship of social role quality to psychological well-being in women with rheumatoid arthritis. *Research in Nursing and Health, 26*(3), 190–202.

Plach, S.K., Stevens, P.E. & Moss, V.A. (2004). Corporeality: Women's experiences of a body with rheumatoid arthritis. *Clinical Nursing Research, 13*(2), 137–155.

Powell, D.A., Furhtgott, E., Henderson, M., Prescott, L., Mitchell, A., Hartis, P. *et al.* (1990). Some determinants of attrition in prospective studies on ageing. *Experimental Ageing Research, 16*, 17–23.

Power, J.D., Perruccio, A.V. & Badley, E.M. (2005). Pain as a mediator of sleep problems in arthritis and other chronic conditions. *Arthritis Care and Research, 53*(6), 911–919.

Pradhan E.K., Baumgarten M., Langenberg P., Handwerger B.H., Gilpin A,K., Magyari T., Hochberg M.C. & Berman B.M. (2007) Effect of mindfulness-based stress reduction in rheumatoid arthritis patients. *Arthritis & Rheumatism. 57*(7), 1134–1142.

Pritchard, M.L. (1989). *Psychological aspects of RA*. New York: Springer.

Prochaska, J., Velicer, W., Rossi, J.S., Goldstein, M.G., Marcus, B.H., Rakowski, W. *et al.* (1994). Stages of change and decisional balance for 12 problem behaviours. *Health Psychology, 13*, 39–46.

Prochaska, T., Peters, K. & Warren, J. (2000). Health behavior: From research to practice. In G.L. Albrecht, R. Fitzpatrick & S.C. Scrimshaw (Eds.) *Handbook of Social Studies in Health and Medicine* (pp.359–373). Thousand Oaks, CA: Sage.

Radloff, L.S. (1977). The CES-D scale: A self-report depression scale for research in the general population. *Applied Psychological Measurement, 1*(3), 385–401.

Radojevic, V., Nicassio, P.M. & Weisman, M.H. (1992). Behavioural intervention with and without family support for rheumatoid arthritis. *Behavior Therapy, 23*(1), 13–30.

Ramsey, S.D.R., Spencer, A.C., Topolski, T.A., Belza, B.L. & Patrick, D.L. (2001). Use of alternative therapies by older adults with osteoarthritis. *Arthritis Care and Research*, 45(3), 222–227.

Rao, J.K., Arick, R., Mihaliak, K.A. & Weinberger, M. (1998). Using focus groups to understand arthritis patients' perceptions about unconventional therapies. *Arthritis Care and Research*, 11(4), 253–260.

Rao, J.K., Kroenke, K., Mihaliak, K.A., Grambow, S.C. & Weinberger, M. (2003). Rheumatology patients' use of complementary therapies: Results from a one-year longitudinal study. *Arthritis & Rheumatism*, 49(5), 619–625.

Rapoff, M.A. & Christopherson, E.R. (1982). Improving compliance in pediatric practice. *Pediatric Clinics of North America*, 29(2), 339–357.

Rapoff, M.A., Purviance, M.R. & Lindsley, C.B. (1988a). Educational and behavioral strategies for improving medication compliance in juvenile rheumatoid arthritis. *Archives of Physical Medicine & Rehabilitation*, 69(6), 439–441.

Rapoff, M.A., Purviance, M.R. & Lindsley, C.B. (1988b). Improving mediation compliance for juvenile rheumatoid arthritis and its effect on clinical outcome: A single-subject analysis. *Arthritis Care and Research*, 1, 12–16.

Reed, G.M., Taylor, S.E. & Kemeny, M.E. (1993). Perceived control and psychological adjustment in gay men with AIDs. *Journal of Applied Social Psychology*, 23(10), 791–824.

Reisine, S. (1995). Marital status and social support in rheumatoid arthritis. *Arthritis & Rheumatism*, 36, 589–592.

Reisine, S., McQuillan, J. & Fifield, J. (1995). Predictors of work disability in rheumatoid arthritis patients. A five-year follow up. *Arthritis & Rheumatism*, 38(11), 1630–1637.

Reisine, S.T., Goodenow, C. & Grady, K.E. (1987). The impact of rheumatoid arthritis on the homemaker. *Social Science and Medicine*, 25(1), 89–95.

Rejeski, W.J., Brawley, L.R. Ettinger, W., Morgan, T. & Thompson, C. (1997). Compliance to exercise therapy in older participants with knee osteoarthritis: Implications for treating disability. *Medicine and Science in Sports and Exercise*, 29(8), 977–985.

Rejeski, W.J. Ettinger, W.H., Jr., Martin, K. & Morgan, T. (1998). Treating disability in knee osteoarthritis with exercise therapy: A central role for self-efficacy and pain. *Arthritis Care and Research*, 11(2), 94–101.

Resch, K.L., Hill, S. & Ernst, E. (1997). Use of complementary therapies by individuals with 'arthritis'. *Clinical Rheumatology*, 16(4), 391–395.

Revenson, T.A. (1993). The role of social support with rheumatic disease. *Baillieres Clinical Rheumatology*, 7(2), 377–396.

Revenson, T.A. & Majerovitz, S.D. (1991). The effects of chronic illness on the spouse. Social resources as stress buffers. *Arthritis Care and Research*, 4(2), 63–72.

Revenson, T.A., Schiaffino, K.A., Majerovitz, D. & Gibofsky, A. (1991). Social support as a double-edged sword: The relation of positive and problematic support to depression among rheumatoid arthritis patients. *Social Science and Medicine, 33,* 807–813.

Rhee, S.H., Parker, J.C., Smarr, K.L., Petroski, G.F., Johnson, J.C., Hewett, J.E. *et al.* (2000). Stress management in rheumatoid arthritis: What is the underlying mechanism? *Arthritis Care and Research, 13*(6), 435–442.

Riemsma, R.P., Kirwan, J.R., Taal, E. & Rasker, J.J. (2002). Patient education for adults with rheumatoid arthritis. *Cochrane Database Systematic Review*(3), CD003688.

Riemsma, R.P., Rasker, J.J., Taal, E., Griep, E.N., Wouters, J.M. & Wiegman, O. (1998). Fatigue in rheumatoid arthritis: The role of self-efficacy and problematic social support. *British Journal of Rheumatology, 37*(10), 1042–1046.

Riemsma, R.P., Taal, E. & Rasker, J.J. (2003). Group education for patients with rheumatoid arthritis and their partners. *Arthritis & Rheumatism, 49*(4), 556–566.

Riemsma, R.P., Taal, E., Rasker, J., Klein, G., Bruyn, G.A.W., Wouters, J.M. *et al.* (1999). The burden of care for informal caregivers of patients with rheumatoid arthritis. *Psychology and Health, 14*(5), 773–794.

Riemsma, R.P., Taal, E., Wiegman, O., Rasker, J., Bruyn, G.A.W. & van Paassen, J.C. (2000). Problematic and positive support in relation to depression in people with rheumatoid arthritis. *Journal of Health Psychology,* 221–230.

Rockport Walking Institute. (1988). *The Rockport Walk Leader Program manual.* Marlboro, MA.

Rosenthal, G.E. & Shannon, S.E. (1997). The use of patient perceptions in the evaluation of healthcare delivery systems. *Medical Care, 35,* 58–68.

Ross, C.K., Lavigne, J.V., Hayford, J.R., Berry, S.L., Sinacore, J.M. & Pachman, L.M. (1993). Psychological factors affecting reported pain in juvenile rheumatoid arthritis. *Journal of Pediatric Psychology, 18*(5), 561–573.

Rupp, I., Boshuizen, H.C., Jacobi, C.E., Dinant, H.J. & van den Bos, G.A. (2004). Impact of fatigue on health-related quality of life in rheumatoid arthritis. *Arthritis & Rheumatism, 51*(4), 578–585.

Russell, M.L. (1985). Ankylosing spondylitis: The case for the underestimated female. *The Journal of Rheumatology, 12*(1), 4–6.

Ryan, S. (1995). Rheumatology: Sharing care in an outpatient clinic. *Nursing Standard, 10*(6), 23–5.

Ryan, S. (1996). Living with rheumatoid arthritis: A phenomenological exploration. *Nursing Standard, 10*(41), 45–48.

Ryff, C.D. & Keyes, C.L. (1995). The structure of psychological well-being revisited. *Journal of Personality and Social Psychology, 69*(4), 719–727.

Sale, J.E., Gignac, M. & Hawker, G. (2006). How 'bad' does the pain have to be? A qualitative study examining adherence to pain medication in older adults with osteoarthritis. *Arthritis & Rheumatism, 55*(2), 272–278.

Sallfors, C., Fasth, A. & Hallberg, L.R. (2002). Oscillating between hope and despair: A qualitative study. *Child Care Health Development, 28*(6), 495–505.

Sangha, O. (2000). Epidemiology of rheumatic diseases. *Rheumatology (Oxford), 39*(suppl. 2), 3–12.

Santos, H., Brophy, S. & Calin, A. (1998). Exercise in ankylosing spondylitis: How much is optimum? *Journal of Rheumatology, 25*(11), 2156–2160.

Savelkoul, M., de Witte, L. & Post, M. (2003). Stimulating active coping in patients with rheumatic diseases: A systematic review of controlled group intervention studies. *Patient Education & Counseling, 50*(2), 133–143.

Savelkoul, M., de Witte, L.P., Candel, M.J., van der Tempel, H. & van den Borne, B. (2001). Effects of a coping intervention on patients with rheumatic diseases: Results of a randomized controlled trial. *Arthritis & Rheumatism, 45*(1), 69–76.

Sawyer, M.G., Carbone, J.A., Whitham, J.N., Roberton, D.M., Taplin, J.E., Varni, J.W. *et al.* (2005). The relationship between health-related quality of life, pain, and coping strategies in juvenile arthritis: A one year prospective study. *Quality of Life Research, 14*(6), 1585–1598.

Schanberg, L.E., Gil, K.M., Anthony, K.K., Yow, E. & Rochon, J. (2005). Pain, stiffness, and fatigue in juvenile polyarticular arthritis: Contemporaneous stressful events and mood as predictors. *Arthritis & Rheumatism, 52*(4), 1196–1204.

Schanberg, L.E., Sandstrom, M.J., Starr, K., Gill, K.M., Lefebvre, J., Keefe, F.J. *et al.* (2000). The relationship between daily mood and stressful events to symptoms in juvenile rheumatic disease. *Arthritis Care and Research, 13*(1), 33–41.

Scharloo, M., Kaptein, A.A., Weinman, J., Hazes, J.M., Willems, L.N., Bergman, W. *et al.* (1998). Illness perceptions, coping and functioning in patients with rheumatoid arthritis, chronic obstructive pulmonary disease and psoriasis. *Journal of Psychosomatic Research, 44*(5), 573–585.

Scheier, M.F. & Carver, C.S. (1992). Effects of optimism on psychological and physical well-being: Theoretical overview and empirical update. *Cognitive Theory and Research, 16*(2), 201–228.

Schiaffino, K.M., Revenson, T.A. & Gibofsky, A. (1991). Assessing the impact of self-efficacy beliefs on adaptation to rheumatoid arthritis. *Arthritis Care and Research, 4*(4), 150–157.

Schneider, S., Schmitt, G., Mau, H., Schmitt, H., Sabo, D. & Richter, W. (2005). Prevalence and correlates of osteoarthritis in Germany: Representative data from the First National Health Survey. *Orthopade, 34*(8), 782–790.

Schoenfeld-Smith, K., Petroski, G.F., Hewett, J.E., Johnson, J.C., Wright, G.E., Smarr, K.L. *et al.* (1996). A biopsychosocial model of disability in rheumatoid arthritis. *Arthritis Care and Research, 9*(5), 368–375.

Schumaker, H.R.E. (1988). *Primer on the rheumatic disease* (9th edn.). Atlanta GA: Arthritis Foundation.

Serbo, B. & Jajic, I. (1991). Relationship of the functional status, duration of the disease and pain intensity and some psychological variables in patients with rheumatoid arthritis. *Clinical Rheumatology, 10*(4), 419–422.

Shapiro, D. (1990). *The bodymind workbook: Exploring how the mind and the body work together*. Shaftesbury: Element.

Sharpe, L., Sensky, T., Brewin, C.R. & Allard, S. (2001). Characteristics of handicap for patients with recent onset rheumatoid arthritis: The validity of the Disease Repercussion Profile. *Rheumatology (Oxford), 40*(10), 1169–1174.

Sharpe, L., Sensky, T., Timberlake, N., Ryan, B., Brewin, C.R. & Allard, S. (2001). A blind, randomised controlled trial of cognitive-behavioural intervention for patients with recent onset rheumatoid arthritis. *Pain, 89*(2–3), 275–283.

Shaw, K. (2001). *A needs assessment of adolescents with juvenile idiopathic arthritis.* Coventry: Coventry University.

Shaw, W.S., Cronan, T.A. & Christie, M.D. (1994). Predictors of attrition in health intervention research among older subjects with osteoarthritis. *Health Psychology, 13*(5), 421–431.

Sheasby, J.E., Barlow, J.H., Cullen, L.A. & Wright, C.C. (2000). Psychometric properties of the Rosenberg Self-Esteem Scale among people with arthritis. *Psychological Reports, 86*(3. pt 2), 1139–1146.

Sheeran, P. & Abraham, C. (1995). The health belief model. In M. Connor & P. Norman (Eds.) *Predicting Health Behaviour* (pp.23–61). Milton Keynes: Open University Press.

Sheeran, P., Abrams, D. & Orbell, S. (1995). Unemployment, self-esteem, and depression: A social comparison theory approach. *Basic and Applied Social Psychology, 17*(1/2), 65–82.

Shifren, K., Park, D.C., Bennett, J.M. & Morrell, R.W. (1999). Do cognitive processes predict mental health in individuals with rheumatoid arthritis? *Journal of Behavioural Medicine, 22*(6), 529–547.

Shuyler, K.S. & Knight, K.M. (2003). What are patients seeking when they turn to the internet? Qualitative content analysis of questions asked by visitors to an orthopaedics website. *Journal of Medical Internet Research, 5*(4), e24.

Silman A.J. & Hochberg M.C. (2001). Rheumatoid arthritis. In A.J. Silman, M.C. Hochberg (Eds.) *Epidemiology of the Rheumatic Diseases* (pp.31–71). Oxford: Oxford University Press.

Silman, A.J., Newman, J. & MacGregor, A.J. (1996). Cigarette smoking increases the risk of rheumatoid arthritis. Results from a nationwide study of disease-discordant twins. *Arthritis & Rheumatism, 39*(5), 732–735.

Silver, E.J., Bauman, L.J. & Ireys, H.T. (1995). Relationships of self-esteem and efficacy to psychological distress in mothers of children with chronic physical illnesses. *Health Psychology, 14*(4), 333–340.

Silvers, I.J., Hovell, M.F., Weisman, M.H. & Mueller, M.R. (1985). Assessing physician/patient perceptions in rheumatoid arthritis. A vital component in patient education. *Arthritis & Rheumatism, 28*(3), 300–307.

Simeoni, E., Bauman, A., Stenmark, J. & O'Brien, J. (1995). Evaluation of a community arthritis program in Australia: Dissemination of a developed program. *Arthritis Care and Research, 8*(2), 102–107.

Sinclair, V.G. & Dowdy, S.W. (2005). Development and validation of the Emotional Intimacy Scale. *Journal of Nursing Measurement, 13*(3), 193–206.

Singer, G.H.S. (2006). Meta-analysis of comparative studies of depression in mothers of children with and without disabilities. *American Journal on Mental Retardation, 111*(3), 155–169.

Skevington, S.M. (1994). Social comparisons in cross-cultural quality of life assessment. *International Journal of Mental Health, 23*(2), 29–47.

Slater, M.A., Doctor, J.N., Pruitt, S.D., Atkinson, J.H. (1997). The clinical significance of behavioral treatment for chronic low back pain: An evaluation of effectiveness. *Pain, 71*(3), 257–263.

Sleath, B., Callahan, L., DeVellis, R.F. & Sloane, P.D. (2005). Patients' perceptions of primary care physicians' participatory decision-making style and communication about complementary and alternative medicine for arthritis. *Journal of Alternative & Complementary Medicine, 11*(3), 449–453.

Sleath, B., Chewning, B., de Vellis, B.M., Weinberger, M., de Vellis, R.F., Tudor, G. *et al.* (2008). Communication about depression during rheumatoid arthritis patient visits. *Arthritis & Rheumatism, 59*(2), 186–191.

Smarr, K.L., Parker, J.C., Wright, G.E., Stucky-Ropp, R.C., Buckelew, S.P., Hoffman, R.W. *et al.* (1997). The importance of enhancing self-efficacy in rheumatoid arthritis. *Arthritis Care and Research, 10*(1), 18–26.

Smedstad, L.M., Moum, T., Vaglum, P. & Kvien, T.K. (1996). The impact of early rheumatoid arthritis on psychological distress. A comparison between 238 patients with RA and 116 matched controls. *Scandinavian Journal of Rheumatology, 25*(6), 377–382.

Smith, B. & Zautra, A.J. (2000). Purpose in life and coping with knee-replacement surgery. *Ocupational Therapy Journal of Research, 20*(S11), 96S–99S.

Smith, B.W. & Zautra, A.J. (2002). The role of personality in exposure and reactivity to interpersonal stress in relation to arthritis disease activity and negative affect in women. *Health Psychology, 21*(1), 81–88.

Smith, B.W. & Zautra, A.J. (2004). The role of purpose in life in recovery from knee surgery. *International Journal of Behavioural Medicine, 11*(4), 197–202.

Smith, C.A. & Wallston, K.A. (1992). Adaptation in patients with chronic rheumatoid arthritis: Application of a general model. *Health Psychology, 11*(3), 151–162.

Smith, T.W., Peck, J.R. & Ward, J.R. (1990). Helplessness and depression in rheumatoid arthritis. *Health Psychology, 9*(4), 377–389.

Smyth, J.M., Stone, A.A., Hurewitz, A. & Kaell, A. (1999). Effects of writing about stressful experiences on symptom reduction in patients with asthma or rheumatoid arthritis: A randomized trial. *Journal of the American Medical Association, 281*(14), 1304–1309.

Soeken, K.L. (2004). Selected CAM therapies for arthritis-related pain: The evidence from systematic reviews. *Clinical Journal of Pain, 20*(1), 13–18.

Southwood, T.R. (writer) (1992). '*Kids Like Us': A disease education video for children with chronic arthritis.* Yorkshire Television Studios.

Southwood, T.R., Barlow, J., Wright, C., Shaw, K., Young, S. & Cheseldine, D. (2000). *Evaluation of disease education for children with chronic arthritis.* Submitted to the Department of Health Physical & Complex Disabilities Programme.

Southwood, T.R. & Malleson, P. (Eds.) (1993). Arthritis in children and adolescents. *Balliere's Clinical Paediatrics. International Practice and Research, 1*(3). London: Bailliere Tindall.

Spector, T.D. & Hochberg, M.C. (1990). The protective effects of the oral contraceptive pill on rheumatoid arthritis: An overview of the analytic epidemiological studies using meta-analysis. *Journal of Clinical Epidemiology, 43*, 1221–1230.

Spector, T.D., Roman, E. & Silman, A.J. (1990). The pill, parity, and rheumatoid arthritis. *Arthritis & Rheumatism, 33*(6), 782–789.

Spector, T.D. & Scott, D.L. (1988). What happens to patients with rheumatoid arthritis? The long-term outcome of treatment. *Clinical Rheumatology, 7*, 315–330.

Spiegel, J.S., Spiegel, T.M., Ward, N.B., Paulus, H.E., Leake, B. & Kane, R.L. (1986). Rehabilitation for rheumatoid arthritis patients. A controlled trial. *Arthritis & Rheumatism, 29*(5), 628–637.

Stefl, M.E., Shear, E.S. & Levinson, J.E. (1989). Summer camps for juveniles with rheumatic disease: Do they make a difference? *Arthritis Care and Research, 2*(1), 10–15.

Stein, D. (1996). *Psychic Healing with Spirit Guides and Angels.* Freedom, CA: The Crossing Press.

Stein, M.B. & Barrett-Connor, E. (2000). Sexual assault and physical health: Findings from a population-based study of older adults. *Psychosomatic Medicine, 62*(6), 838–843.

Stenstrom, C.H., Arge, B. & Sundbom, A. (1997). Home exercise and compliance in inflammatory rheumatic diseases – a prospective clinical trial. *Journal of Rheumatology, 24*(3), 470–476.

Stephens, M.A.P., Martire, L.M., Cremeans-Smith, J.K., Druley, J.A. & Wojno, W.C. (2006). Older women with osteoarthritis and their caregiving husbands: Effects of pain and pain expression on husbands' well-being and support. *Rehabilitation Psychology, 51*(1), 3–12.

Stiles, T.C. (1993). Personal communication. Department of Psychology, Trondheim University, Norway.

Stone, A.A., Smyth, J.M., Kaell, A. & Hurewitz, A. (2000). Structured writing about stressful events: Exploring potential psychological mediators of positive health effects. *Health Psychology, 19*(6), 619–624.

Stone, S.D. (1995). The myth of bodily perfection. *Disability & Society, 10*(4), 413–424.

Straughair, S. & Fawcitt, S. (1992). *The road towards independence: The experiences of young people with arthritis.* London: Arthritis Care.

Sullivan, T., Allegrante, J.P., Peterson, M.G., Kovar, P.A. & MacKenzie, C.R. (1998). One-year follow-up of patients with osteoarthritis of the knee who participated in a program of supervised fitness walking and supportive patient education. *Arthritis Care and Research, 11*, 228–233.

Summers, M.N., Haley, W.E., Reveille, J.D. & Alarcon, G.S. (1988). Radiographic assessment and psychologic variables as predictors of pain and functional impairment in osteoarthritis of the knee or hip. *Arthritis & Rheumatism, 31*(2), 204–209.

Superio-Cabuslay, E., Ward, M.M. & Lorig, K.R. (1996). Patient education interventions in osteoarthritis and rheumatoid arthritis: A meta-analytic comparison with nonsteroidal anti-inflammatory drug treatment. *Arthritis Care and Research, 9*(4), 292–301.

Suurmeijer, T.P., Waltz, M., Moum, T., Guillemin, F., van Sonderen, F.L., Briancon, S. *et al.* (2001). Quality of life profiles in the first years of rheumatoid arthritis: Results from the EURIDISS longitudinal study. *Arthritis & Rheumatism, 45*(2), 111–121.

Suurmeijer, T.P.B.M., Van Sonderen, F.L.P., Krol, B., Doeglas, D.M., Van Den Heuvel, W.J.A. & Sanderman, R. (2005). The relationship between personality, supportive transactions and support satisfaction, and mental health of patients with early rheumatoid arthritis: Results from the Dutch part of the Euridiss study. [peer reviewed]. *Social Indicators Research, 73*(2), 179.

Sweeney, S., Taylor, G. & Calin, A. (2002). The effect of a home based exercise intervention package on outcome in ankylosing spondylitis: A randomized controlled trial. *Journal of Rheumatology, 29*(4), 763–766.

Symmons, D.P., Jones, M., Osborne, J., Sills, J., Southwood, T.R. & Woo, P. (1996). Pediatric rheumatology in the United Kingdom: Data from the British Pediatric Rheumatology Group National Diagnostic Register. *Journal of Rheumatology, 23*(11), 1975–1980.

Taal, E., Johannes, M.A., Rasker. J. *et al.* (1993). Health status, adherence with health recommendations, self-efficacy and social support in patients with rheumatoid arthritis. *Patient Education & Counseling, 20*, 63–76.

Taal, E., Rasker, J.J., Seydel, E.R. & Wiegman, O. (1993). Health status, adherence with health recommendations, self-efficacy and social support in patients with rheumatoid arthritis. *Patient Education & Counseling, 20*(2–3), 63–76.

Taal, E., Rasker, J.J. & Wiegman, O. (1996). Patient education and self-management in the rheumatic diseases: A self-efficacy approach. *Arthritis Care and Research, 9*(3), 229–238.

Taal, E., Riemsma, R.P., Brus, H.L., Seydel, E.R., Rasker, J.J. & Wiegman, O. (1993). Group education for patients with rheumatoid arthritis. *Patient Education & Counseling, 20*(2–3), 177–187.

Taal, E., Seydel, E.R., Rasker, J.J. & Wiegman, O. (1993). Psychosocial aspects of rheumatic diseases: Introduction. *Patient Education & Counseling, 20*(2–3), 55–61.

Tak, S.H. (2006). An insider perspective of daily stress and coping in elders with arthritis. *Orthopaedic Nursing, 25*(2), 127–132.

Tak, S.H. & Hong, S.H. (2005). Use of the internet for health information by older adults with arthritis. *Orthopaedic Nursing, 24*(2), 134–138.

Tak, S.H. & Laffrey, S.C. (2003). Life satisfaction and its correlates in older women with osteoarthritis. *Orthopaedic Nursing, 22*(3), 182–189.

Tallon, D., Chard, J. & Dieppe, P. (2000). Exploring the priorities of patients with osteoarthritis of the knee. *Arthritis Care and Research, 13*(5), 312–319.

Taylor, B. (2001). Promoting self-help strategies by sharing the lived experience of arthritis. *Contemporary Nurse, 10*(1–2), 117–125.

Taylor, L.F., Kee, C.C., King, S.V. & Ford, T.A. (2004). Evaluating the effects of an educational symposium on knowledge, impact, and self-management of older African Americans living with osteoarthritis. *Journal of Community Health & Nursing, 21*(4), 229–238.

Taylor, S.E., Lichtman, R.R. & Wood, J.V. (1984). Attributions, beliefs about control, and adjustment to breast cancer. *Journal of Personality and Social Psychology, 46*(3), 489–502.

Templeton, C.L., Petty, B.J. & Harter, J.L. (1978). Weight-control: A group approach for arthritis clients. *Journal of Nutrition Education, 10*, 33–35.

Tennen, H., Affleck, G., Armeli, S. & Carney, M.A. (2000). A daily process approach to coping. Linking theory, research, and practice. *American Psychologist, 55*(6), 626–636.

Thompson, P.W., Kirwan, J.R. & Barnes, C.G. (1985). Practical results of treatment with disease-modifying antirheumatoid drugs. *British Journal of Rheumatology, 24*(2), 167–175.

Thompson, R.J., Jr., Gustafson, K.E., George, L.K. & Spock, A. (1994). Change over a 12-month period in the psychological adjustment of children and adolescents with cystic fibrosis. *Journal of Pediatric Psychology, 19*(2), 189–203.

Tijhuis, G.J., Zwinderman, A.H., Hazes, J.M., van den Hout, W.B., Breedveld, F.C. & Vliet Vlieland, T.P.M. (2002). A randomised comparison of care provided by a clinical nurse specialist, an inpatient team and a day patient team in rheumatoid arthritis. *Arthritis Care and Research, 47*(5), 525–531.

Timko, C., Stovel, K.W. & Moos, R.H. (1992). Functioning among mothers and fathers of children with juvenile rheumatic disease: A longitudinal study. *Journal of Pediatric Psychology, 17*, 705–724.

Timko, C., Stovel, K.W., Moos, R.H. & Miller, J.J. III. (1992). Adaptation to juvenile rheumatic disease: A controlled evaluation of functional disability with a one-year follow-up. *Health Psychology, 11*(1), 67–76.

Tomlinson, M., Barefoot, J. & Dixon, A. (1986). Intensive in-patient physiotherapy courses improve movement and posture in ankylosing spondylitis. *Physiotherapy, 75*(S).

Tonnes, K.M.A. (1990). Why theorise? Ideology in health education. *Health Education Journal, 49*, 2–6.

Toye, F. (2003). *Need and priority for total knee replacement among people with osteoarthritis.* Coventry: Coventry University.

Treharne, G.J., Kitas, G.D., Lyons, A.C. & Booth, D.A. (2005). Well-being in rheumatoid arthritis: The effects of disease duration and psychosocial factors. *Journal of Health Psychology, 10*(3), 457–474.

Tsai, P.F. (2005). Predictors of distress and depression in elders with arthritic pain. *Journal of Advanced Nursing, 51*(2), 158–165.

Turner, A. (2001) The long term physical and psychosocial consequences of playing professional football. Ph.D. thesis, Coventry University.

Turner, A. (2003). *Osteoarthritis among ex-professional footballers.* Coventry: Coventry University.

Turner, A. & Barlow, J. (2001). Residential workshops for parents of adolescents with juvenile idiopathic arthritis: A preliminary evaluation. *Psychology, Health & Medicine, 6*(4), 447–461.

Turner, A., Williams, R.B. & Barlow, J. (2002). Learning to live with arthritis: The impact of attending a community based arthritis self-management programme on psychological wellbeing. *Health Education, 102*(3), 95–105.

Turner, A.P., Barlow, J.H. & Heathcote-Elliott, C. (2000). Long-term health impact of playing professional football in the United Kingdom. *British Journal of Sports Medicine, 34*(5), 332–336.

Uhlig, T., Smedstad, L.M., Vaglum, P., Moum, T., Gérard, N. & Kvien, T.K. (2000). The course of rheumatoid arthritis and predictors of psychological, physical and radiographic outcome after 5 years of follow-up. *Rheumatology, 39*, 732–741.

Ungerer, J.A., Horgan, B., Chaitow, J. & Champion, G.D. (1988). Psychosocial functioning in children and young adults with juvenile arthritis. *Pediatrics, 81*(2), 195–202.

van der Heide, A., Jacobs, J.W., van Albada-Kuipers, G.A., Kraaimaat, F.W., Geenen, R. & Bijlsma, J.W. (1994). Physical disability and psychological well being in recent onset rheumatoid arthritis. *Journal of Rheumatology, 21*(1), 28–32.

van Dyke, M.M., Parker, J.C., Smarr, K.L., Hewett, J.E., Johnson, G.E., Slaughter, J.R. *et al.* (2004). Anxiety in rheumatoid arthritis. *Arthritis & Rheumatism, 51*(3), 408–412.

van Tubergen, A. & Hidding, A. (2002). Spa and exercise treatment in ankylosing spondylitis: Fact or fancy? *Best Practice & Research Clinical Rheumatology, 16,* 653–666.

van Uden-Kraan, C.F., Drossaert, C.H., Taal, E., Lebrun, C.E.I., Drossaers-Bakker, K.W., Smit, W.M. *et al.* (2008). Coping with somatic illnesses in online support groups: Do the feared disadvantages actually occur? *Computers in Human Behaviour, 24,* 309–324.

van Uden-Kraan, C.F., Drossaert, C.H., Taal, E., Shaw, B.R., Seydel, E.R. & van de Laar, M.A. (2008). Empowering processes and outcomes of participation in online support groups for patients with breast cancer, arthritis, or fibromyalgia. *Qualitative Health Research, 18*(3), 405–417.

Vandenbroucke, J.P., Hazevoet, H.M. & Cats, A. (1984). Survival and cause of death in rheumatoid arthritis: A 25-year prospective followup. *Journal of Rheumatology, 11*(2), 158–161.

Vandvik, I. H. (1990). Mental health and psychosocial functioning in children with recent onset of rheumatic disease. *Journal of Child Psychology and Psychiatry, 31,* 961–971.

Vandvik, I.H. & Eckblad, G. (1991). Mothers of children with recent onset of rheumatic disease: Associations between maternal distress, psychosocial variables, and the disease of the children. *Journal of Development & Behavioural Paediatrics, 12*(2), 84–91.

Varni, J.W. & Wallander, J.L. (1984). Adherence to health-related regimens for pediatric chronic disorders. *Clinical Psychology Review, 4,* 585–596.

Varni, J.W., Wilcox, K.T. & Hanson, V. (1988). Mediating effects of family social support on child psychological adjustment in juvenile rheumatoid arthritis. *Health Psychology, 7*(5), 421–431.

Vaughan, S., Schumm, J.S. & Sinagub, J. (1996). *Focus group interviews in education and psychology.* Thousand Oaks, CA: Sage.

Vecchio, P.C. (1994). Attitudes to alternative medicine by rheumatology outpatient attenders. *Journal of Rheumatology, 21*(1), 145–147.

Vingard, E. (1994). Sport and the development of osteoarthrosis of the hip. *Sports Medicine, 18*(1), 1–3.

Vinokur, A.D., Price, R.H. & Caplan, R.D. (1996). Hard times and hurtful partners: How financial strain affects depression and relationship satisfaction of unemployed persons and their spouses. *Journal of Personality and Social Psychology, 71*(1), 166–179.

von Weiss, R.T., Rapoff, M.A., Varni, J.W., Lindsley, C.B., Olson, N.Y., Madson, K.L. *et al.* (2002). Daily hassles and social support as predictors of adjustment in children with pediatric rheumatic disease. *Journal of Pediatric Psychology, 27*(2), 155–165.

Wainapel, S.F., Thomas, A.D. & Kahan, B.S. (1998). Use of alternative therapies by rehabilitation outpatients. *Archives of Physical Medicine Rehabilitation, 79*, 1003–1005.

Waite-Jones, J.M. & Madill, A. (2007). Amplified ambivalence: Having a sibling with juvenile idiopathic arthritis. *Psychology and Health* (iFirst), 1–16.

Walco, G.A., Varni, J.W. & Ilowite, N. (1992). Cognitive-behavioural pain management in children with juvenile rheumatoid arthritis. *Pediatrics, 2*(89), 1075–1079.

Walker, L.S., Ford, M.B. & Donald, W.D. (1987). Cystic fibrosis and family stress: Effects of age and severity of illness. *Pediatrics, 79*(2), 239–246.

Wallander, J.L. & Varni, J.W. (1989). Social support and adjustment in chronically ill and handicapped children. *American Journal of Community Psychology, 17*(2), 185–201.

Wallston, K.A. (1989). Assessment of control in health care settings. In A. Steptoe and A. Appels (Eds.) *Stress, Personal Control and Health* (pp.85–106). London: John Wiley.

Wallston, K.A. (1992). Hocus-pocus, the focus isn't strictly on locus: Rotter's social learning theory modified for health. *Cognitive Theory and Research, 16*(2), 183–199.

Wallston, K.A. (1993). Psychological control and its impact in the management of rheumatological disorders. *Baillieres Clinical Rheumatology, 7*(2), 281–295.

Wallston, K.A., Wallston, B.S. & deVellis, B.M. (1978). Development of a multidimensional health locus of control (MHLC) scale. *Health Education Monographs, 6*, 160–170.

Wallston, K.A., Wallston, B.S., Smith, S. & Dobbins, C.J. (1987). Perceived control and health. *Current Psychological Research and Reviews, 6*, 5–25.

Walsh, J.D., Blanchard, E.B., Kremer, J.M. & Blanchard, C.G. (1999). The psychosocial effects of rheumatoid arthritis on the patient and the well partner. *Behaviour Research & Therapy, 37*(3), 259–271.

Ward, M.M. & Leigh, J.P. (1993). Marital status and the progression of functional disability in patients with rheumatoid arthritis. *Arthritis and Rheumatism, 36*(5), 581–588.

Ware, J.E., Snow, K.K., Kosinski, M. & Gandek, B. (1993). *SF-36® Health Survey Manual and Interpretation Guide*. Boston, MA: New England Medical Center, the Health Institute.

Warsi, A., LaValley, M.P., Wang, P.S., Avorn, J. & Solomon, D.H. (2003). Arthritis self-management education programs: A meta-analysis of the effect on pain and disability. *Arthritis & Rheumatism, 48*(8), 2207–2213.

Wegener, S.T. (1991). Psychosocial aspects of rheumatic disease: The developing biopsychosocial framework. *Current Opinion in Rheumatology, 3*(2), 300–304.

Wehmeyer, M.L., Sands, D.J., Doll, B. & Palmer, S. (1997). The development of self-determination and implications for educational interventions with students with disabilities. *International Journal of Disability, Development and Education, 44*(4), 305–328.

Weinberger, M., Tierney, W.M. & Booher, P. (1989). Common problems experienced by adults with osteoarthritis. *Arthritis Care and Research, 2*(3), 94–100.

Weinberger, M., Tierney, W.M., Booher, P. & Katz, B.P. (1989). Can the provision of information to patients with osteoarthritis improve functional status? A randomized, controlled trial. *Arthritis and Rheumatism, 32,* 1577–1583.

Weiner, C.L. (1975). The burden of rheumatoid arthritis. In A.L. Strauss (Ed.) *Chronic illness and the quality of life* (pp.88–98). St Louis: C.V. Mosby.

Weinman, J. (1990). Providing written information for patients: Psychological considerations. *Journal of the Royal Society of Medicine, 83*(5), 303–305.

Weiss, K.A., Schiaffino, K.M. & Ilowite, N. (2001). Predictors of sibling relationship characteristics in youth with juvenile chronic arthritis. *Children's Health Care, 30,* 67–77.

Wells, K.B., Golding, J.M. & Burnam, M.A. (1988). Psychiatric disorder in a sample of the general population with and without chronic medical conditions. *American Journal of Psychiatry, 145*(8), 976–981.

Wells, K.B., Golding, J.M. & Burnam, M.A. (1989). Affective, substance use, and anxiety disorders in persons with arthritis, diabetes, heart disease, high blood pressure, or chronic lung conditions. *General Hospital Psychiatry, 11*(5), 320–327.

Wetherall, M.A., Byrne-Davis, L., Dieppe, P., Donovan, J., Brookes, S., Byron, M. *et al.* (2005). Effects of emotional disclosure on psychological and physiological outcomes in patients with rheumatoid arthritis: An exploratory home-based study. *Journal of Health Psychology, 10*(2), 277–285.

White, P.H. & Shear, E.S. (1992). Transition/job readiness for adolescents with juvenile arthritis and other chronic illness. *Journal of Rheumatology Supplement, 33,* 23–27.

WHO. (1993). *The ICD–10 classification of mental and behavioural disorders: Diagnostic criteria for research (DCR–10).* Geneva: World Health Organization.

Wilkins, K.E. (200). *A psychological model for the impact of rheumatoid arthritis on well-being.* Detroit: Wayne State University Press.

Williams, G.H. (1989). Hope for the humblest? The role of self-help in chronic illness: The case of ankylosing spondylitis. *Sociology of Health & Illness, 11*(2), 135–159.

Wolfe, F., Anderson, J.J. & Hawley, D.J. (1994). Rates and predictors of work disability in rheumatoid arthritis: Importance of disease, psychological and workplace factors (abstract). *Arthritis and Rheumatism, 37*(S9), S231.

Wolfe, F., Hawley, D.J. & Wilson, K. (1996). The prevalence and meaning of fatigue in rheumatic disease. *Journal of Rheumatology, 23,* 1407–1417.

Wolfe, F., Mitchell, D.M., Sibley, J.T., Fries, J.F., Bloch, D.A., Williams, C.A. *et al.* (1994). The mortality of rheumatoid arthritis. *Arthritis & Rheumatism, 37*(4), 481–494.

Wolfe, F., Zhao, S. & Lane, N. (2000). Preference for nonsteroidal anti-inflammatory drugs over acetaminophen by rheumatic disease patients: A survey of 1,799 patients with osteoarthritis, rheumatoid arthritis, and fibromyalgia. *Arthritis & Rheumatism, 43*(2), 378–385.

Wong, A.L., Harker, J.O., Lau, V.P., Shatzel, S. & Port, L.H. (2004). Spanish Arthritis Empowerment Program: A dissemination and effectiveness study. *Arthritis & Rheumatism, 51*(3), 332–336.

Woolhead, G.M., Carr, A., Wilkinson, M. *et al.* (1996). Expectations of treatment and its outcome in patients awaiting joint replacement surgery and general orthopaedic outpatient referrals. *Arthritis and Rheumatism, 38,* S174.

Wordsworth, B.P. & Mowat, A.G. (1986). A review of 100 patients with ankylosing spondylitis with particular reference to socio-economic effects. *British Journal of Rheumatology, 25*(2), 175–180.

Wright, G.E., Parker, J.C., Smarr, K.L., Schoenfeld-Smith, K., Buckelew, S.P., Slaughter, J.R. *et al.* (1996). Risk factors for depression in rheumatoid arthritis. *Arthritis Care and Research, 9*(4), 264–272.

Wright, V. & Hopkins, R. (1990). Patients' perceptions of staff in a department of rheumatology. *British Journal of Rheumatology, 29*(5), 374–376.

Xin, L. (2006). The indirect costs of arthritis resulting from unemployment, reduced performance, and occupational changes while at work. *Medical Care, 44*(4), 304–310.

Yelin, E. (1992). Arthritis: The cumulative impact of a common chronic condition. *Arthritis & Rheumatism, 35*(5), 489–497.

Yelin, E. (1998). The economics of osteoarthritis. In K. Brandt, L. Doherty & L. Lomander (Eds.) *Osteoarthritis* (pp.23–30). New York: Oxford University Press.

Yelin, E., Henke, C. & Epstein, W. (1987). The work dynamics of the person with rheumatoid arthritis. *Arthritis & Rheumatism, 30*(5), 507–512.

Yelin, E., Lubeck, D., Holman, H. & Epstein, W. (1987). The impact of rheumatoid arthritis and osteoarthritis: The activities of patients with rheumatoid arthritis and osteoarthritis compared to controls. *Journal of Rheumatology, 14*(4), 710–717.

Yip, Y.B., Sit, J.W., Fung, K.K., Wong, D.Y., Chong, S.Y., Chung, L.H. *et al.* (2007). Impact of an arthritis self-management programme with an added exercise component for osteoarthritic knee sufferers on improving pain, functional outcomes, and use of health care services: An experimental study. *Patient Education & Counseling, 65*(1), 113–121.

Young, L.D. (1992). Psychological factors in rheumatoid arthritis. *Journal of Consulting & Clinical Psychology, 60*(4), 619–627.

Zaadstra, B.M., Seidell, J.C., Van Noord, P.A., te Velde, E.R., Habbema, J.D., Vrieswijk, B. *et al.* (1993). Fat and female fecundity: Prospective study of effect of body fat distribution on conception rates. *British Medical Journal, 306*(6876), 484–487.

Zant, J.L., Dekker-Saeys, A.J., Van den Burgh, I.C., Kolman, A. & Van der Stadt, R.J. (1982). Sthenia, ambition and educational level in patients suffering from ankylosing spondylitis: A controlled study of personality features as compared to rheumatoid arthritis and unspecified low back pain. *Clinical Rheumatology, 1*(4), 243–250.

Zautra, A.J., Burleson, M.H., Smith, C.A., Blalock, S.J., Wallston, K.A., DeVellis, R.F. *et al.* (1995). Arthritis and perceptions of quality of life: An examination of positive and negative affect in rheumatoid arthritis patients. *Health Psychology, 14*(5), 399–408.

Zautra, A.J., Hamilton, N.A. & Burke, H.M. (1999). Comparison of stress responses in women with two types of chronic pain: Fibromyalgia and osteoarthritis. *Cognitive Theory and Research, 23*(2), 209–230.

Zautra, A.J., Hoffman, J.M., Matt, K.S., Yocum, D., Potter, P.T., Castro, W.L. *et al.* (1998). An examination of individual differences in the relationship between interpersonal stress and disease activity among women with rheumatoid arthritis. *Arthritis Care and Research, 11*(4), 271–279.

Zautra, A.J., Johnson, L.M. & Davis, M.C. (2005). Positive affect as a source of resilience for women in chronic pain. *Journal of Consulting & Clinical Psychology, 73*(2), 212–220.

Zautra, A.J., Okun, M.A., Robinson, S.E., Lee, D., Roth, S.H. & Emmanual, J. (1989). Life stress and lymphocyte alterations among patients with rheumatoid arthritis. *Health Psychology, 8*(1), 1–14.

Zautra, A.J. & Smith, B.W. (2001). Depression and reactivity to stress in older women with rheumatoid arthritis and osteoarthritis. *Psychosomatic Medicine, 63*(4), 687–696.

Zautra, A.J., Yocum, D.C., Villanueva, I., Smith, B., Davis, M.C., Attrep, J. *et al.* (2004). Immune activation and depression in women with rheumatoid arthritis. *Journal of Rheumatology, 31*(3), 457–463.

Zigmond, A.S. & Snaith, R.P. (1983). The hospital anxiety and depression scale. *Acta Psychiatrica Scandinavica, 67*(6), 361–370.

Zimmerman, M.A. (1990). Toward a theory of learned hopefulness: A structural model analysis of participation and empowerment. *Journal of Research in Personality, 24*, 71–86.

Zochling, J., March, L., Lapsley, H., Cross, M., Tribe, K. & Brooks, P. (2004). Use of complementary medicines for osteoarthritis: A prospective study. *Annals of the Rheumatic Diseases, 63*(5), 549–554.

Zochling, J., van der Heijde, D., Dougados, M. & Braun, J. (2006). Current evidence for the management of ankylosing spondylitis: A systematic literature review for the ASAS/EULAR management recommendations in ankylosing spondylitis. *Annals of the Rheumatic Diseases, 65*(4), 423–432.

Index of Citations

Abbott, C.A., Helliwell, P.S. &
    Chamberlain, M.A. (1994) 16
Abdel-Nasser, A.M., Abd El-Azim, S.,
    Taal, E., El-Badawy, S.A.,
    Rasker, J.J. & Valkenburg, H.A.
    (1998) 110
Achenbach, T.M. & Edelbrock, C.S.
    (1983) 90
Adab, P., Rankin, E.C., Witney, A.G.,
    Miles, K.A., Bowman, S., Kitas,
    G.D. et al. (2004) 153
Adam, V., St-Pierre, Y., Fautrel, B.,
    Clarke, A.E., Duffy, C.M. &
    Penrod, J.R. (2005) 89
Affleck, G. & Tennen, H. (1991) 50
Affleck, G., Tennen, H. & Apter, A.
    (2001) 30
Affleck, G., Tennen, H., Pfeiffer, C. &
    Fifield, J. (1987) 74
Affleck, G., Tennen, H., Pfeiffer, C. &
    Fifield, J. (1998) 108
Affleck, G., Tennen, H., Urrows, S. &
    Higgins, P. (1994) 34
Affleck, G., Urrows, S., Tennen, H. &
    Higgins, P. (1992) 23
Al-Allaf, A.W., Sanders, P.A., Ogston,
    S.A. & Marks, J.S. (2001) 11
Albers, J.M., Kuper, H.H., van Riel,
    P.L., Prevoo, M.L., van 't Hof,

M.A., van Gestel, A.M. et al.
    (1999) 117
Allaire, S., Wolfe, F., Niu, J., Lavalley,
    M. & Michaud, K. (2005) 119
Allegrante, J.P., Kovar, P.A.,
    MacKenzie, C.R., Peterson, M.G.
    & Gutin, B. (1993) 168, 198
Anderson, K.O., Bradley, L.A.,
    Young, L.D., McDaniel, L.K. &
    Wise, C.M. (1985) 32, 43
Andersson, S., Nilsson, B., Hessel, T.,
    Saraste, M., Noren, A., Stevens-
    Andersson, A. et al. (1989) 8
Ang, D.C., Choi, H., Kroenke, K. &
    Wolfe, F. (2005) 69
Ansani, N.T., Fedutes-Henderson, B.,
    Weber, R., Smith, R., Dean, J.,
    Vogt, M. et al. (2006) 157
Ansani, N.T., Vogt, M., Henderson,
    B.A., McKaveney, T.P., Weber,
    R.J., Smith, R.B. et al. (2005)
    157
Applebaum, K.A., Blanchar, E.B.,
    Hickling, E.J. & Alfonso, M.
    (1988) 162
April, K.T., Feldman, D.E., Platt, R.W.
    & Duffy, C.M. (2006) 91
Arnett, F.C. (1989) 14
Arthritis Foundation (1999) 218

Backman, C.L., Kennedy, S.M.,
    Chalmers, A. & Singer, J.
    (2004) 118
Badley, E.M. & Tennant, A. (1993) 2
Badley, E.M. & Wood, P.H.
    (1979) 113–14
Bandura, A. (1977) 75–6, 79, 147, 176,
    177
Barlow, J. & Cullen, L. (1996) 36
Barlow, J., Cullen, L.A., Davis, S. &
    Williams, R.B. (1997) 52, 114
Barlow, J., Cullen, L.A. & Rowe, I.F.
    (1999) 40
Barlow, J., Cullen, L.A. & Rowe, I.F.
    (2001) 67
Barlow, J. & Harrison, K. (1996) 113,
    120, 150
Barlow, J., Harrison, K. & Shaw, K.
    (1998) 1, 38, 56, 57, 60, 62, 88, 92,
    97, 114, 155
Barlow, J., Macey, S.J., Pugh, M. &
    Struthers, G. (1994) 74
Barlow, J., Macey, S.J. & Struthers, G.
    (1993) 7, 37, 42, 66, 69, 77, 118
Barlow, J. & Pennington, D.C.
    (1996) 153
Barlow, J., Pennington, D.C. &
    Bishop, P.E. (1997) 2, 151, 153, 155
Barlow, J., Shaw, K.L. & Southwood,
    T.R. (1998) 147
Barlow, J., Turner, A. & Wright, C.
    (1998a) 123, 180
Barlow, J., Turner, A. & Wright, C.
    (1998b) 180
Barlow, J. & Williams, B. (1999). 53, 189
Barlow, J., Williams, R.B. & Wright, C.
    (1997a) 179, 181
Barlow, J., Wright, C., Carr, A.,
    Hughes, R., Sheasby, J.E. &
    Stowers, K. (2001) 135, 138
Barlow, J., Wright, C. & Krol, T.
    (2001) 43, 66, 121, 123, 191

Barlow, J., Wright, C., Shaw, K.,
    Luqmani, R. & Wyness, I.J.
    (2002) 94, 97
Barlow, J., Wright, S. & Wright, C.
    (2000) 193
Barlow, J.H. (1998) 139, 170, 211
Barlow, J.H. (2001) 174
Barlow, J.H. & Barefoot, J. (1996) 37,
    52, 79, 118, 144, 145, 171, 172
Barlow, J.H., Bishop, P.E. &
    Pennington, D.C. (1996) 26, 154,
    155, 200
Barlow, J.H. & Cullen, L. (1996) 114
Barlow, J.H., Cullen, L.A., Foster,
    N.E., Harrison, K. & Wade, M.
    (1999) 37, 66, 102, 111
Barlow, J.H., Cullen, L.A. & Rowe, I.F.
    (1999) 67, 151
Barlow, J.H. & Ellard, D.R. (2006) 91
Barlow, J.H. & Ellard, D.R. (2007)
    212
Barlow, J.H., Shaw, K.L. & Harrison,
    K. (1999) 56, 62, 63, 64, 130, 154
Barlow, J.H., Shaw, K.L. & Wright,
    C.C. (2000) 96
Barlow, J.H., Shaw, K.L. & Wright,
    C.C. (2001) 57, 95
Barlow, J.H., Turner, A.P. & Wright,
    C.C. (1998) 123
Barlow, J.H., Turner, A.P. & Wright,
    C.C. (2000) 123, 180, 181
Barlow, J.H., Williams, B. & Wright,
    C.C. (1999) 177, 179, 214
Barlow, J.H., Wright, C.C., Williams,
    B. & Keat, A. (2001) 46, 49, 77,
    116, 118, 119, 122, 124–5
Baron, R.M. & Kenny, D.A. (1986) 72
Barrett, E.M., Scott, D.G., Wiles, N.J.
    & Symmons, D.P. (2000) 2
Basler, H.D. (1993) 144, 162, 185
Beales, J.G., Holt, P.J., Keen, J.H. &
    Mellor, V.P. (1983) 58

Beckham, J.C., Burker, E.J., Rice, J.R.
& Talton, S.L. (1995) 107
Beckham, J.C., Rice, J.R., Talton, S.L.
& Helms, M.J. (1994) 76
Bediako, S.M. & Friend, R. (2004)
105
Belot, H. (1999) 20
Belza, B.L., Henke, C.J., Yelin, E.H.,
Epstein, W.V. & Gilliss, C.L.
(1993) 68
Benjamin, C.M. (1990) 16
Beresford, B. (1995) 146
Berkanovic, E., Oster, P. & Wong,
W.K. (1996) 11
Bermas, B.L., Tucker, J.S., Winkelman,
D.K. & Katz, J.N. (2000) 84, 109
Billings, A.G., Moos, R.H., Miller, J.J.
& Gottlieb, J. (1987) 41, 88, 91
Blalock, S.J., deVellis, B.M. & deVellis,
R.F. (1989) 50
Blalock, S.J., deVellis, B.M., deVellis,
R.F. & Sauter, S.H. (1988) 86
Blalock, S.J., deVellis, B.M., Holt, K. &
Hahn, P.M. (1993) 85
Blalock, S.J., deVellis, R.F., Brown,
G.K. & Wallston, K.A. (1989) 67
Blaxter, M. (1983) 64, 65, 213
Boonen, A. (2002) 119
Boonen, A., Chorus, A., Miedema, H.,
van der Heijde, D., van der
Tempel, H. & van der Linden, S.
(2001) 119
Booth, G.C. (1937) 28
Bradford, R. (1994) 94, 98
Bradley, L.A. (1989) 34, 141
Bradley, L.A. (1996) 162
Bradley, L.A., Young, L.D., Anderson,
K.O., Turner, R.A., Agudelo,
C.A., McDaniel, L.K. *et al.*
(1987) 162
Brekke, M., Hjortdahl, P. & Kvien,
T.K. (2001a) 76

Brekke, M., Hjortdahl, P. & Kvien,
T.K. (2001b) 137
Brekke, M., Hjortdahl, P., Thelle, D.S.
& Kvien, T.K. (1999) 77
Brenner, G.F., Melamed, B.G. &
Panush, R.S. (1994) 29–30
Breuer, G.S., Orbach, H., Elkayam,
O., Berkun, Y., Paran, D., Mates,
M. *et al.* (2005) 26
Breuer, G.S., Orbach, H., Elkayam,
O., Berkun, Y., Paran, D., Mates,
M. *et al.* (2006) 23, 25
Brewerton, D.A., Hart, F.D., Nicholls,
A., Caffrey, M., James, D.C. &
Sturrock, R.D. (1973) 14
Britton, C. (2000) 160
Britton, C. & Moore, A. (2002a) 113,
130
Britton, C. & Moore, A. (2002b) 113,
130
Brown, G.K. (1990) 69
Brown, G.K., Wallston, K.A. &
Nicassio, P.M. (1989) 81, 107
Brus, H., van de Laar, M., Taal, E.,
Rasker, J. & Wiegman, O.
(1999) 143
Buckelew, S.P., Shutty, M.S., Jr.,
Hewett, J., Landon, T., Morrow,
K. & Frank, R.G. (1990) 74
Bulstrode, S.J., Barefoot, J., Harrison,
R.A. & Clarke, A.K. (1987) 15
Burckhardt, C.S. (1985) 110
Burckhardt, C.S., Lorig, K., Moncur,
C., Melvin, J., Beardmore, T.,
Boyd, M. *et al.* (1994) 147–8
Burton, W., Morrison, A., Maclean, R.
& Ruderman, E. (2006) 116, 117
Bury, M. (1991) 51
Buszewicz, M., Rait, G., Griffin, M.,
Nazareth, I., Patel, A., Atkinson,
A. *et al.* (2006) 180, 181
Buunk, B.P. (1995) 178

Callahan, L. & Pincus, T. (1988) 11
Callahan, L.F., Bloch, D.A. & Pincus,
    T. (1992) 66, 119
Callahan, L.F., Kaplan, M.R. &
    Pincus, T. (1991) 69
Carette, S., Graham, D., Little, H.,
    Rubenstein, J. & Rosen, P.
    (1983) 118
Carlisle, A.C., John, A.M., Fife-Schaw,
    C. & Lloyd, M. (2005) 81
Cassidy, J. & Petty, R. (1990) 16
Cassileth, B.R., Lusk, E. J., Strouse,
    T.B., Miller, D.S., Brown, L.L.,
    Cross, P.A. *et al.* (1984) 67
Castenada, D., Bigatti, S. & Cronan,
    T.A. (1998) 29
Chandrashekara, S., Anilkumar, T. &
    Jamuna, S. (2002) 25
Chaney, J.M., Uretsky, D., Mullins, L.,
    Doppler, M., Palmer, W., Wees, S.
    et al. (1996) 39
Charles, C., Whelan, T. & Gafni, A.
    (1999) 128
Chehata, J.C., Hassell, A.B., Clarke,
    S.A., Mattey, D.L., Jones, M.A.,
    Jones, P.W. *et al.* (2001) 12
Chipperfield, J. & Greenslade, L.
    (1999) 75
Chorus, A.M., Miedema, H.S.,
    Boonen, A. & van der Linden, S.
    (2003) 124
Clark, N., Becker, M., Janz, N. &
    Lorig, K. (1991) 174
Claudpierre, P. (2005) 16
Cohen, J.L., Sauter, S.V., deVellis, R.F.
    & deVellis, B.M. (1986) 175
Conrad, P. (1990) 43
Crawford, J.R., Henry, J.D., Crombie,
    C. & Taylor, E.P. (2001) 95
Creed, F. & Ash, G. (1992) 7, 37, 66, 69
Croft, P., Cooper, C., Wickham, C. &
    Coggon, D. (1992) 8

Cronan, T.A., Hay, M., Groessl, E.,
    Bigatti, S., Gallagher, R. &
    Tomita, M. (1998) 166, 205
Cullen, L.A. & Barlow, J.H.
    (1998) 193
Curtis, R., Groarke, A., Coughlan, R.
    & Gsel, A. (2005) 87
Dagfinrud, H., Kjeken, I., Mowinckel,
    P., Hagen, K.B. & Kvien, T.K.
    (2005) 47
Daltroy, L.H., Eaton, L., Hashimoto,
    H. & Liang, M.H. (1995) 142
Daltroy, L.H., Larson, M.G., Eaton,
    H.M., Partridge, A.J., Pless, I.B.,
    Rogers, M.P. *et al.* (1992) 41, 92,
    94
Damush, T.M., Perkins, S.M.,
    Mikesky, A.E., Roberts, M. &
    O'Dea, J. (2005) 145
Danoff-Burg, S., Agee, J.D.,
    Romanoff, N.R., Kremer, J.M. &
    Strosberg, J.M. (2006) 164
Danoff-Burg, S. & Revenson, T.A.
    (2005) 106
Danoff-Burg, S., Revenson, T.A.,
    Trudeau, K.J. & Paget, S.A.
    (2004) 29, 84
De Jong, O., Hopman-Rock, M., Tak,
    E. & Klazinga, N. (2004) 217
De Roos, A.J. & Callahan, L.F.
    (1999) 117
Dekker, J., Boot, B., van der Woude,
    L.H. & Bijlsma, J.W. (1992) 82,
    128
Dekker, J., Tola, P., Aufdemkampe, G.
    & Winckers, M. (1993) 70
Dekker-Saeys, A.J. (1976) 37
Dekkers, J.C., Geenen, R., Evers,
    A.W., Kraaimaat, F.W., Bijlsma,
    J.W. & Godaert, G.L. (2001)
    35–6

Demange, V., Guillemin, F.,
Baumann, M., Suurmeijer, T.P.,
Moum, T., Doeglas, D. et al.
(2004) 106
Deyo, R.A. (1982) 142
Dickens, C. & Creed, F. (2001) 68, 70,
215
Dickens, C., McGowan, L., Clark-
Carter, D. & Creed, F. (2002) 67
Diehl, S.F., Moffitt, K.A. & Wade, S.M.
(1991) 146
Dildy, S.M.P. (1992) 55
DiMatteo, M., Lepper, H. & Croghan,
T. (2000) 143
Dishman, R.K. (1982) 142
Dixon, K.E., Keefe, F.J., Scipio, C.D.,
Perri, L.M. & Abernethy, A.P.
(2007) 200, 201, Tab. 8.2
Doeglas, D., Suurmeijer, T., Krol, B.,
Sanderman, R., van Rijswijk, M.
& van Leeuwen, M. (1994) 108
Doeglas, D., Suurmeijer, T., Krol, B.,
Sanderman, R., van Leeuwen, M.
& van Rijswijk, M. (1995) 117
Doeglas, D.M., Suurmeijer, T.P., van
den Heuvel, W.J., Krol, B., van
Rijswijk, M.H., van Leeuwen,
M.A. et al. (2004) 108
Donovan, J.L. & Blake, D.R.
(1992) 142
Doyle, D. (1999) 204
Duff, I.F., Carpenter, J.O. & Neukom,
J.E. (1974) 131
Duffy, C.M. (2005) 17
Dwyer, K.A. (1997) 76

Eberhardt, K., Larsson, B.M. &
Nived, K. (1993) 39
Edwards, J., Mulherin, D., Ryan, S. &
Jester, R. (2001) 132, 133
Edwards, S. (2002) 199
Eiser, C. (1993) 210

Elder, R.G. (1973) 9
Elfant, E., Gali, E. & Perlmuter, L.
(1999) 96
Emmons, R.A. & McCullough, M.E.
(2003) 214
Ennett, S.T., DeVellis, B.M., Earp, J.A.,
Kredich, D., Warren, R.W. &
Wilhelm, C.L. (1991) 41
Eskanazi, D. (1998) 22
Evers, A.W., Kraaimaat, F.W., Geenen,
R. & Bijlsma, J.W. (1997) 40
Evers, A.W., Kraaimaat, F.W.,
Geenen, R., Jacobs, J.W. &
Bijlsma, J.W. (2002) 29, 106
Evers, A.W., Kraaimaat, F.W.,
Geenen, R., Jacobs, J.W. &
Bijlsma, J.W. (2003) 106

Falkenbach, A. (2003) 145
Faucett, J. & Levine, J. (1991) 105
Fautrel, B., Adam, V., St-Pierre, Y.,
Joseph, L., Clarke, A.E. &
Penrod, J.R. (2002) 25
Feifel, H., Strack, S. & Nagy, V.T.
(1987) 78
Feldman, D.E., Duffy, C., De Civita,
M., Malleson, P., Philibert, L.,
Gibbon, M. et al. (2004) 23, 25
Felson, D. (1994) 8, 119
Felson, D., Anderson, J.J., Naimark,
A., Hannan, M., Kannel, W. &
Meenan, R.F. (1989) 9
Felson, D.T., Zhang, Y., Anthony, J.M.,
Naimark, A. & Anderson, J.J.
(1992) 9
Felton, B.J. & Revenson, T.A.
(1984) 81
Felton, B.J., Revenson, T.A. &
Hinrichsen, G.A. (1984) 40
Fifield, J., McQuillan, J., Armeli, S.,
Tennen, H., Reisine, S. & Affleck,
G. (2004) 122

Fisher, P. & Ward, A. (1994) 23
Fitzpatrick, R., Newman, S., Archer,
    R. & Shipley, M. (1991) 43
Fitzpatrick, R., Newman, S., Lamb, R.
    & Shipley, M. (1988) 108, 111
Flor, H., Haag, G. & Turk, D.C. (1986)
    22
Focht, B.C., Gauvin, L. & Rejeski, W.J.
    (2004) 144
Foster, H.E., Eltringham, M.S., Kay,
    L.J., Friswell, M., Abinun, M. &
    Myers, A. (2007) 38
Foster, H.E., Marshall, N., Myers, A.,
    Dunkley, P. & Griffiths, I.D.
    (2003) 90
Fries, J.F., Carey, C. & McShane, D.J.
    (1997) 185
Fries, J.F., Spitz, P., Kraines, R.G. &
    Holman, H.R. (1980) 2
Fries, J.F., Williams, C.A., Morfeld,
    D., Singh, G. & Sibley, J. (1996)
    2
Fyrand, L., Moum, T., Finset, A. &
    Glennas, A. (2002) 106

Geenen, R., Van Middendorp, H. &
    Bijlsma, J.W. (2006) 36
Geirdal, O. (1990) 102
Gignac, M.A., Badley, E.M., Lacaille,
    D., Cott, C.C., Adam, P. & Anis,
    A.H. (2004) 123
Gignac, M.A., Cott, C. & Badley, E.M.
    (2000) 85
Gignac, M.A., Sutton, D. & Badley,
    E.M. (2006) 123
Glazier, R.H., Badley, E.M., Lineker,
    S.C., Wilkins, A.L. & Bell, M.J.
    (2005) 134
Goemaere, S., Ackerman, C.,
    Goethals, K., De Keyser, F., Van
    der Straeten, C., Verbruggen, G.
    et al. (1990) 7

Goeppinger, J., Armstrong, B.,
    Schwartz, T., Ensley, D. & Brady,
    T.J. (2007) 184
Gonzalez, A., Maradit Kremers, H.,
    Crowson, C.S., Nicola, P.J.,
    Davis, J.M. III, Therneau, T.M.
    et al. (2007) 12
Gonzalez, V.M., Goeppinger, J. &
    Lorig, K. (1990) 176
Gorter, S., van der Linden, S. &
    Brauer, J. (2001) 136
Gran, J.T. & Husby, G. (1990) 15
Gran, J.T. & Husby, G. (2003) 14
Grant, M. & Barlow, J. (2000) 104
Griffin, K.W., Friend, R., Kaell, A.T. &
    Bennett, R.S. (2001) 83, 109

Hackett, J. (2003) 113
Hagen, L.E., Schneider, R., Stephens,
    D., Modrusan, D. & Feldman,
    B.M. (2003) 25
Hainsworth, J. & Barlow, J.
    (2003) 214
Hakkinen, A., Kautiainen, H.,
    Hannonen, P., Ylinen, J.,
    Makinen, H. & Sokka, T.
    (2006) 13
Hall, J.A., Milburn, M.A., Roter, D.L.
    & Daltroy, L.H. (1998) 137
Hamilton-West, K.E. & Quine, L.
    (2007) 164
Hampson, S.E., Glasgow, R.E. &
    Zeiss, A.M. (1994) 54
Harris, J.A., Newcomb, A.F. &
    Gewanter, H.L. (1991) 93
Harrison, H. & Barlow, J. (1996) 57
Haugli, L., Strand, E. & Finset, A.
    (2004) 129
Hawley, D.J. & Wolfe, F. (1993) 67
Hay, L. (1984) 19
Haynes, R.B., Taylor, W.D. & Sackett,
    D.L. (Eds.) (1979) 141

Hazes, J.M. & Silman, A.J. (1990) 11
Heckhausen, J. & Schulz, R. (1995) 190
Heiberg, T. & Kvien, T.K. (2002) 128
Hendry, M., Williams, N.H.,
Markland, D., Wilkinson, C. &
Maddison, P. (2006) 145
Herman, C.J., Allen, P., Hunt, W.C.,
Prasad, A. & Brady, T.J.
(2004) 23, 25
Hidding, A., van der Linden, S.,
Boers, M., Gielen, X., de Witte,
L., Kester, A. *et al.* (1993) 15
Hill, J. (1992) 134
Hill, J. (1997) 134, 138
Hill, J., Bird, H.A., Hopkins, R.,
Lawton, C. & Wright, V.
(1991) 151
Hirano, P.C., Laurent, D.D. & Lorig,
K. (1994) 198
Hirsch, B.J., Moos, R.H. & Reischl,
T.M. (1985) 111
Hollander, J. & Comroe, B. (1949) 7
Holman, H. & Lorig, K. (1992) 176
Hughes, S.L., Dunlop, D., Edelman, P.,
Chang, R.W. & Singer, R.H.
(1994) 71
Hutton, C.W. (1995) 9
Huygen, A.C., Kuis, W. & Sinnema,
G. (2000) 88
Huyser, B.A., Parker, J.C., Thoreson,
R., Smarr, K.L., Johnson, J.C. &
Hoffman, R. (1998) 106

Ireys, H.T., Sills, E.M., Kolodner, K.B.
& Walsh, B.B. (1996) 196
Ishii, H., Nagashima, M., Tanno, M.,
Nakajima, A. & Yoshino, S.
(2003) 35

Jacobi, C.E., Rupp, I., Boshuizen,
H.C., Triemstra, M., Dinant, H.J.
& van den Bos, G.A. (2004) 136

Jacoby, R.K., Newell, R.L. & Hickling,
P. (1985) 15
Jahn, L. (1997) 32
James, N.T., Miller, C.W., Brown, K.C.
& Weaver, M. (2005) 69
Janse, A.J., Sinnema, G., Uiterwaal,
C.S., Kimpen, J.L. & Gemke, R.J.
(2005) 130, 215
Jenkinson, C., Wright, L. & Coulter,
A. (1993) 97
Jones, R.L. (1909) 28
Jordan, J.M., Luta, G., Renner, J.B.,
Linder, G.F., Dragomir, A.,
Hochberg, M.C. *et al.* (1996) 70,
71

Kaarela, K., Lehtinen, K. &
Luukkainen, R. (1987) 118, 119
Kaboli, P.J., Doebbeling, B.N., Saag,
K.G. & Rosenthal, G.E. (2001) 23
Kahn, A.N. & van der Linden, S.
(1990) 14
Katz, P.P. (2005) 85
Katz, P.P. & Alfieri, W.S. (1997) 86
Katz, P.P. & Neugebauer, A. (2001) 86
Katz, P.P., Pasch, L.A. & Wong, B.
(2003) 104
Katz, P.P. & Yelin, E.H. (1993) 67, 70
Katz, P.P. & Yelin, E.H. (1994) 101
Katz, P.P. & Yelin, E.H. (1995) 70, 86
Kavale, S. (1996) 44
Kay, E.A. & Punchak, S.S. (1988) 153
Kazis, L.E., Anderson, J.J. & Meenan,
R.F. (1989) 181
Kean, W.F., Hart, L. & Buchanan,
W.W. (1997) 1
Keefe, F.J., Affleck, G., Lefebvre, J.,
Underwood, L., Caldwell, D.S.,
Drew, J. *et al.* (2001) 87
Keefe, F.J., Caldwell, D.S., Martinez,
S., Nunley, J., Beckham, J. &
Williams, D.A. (1991) 13, 56, 83

Keefe, F.J., Caldwell, D.S., Queen,
    K.T., Gil, K.M., Martinez, S.,
    Crisson, J.E. *et al.* (1987) 83
Keefe, F.J., Caldwell, D.S., Williams,
    D.A., Gil, K.M., Mitchell, D.M.
    et al. (1990) 162
Keefe, F.J., Lefebvre, J.C., Egert, J.R.,
    Affleck, G., Sullivan, M.J. &
    Caldwell, D.S. (2000) 83, 203, 204
Keefe, F.J., Lefebvre, J.C., Maixner,
    W., Salley, A.N., Jr. & Caldwell,
    D.S. (1997) 77
Kelley, J.E., Lumley, M.A. & Leisen,
    J.C. (1997) 35, 163
Kessler, R.C., Berglund, P., Demler,
    O., Jin, R., Koretz, D.,
    Merikangas, K.R. *et al.* (2003) 67
Kim, S., Drabinski, A., Williams, G. &
    Formica, C. (2001) 123, 156
King, L., Hawe, P. & Wise, M.
    (1998) 217
Kitzinger, J. (1995) 56
Kocher, M. (1994) 102
Konkol, L., Lineberry, J., Gottlieb, J.,
    Shelby, P.E., Miller, J.J. III &
    Lorig, K. (1989) 94
Kopec, J.A. & Sayre, E.C. (2004) 32, 212
Kovar, P.A., Allegrante, J.P.,
    MacKenzie, C.R., Peterson, M.G.,
    Gutin, B. & Charlson, M.E.
    (1992) 169
Kraag, G.R., Gordon, D.A., Menard,
    H.A., Russell, A.S. & Kalish,
    G.H. (1994) 145
Kraimaat, F.W., van Dam-Baggen,
    C.M.J. & Bijlsma, J.W. (1995) 105,
    109
Kralik, D., Koch, T., Price, K. &
    Howard, N. (2004) 53
Krol, B., Sanderman, R., Suurmeijer,
    T.P., Doeglas, D., van Sonderen,
    E., Rijswijk *et al.* (1998) 29, 40

Krol, T., Barlow, J.H. & Shaw, K.
    (1999) 18
Krol, T. & Peake, S. (1996) 121
Kruger, J.M., Helmick, C.G.,
    Callahan, L.F. & Haddix, A.C.
    (1998) 179
Kujala, U.M., Kettunen, J., Paananen,
    H., Aalto, T., Battie, M.C.,
    Impivaara, O. *et al.* (1995) 8
Kyngas, H. (2004) 113

La Montagna, G., Tirri, G., Cacace, E.,
    Perpignano, G., Covelli, M.,
    Pipitone, V. *et al.* (1998) 141
La Plante, M.P. (1988) 8
Lacaille, D., Sheps, S., Spinelli, J.J.,
    Chalmers, A. & Esdaile, J.M.
    (2004) 117
Lacaille, D., White, M.A., Backman,
    C.L. & Gignac, M.A. (2007) 121
Latman, N.S. & Walls, R. (1996) 28
Lavigne, J.V., Ross, C.K., Berry, S.L.,
    Hayford, J.R. & Pachman, L.M.
    (1992) 195, 197
Lawrence, J.S., Bremner, J.M. & Bier,
    F. (1966) 8
Lazarus, R.S. & Folkman, S. (1984)
    79
LeBovidge, J.S., Lavigne, J.V.,
    Donenberg, G.R. & Miller, M.L.
    (2003) 90
LeBovidge, J.S., Lavigne, J.V. &
    Miller, M.L. (2005) 33–4
Lehtinen, K. (1981) 118
Lempp, H., Scott, D.L. & Kingsley,
    G.H. (2006) 133
Lenker, S.L., Lorig, K. & Gallagher, D.
    (1984) 176
Leventhal, H., Meyer, D. & Nerenz,
    D. (1980) 81
Li, J., Schiottz-Christensen, B. &
    Olsen, J. (2005) 32

Lichtenberg, P.A., Skehan, M.W. &
Swensen, C.H. (1984) 29
Lim, H.J., Lee, M.S. & Lim, H.S.
(2005) 144
Lin, E.H., Katon, W., Von Korff, M.,
Tang, L., Williams, J.W., Jr.,
Kroenke, K. *et al.* (2003) 68
Lindroth, Y., Bauman, A., Brooks, P.M.
& Priestley, D. (1995) 185, 187,
201
Lindroth, Y., Brattström, M., Bellman,
I., Ekestaf, G., Olofsson, Y.,
Strömbeck, B., Stenshed, B.,
Wikström, I., Nilsson, J.A.,
Wollheim, F.A. (1997) 188
Lineker, S.C., Hughes, A. & Badley,
E.M. (1995) 151
Locker, D. (1983) 53
Loffer, S.L. (2000) 55
Lorig, K., Chastain, R.L., Ung, E.,
Shoor, S. & Holman, H.R.
(1989) 176
Lorig, K., Feigenbaum, P., Regan, C.,
Ung, E., Chastain, R.L. &
Holman, H.R. (1986) 175
Lorig, K. & Fries, J.F. (1990) 166
Lorig, K. & Gonzalez, V. (1992) 174, 206
Lorig, K., Gonzalez, V.M., Laurent,
D.D., Morgan, L. & Laris, B.A.
(1998) 202
Lorig, K. & Holman, H.R. (1989) 179
Lorig, K. & Holman, H.R. (1993) 27,
79, 169, 179, 182
Lorig, K., Ritter, P.L. & Plant, K.
(2005) 184
Lorig, K., Seleznick, M., Lubeck, D.,
Ung, E., Chastain, R.L. &
Holman, H.R. (1989) 76, 78
Lorig, K., Sobel, D., Stewart, A.,
Brown, B., Bandura, A., Ritter, P.,
Gonzalez, V., Laurent, D. &
Holman, H. (1999) 183

Lorig, K.R., Mazonson, P.D. &
Holman, H.R. (1993) 179
Lorig, K.R., Ritter, P.L., Laurent, D.D.
& Fries, J.F. (2004) 186
Lovell, D.J., Athreya, B., Emery, H.M.,
Gibbas, D.L., Levinson, J.E.,
Lindsley, C.B., Spencer, C.H. &
White, P.H. (1990) 115
Lowe, R., Cockshott, Z., Greenwood,
R., Kirwan, J.R., Almeida, C.,
Richards, P. *et al.* (2008) 77
Lubeck, D.P. (1995) 43, 66
Lustig, J.L., Ireys, H.T., Sills, E.M. &
Walsh, B.B. (1996) 96, 112

MacFarland, L. (2007) 163
MacKinnon, J.R., Avison, W.R. &
McCain, G.A. (1994) 69
Maggs, F.M., Jubb, R.W. & Kemm,
J.R. (1996) 155
Mancuso, C.A., Rincon, M., Sayles,
W. & Paget, S.A. (2006) 71
Manne, S.L. & Zautra, A.J. (1989) 81,
105, 109
Manne, S.L. & Zautra, A.J. (1990) 109
Manninen, P., Riihimaki, H.,
Heliovaara, M. & Suomalainen,
O. (2001) 144
Manuel, J.C. (2001) 34
March, L.M. & Bachmeier, C.J.
(1997) 2
Marinker, M., Blenkinsopp, A., Bond,
C. *et al.* (1997) 18
Marks, R. & Allegrante, J.P. (2005) 146
Martin, J., Meltzer, H. & Elliott, D.
(1988) 2
Martire, L.M., Keefe, F.J., Schulz, R.,
Ready, R., Beach, S.R., Rudy, T.E.
et al. (2006) 107
Martire, L.M., Schulz, R., Keefe, F.J.,
Starz, T.W., Osial, T.A., Jr., Dew,
M.A. *et al.* (2003) 202

Masdottir, B., Jonsson, T.,
   Manfredsdottir, V., Vikingsson,
   A., Brekkan, A. & Valdimarsson,
   H. (2000) 11
Mau, W., Bornmann, M., Weber, H.,
   Weidemann, H.F., Hecker, H. &
   Raspe, H.H. (1996) 117, 119
McAnarney, E.R., Pless, I.B.,
   Satterwhite, B. & Friedman, S.B.
   (1974) 88
McCauley, J., Tarpley, M.J., Haaz, S. &
   Bartlett, S.J. (2008) 88
McDougall, J., Bruce, B., Spiller, G.,
   Westerdahl, J. & McDougall, M.
   (2002) 26
McFarlane, A.C. & Brooks, P.M.
   (1988) 70
McGuigan, L.E., Hart, H.H., Gow,
   P.J., Kidd, B.L., Grigor, R.R. &
   Moore, T.E. (1984) 118
McIntosh, E. (1996) 12, 117
McMurray, R., Heaton, J., Sloper, P. &
   Nettleton, S. (1999) 10
McPherson, K.M., Brander, P., Taylor,
   W.J. & McNaughton, H.K.
   (2001) 52
McVeigh, C.M. & Cairns, A.P.
   (2006) 15–16
Meenan, R.F., Kazis, L.E., Anthony,
   J.M. & Wallin, B.A. (1991) 12,
   39
Meenan, R.F., Mason, J.H., Anderson,
   J.J., Guccione, A.A. & Kazis, L.E.
   (1992) 110
Miller, J.J. (1993) 88, 96, 112, 115
Miller, J.J. III, Spitz, P.W., Simpson, U.
   & Williams, G.F. (1982) 115
Mindham, R.H., Bagshaw, A., James,
   S.A. & Swannell, A.J. (1981) 71
Minor, M.A., Hewett, J.E., Webel,
   R.R., Anderson, S.K. & Kay, D.R.
   (1989) 168

Moll, J.M. (1986) 155
Moos, R.H. (1964) 28
Morgan, M. (1989) 51
Morrill, J.A. (2004) 94
Moussavi, S., Chatterji, S., Verdes, E.,
   Tandon, A., Patel, V. & Ustun, B.
   (2007) 66, 199
Muller-Godeffroy, E., Lehmann, H.,
   Kuster, R.M. & Thyen, U. (2005) 89
Mullick, M.S., Nahar, J.S. & Haq, S.A.
   (2005) 41, 89
Munthe, E. (1990) 16
Murphy, H., Dickens, C., Creed, F. &
   Bernstein, R. (1999) 143

Nagyova, I., Stewart, R.E., Macejova,
   Z., van Dijk, J.P. & van den
   Heuvel, W.J. (2005) 82
Naidoo, P. & Pretorius, T.B. (2006) 73
Nasser-Abdel, A. (1996) 32
Neame, R. & Hammond, A. (2005) 143
Neugebauer, A. & Katz, P.P.
   (2004) 110
Neugebauer, A., Katz, P.P. & Pasch,
   L.A. (2003) 86
Neville, C., Fortin, P.R., Fitzcharles,
   M.A., Baron, M., Abrahamowitz,
   M., Du Berger, R. *et al.* (1999) 152
Newman, S.P., Fitzpatrick, R., Lamb,
   R. & Shipley, M. (1989) 39, 42, 70
Newman, S.P., Fitzpatrick, R., Lamb,
   R. & Shipley, M. (1990) 81, 84
Nicassio, P.M. (2008) 68, 216
Nicassio, P.M. & Wallston, K.A.
   (1992) 42, 69

O'Leary, A., Shoor, S., Lorig, K. &
   Holman, H.R. (1988) 162
Oliver, M. (1992) 56
Oliveria, S.A., Felson, D.T., Cirillo,
   P.A., Reed, J.I. & Walker, A.M.
   (1999) 9

Ong, L.M., de Haes, J.C., Hoos, A.M. & Lammes, F.B. (1995) 155
Orbell, S., Espley, A., Johnston, M. & Rowley, D. (1998) 10
Orbell, S., Johnston, M., Rowley, D., Davey, P. & Espley, A. (1998) 10
Orbell, S., Johnston, M., Rowley, D., Davey, P. & Espley, A. (2001) 78
O'Reilly, S.C., Muir, K.R. & Doherty, M. (1999) 142
Osborn, C.E. (2001) 23, 24, 25
Osborne, R.H., Wilson, T., Lorig, K.R. & McColl, G.J. (2007) 217, 218

Packham, J.C. & Hall, M.A. (2002) 17
Palermo, T.M. & Kiska, R. (2005) 92
Palermo, T.M., Zebracki, K., Cox, S., Newman, A.J. & Singer, N.G. (2004) 91
Pariser, D.A. (2004) 186
Parker, J.C., Buckelew, S.P., Smarr, K.L., Buescher, K.L., Beck, N.C., Frank, R.G. *et al.* (1990) 12
Parker, J.C., Frank, R.G., Beck, N.C., Smarr, K.L., Buescher, K.L., Phillips, L.R. *et al.* (1988) 162
Parker, J.C., Smarr, K.L., Angelone, E.O., Mothersead, P.K., Lee, B.S., Walker, S.E. *et al.* (1992) 69
Parker, J.C., Smarr, K.L., Slaughter, J.R., Johnston, S.K., Priesmeyer, M.L., Hanson, K.D. *et al.* (2003) 68
Pashler, H.E. (2002) 180
Perrin, J.M., MacLean, W.E. & Perrin, E.C. (1989) 98
Persson, L.O., Larsson, B.M., Nived, K. & Eberhardt, K. (2005) 69
Persson, L.O. & Sahlberg, D. (2002) 29
Peterson, M.G., Kovar-Toledano, P.A., Otis, J.C., Allegrante, J.P., Mackenzie, C.R., Gutin, B. *et al.* (1993) 169

Pincus, T. & Callahan, L.F. (1986) 12
Pincus, T. & Callahan, L.F. (1993) 2
Pincus, T., Swearingen, C., Cummins, P. & Callahan, L.F. (2000) 10
Pisters, M.F., Veenhof, C., van Meeteren, N.L., Ostelo, R.W., de Bakker, D.H., Schellevis, F.G. *et al.* (2007) 10
Plach, S.K., Heidrich, S.M. & Waite, R.M. (2003) 110
Plach, S.K., Stevens, P.E. & Moss, V.A. (2004) 48
Powell, D.A., Furhtgott, E., Henderson, M., Prescott, L., Mitchell, A., Hartis, P. *et al.* (1990) 205
Power, J.D., Perruccio, A.V. & Badley, E.M. (2005) 71
Pradhan, E.K., Baumgarten, M., Langenberg, P., Handwerger, B.H., Gilpin, A.K., Magyari, T., Hochberg, M.C. & Berman, B.M. (2007) 216
Pritchard, M.L. (1989) 105
Prochaska, J., Velicer, W., Rossi, J.S., Goldstein, M.G., Marcus, B.H., Rakowski, W. *et al.* (1994) 203, 204, Tab. 8.3
Prochaska, T., Peters, K. & Warren, J. (2000) 217

Radojevic, V., Nicassio, P.M. & Weisman, M.H. (1992) 162
Ramsey, S.D.R., Spencer, A.C., Topolski, T.A., Belza, B.L. & Patrick, D.L. (2001) 24
Rao, J.K., Arick, R., Mihaliak, K.A. & Weinberger, M. (1998) 25
Rao, J.K., Kroenke, K., Mihaliak, K.A., Grambow, S.C. & Weinberger, M. (2003) 26
Rapoff, M.A. & Christopherson, E.R. (1982) 18

Rapoff, M.A., Purviance, M.R. &
    Lindsley, C.B. (1988a) 194
Rapoff, M.A., Purviance, M.R. &
    Lindsley, C.B. (1988b) 194
Reed, G.M., Taylor, S.E. & Kemeny,
    M.E. (1993) 74
Reisine, S. (1995) 66, 95, 105, 109
Reisine, S., McQuillan, J. & Fifield, J.
    (1995) 119
Reisine, S.T., Goodenow, C. & Grady,
    K.E. (1987) 101, 102
Rejeski, W.J., Brawley, L.R. Ettinger,
    W., Morgan, T. & Thompson, C.
    (1997) 145
Rejeski, W.J. Ettinger, W.H., Jr.,
    Martin, K. & Morgan, T.
    (1998) 77
Resch, K.L., Hill, S. & Ernst, E.
    (1997) 23
Revenson, T.A. (1993) 111
Revenson, T.A. & Majerovitz, S.D.
    (1991) 106, 110
Revenson, T.A., Schiaffino, K.A.,
    Majerovitz, D. & Gibofsky, A.
    (1991) 43, 110
Riemsma, R.P., Kirwan, J.R., Taal, E.
    & Rasker, J.J. (2002) 198, 199
Riemsma, R.P., Rasker, J.J., Taal, E.,
    Griep, E.N., Wouters, J.M. &
    Wiegman, O. (1998) 51, 77
Riemsma, R.P., Taal, E. & Rasker, J.J.
    (2003) 182–3
Riemsma, R.P., Taal, E., Rasker, J.,
    Klein, G., Bruyn, G.A.W.,
    Wouters, J.M. *et al.* (1999) 106
Riemsma, R.P., Taal, E., Wiegman, O.,
    Rasker, J., Bruyn, G.A.W. & van
    Paassen, J.C. (2000) 109
Rockport Walking Institute
    (1988) 169
Rosenthal, G.E. & Shannon, S.E.
    (1997) 137

Ross, C.K., Lavigne, J.V., Hayford,
    J.R., Berry, S.L., Sinacore, J.M. &
    Pachman, L.M. (1993) 93
Russell, M.L. (1985) 14
Ryan, S. (1995) 135
Ryan, S. (1996) 47, 50, 54, 129
Sale, J.E., Gignac, M. & Hawker, G.
    (2006) 143
Sallfors, C., Fasth, A. & Hallberg, L.R.
    (2002) 61
Sangha, O. (2000) 7, 8, 10, 11, 14
Santos, H., Brophy, S. & Calin, A.
    (1998) 145
Savelkoul, M., de Witte, L.P., Candel,
    M.J., van der Tempel, H. & van
    den Borne, B. (2001) 165, 166
Sawyer, M.G., Carbone, J.A.,
    Whitham, J.N., Roberton, D.M.,
    Taplin, J.E., Varni, J.W. *et al.*
    (2005) 91
Schanberg, L.E., Gil, K.M., Anthony,
    K.K., Yow, E. & Rochon, J.
    (2005) 91
Schanberg, L.E., Sandstrom, M.J.,
    Starr, K., Gill, K.M., Lefebvre, J.,
    Keefe, F.J. *et al.* (2000) 33
Scharloo, M., Kaptein, A.A.,
    Weinman, J., Hazes, J.M.,
    Willems, L.N., Bergman, W. *et al.*
    (1998) 82
Schiaffino, K.M., Revenson, T.A. &
    Gibofsky, A. (1991) 79
Schneider, S., Schmitt, G., Mau, H.,
    Schmitt, H., Sabo, D. & Richter,
    W. (2005) 8
Schoenfeld-Smith, K., Petroski, G.F.,
    Hewett, J.E., Johnson, J.C.,
    Wright, G.E., Smarr, K.L. *et al.*
    (1996) 73
Schumaker, H.R.E. (1988) 11
Serbo, B. & Jajic, I. (1991) 40

Shapiro, D. (1990) 19, 20, 21
Sharpe, L., Sensky, T., Brewin, C.R. &
    Allard, S. (2001) 39
Sharpe, L., Sensky, T., Timberlake, N.,
    Ryan, B., Brewin, C.R. & Allard,
    S. (2001) 39
Shaw, K. (2001) 58–9, 60, 88, 89, 93,
    114, 115
Shaw, W.S., Cronan, T.A. & Christie,
    M.D. (1994) 205
Sheeran, P. & Abraham, C. (1995) 147
Sheeran, P., Abrams, D. & Orbell, S.
    (1995) 122
Shifren, K., Park, D.C., Bennett, J.M.
    & Morrell, R.W. (1999) 77
Shuyler, K.S. & Knight, K.M.
    (2003) 156
Silman, A.J. & Hochberg, M.C.
    (2001) 11
Silman, A.J., Newman, J. &
    MacGregor, A.J. (1996) 11
Silver, E.J., Bauman, L.J. & Ireys, H.T.
    (1995) 96
Silvers, I.J., Hovell, M.F., Weisman,
    M.H. & Mueller, M.R. (1985) 152
Singer, G.H.S. (2006) 210
Slater, M.A., Doctor, J.N., Pruitt, S.D.,
    Atkinson, J.H. (1997) 185
Sleath, B., Callahan, L., DeVellis, R.F.
    & Sloane, P.D. (2005) 25
Sleath, B., Chewning, B., de Vellis,
    B.M., Weinberger, M., de Vellis,
    R.F., Tudor, G. *et al.* (2008) 68
Smedstad, L.M., Moum, T., Vaglum,
    P. & Kvien, T.K. (1996) 67
Smith, B. & Zautra, A.J. (2000) 83
Smith, B.W. & Zautra, A.J. (2002) 29
Smith, B.W. & Zautra, A.J. (2004) 87
Smith, C.A. & Wallston, K.A.
    (1992) 73
Smith, T.W., Peck, J.R. & Ward, J.R.
    (1990) 73

Smyth, J.M., Stone, A.A., Hurewitz,
    A. & Kaell, A. (1999) 35, 163,
    164
Southwood, T.R. (writer) (1992) 131,
    195
Southwood, T.R., Barlow, J., Wright,
    C., Shaw, K., Young, S. &
    Cheseldine, D. (2000) 195
Southwood, T.R. & Malleson, P.
    (Eds.) (1993) 18
Spector, T.D. & Hochberg, M.C.
    (1990) 11
Spector, T.D. & Scott, D.L. (1988) 12
Spiegel, J.S., Spiegel, T.M., Ward, N.B.,
    Paulus, H.E., Leake, B. & Kane,
    R.L. (1986) 131
Stefl, M.E., Shear, E.S. & Levinson,
    J.E. (1989) 195
Stein, D. (1996) 21
Stein, M.B. & Barrett-Connor, E.
    (2000) 33, 212
Stenstrom, C.H., Arge, B. &
    Sundbom, A. (1997) 143
Stephens, M.A.P., Martire, L.M.,
    Cremeans-Smith, J.K., Druley,
    J.A. & Wojno, W.C. (2006) 107
Stiles, T.C. (1993) 31
Stone, A.A., Smyth, J.M., Kaell, A. &
    Hurewitz, A. (2000) 35
Straughair, S. & Fawcitt, S. (1992)
    121
Sullivan, T., Allegrante, J.P., Peterson,
    M.G., Kovar, P.A. & MacKenzie,
    C.R. (1998) 169
Summers, M.N., Haley, W.E.,
    Reveille, J.D. & Alarcon, G.S.
    (1988) 70
Superio-Cabuslay, E., Ward, M.M. &
    Lorig, K.R. (1996) 198
Suurmeijer, T.P., Waltz, M., Moum, T.,
    Guillemin, F., van Sonderen, F.L.,
    Briancon, S. *et al.* (2001) 41

Suurmeijer, T.P.B.M., Van Sonderen, F.L.P., Krol, B., Doeglas, D.M., Van Den Heuvel, W.J.A. & Sanderman, R. (2005) 29

Sweeney, S., Taylor, G. & Calin, A. (2002) 171

Taal, E., Johannes, M.A., Rasker, J. *et al.* (1993) 1

Taal, E., Rasker, J.J. & Wiegman, O. (1996) 76

Taal, E., Riemsma, R.P., Brus, H.L., Seydel, E.R., Rasker, J.J. & Wiegman, O. (1993) 182

Taal, E., Seydel, E.R., Rasker, J.J. & Wiegman, O. (1993) 1

Tak, S.H. (2006) 54

Tak, S.H. & Hong, S.H. (2005) 157

Tak, S.H. & Laffrey, S.C. (2003) 83, 87

Tallon, D., Chard, J. & Dieppe, P. (2000) 45, 146

Taylor, B. (2001) 54

Taylor, S.E., Lichtman, R.R. & Wood, J.V. (1984) 74

Tennen, H., Affleck, G., Armeli, S. & Carney, M.A. (2000) 81

Thompson, P.W., Kirwan, J.R. & Barnes, C.G. (1985) 1

Tijhuis, G.J., Zwinderman, A.H., Hazes, J.M., van den Hout, W.B., Breedveld, F.C. & Vliet Vlieland, T.P.M. (2002) 138

Timko, C., Stovel, K.W. & Moos, R.H. (1992) 41, 93, 94

Timko, C., Stovel, K.W., Moos, R.H. & Miller, J.J. III (1992) 41, 93, 94

Tomlinson, M., Barefoot, J. & Dixon, A. (1986) 15

Tonnes, K.M.A. (1990) 147

Toye, F. (2003) 44–5, 46

Treharne, G.J., Kitas, G.D., Lyons, A.C. & Booth, D.A. (2005) 30

Tsai, P.F. (2005) 110

Turner, A. (2003) 83

Turner, A. & Barlow, J. (2001) 196

Turner, A., Williams, R.B. & Barlow, J. (2002) 44, 46, 47, 51, 52, 54, 177, 178, 214, 218, 225

Turner, A.P., Barlow, J.H. & Heathcote-Elliott, C. (2000) 8, 225

Uhlig, T., Smedstad, L.M., Vaglum, P., Moum, T., Gérard, N. & Kvien, T.K. (2000) 67

Ungerer, J.A., Horgan, B., Chaitow, J. & Champion, G.D. (1988) 88, 91, 92

van der Heide, A., Jacobs, J.W., van Albada-Kuipers, G.A., Kraaimaat, F.W., Geenen, R. & Bijlsma, J.W. (1994) 42

van Dyke, M.M., Parker, J.C., Smarr, K.L., Hewett, J.E., Johnson, G.E., Slaughter, J.R. *et al.* (2004) 40

van Tubergen, A. & Hidding, A. (2002) 15

van Uden-Kraan, C.F., Drossaert, C.H., Taal, E., Lebrun, C.E.I., Drossaers-Bakker, K.W., Smit, W.M. *et al.* (2008) 167

van Uden-Kraan, C.F., Drossaert, C.H., Taal, E., Shaw, B.R., Seydel, E.R. & van de Laar, M.A. (2008) 167

Vandenbroucke, J.P., Hazevoet, H.M. & Cats, A. (1984) 12

Vandvik, I. H. (1990) 88, 92

Vandvik, I.H. & Eckblad, G. (1991) 93, 94

Varni, J.W. & Wallander, J.L. (1984) 18

Varni, J.W., Wilcox, K.T. & Hanson, V. (1988) 93

Vaughan, S., Schumm, J.S. & Sinagub,
 J. (1996) 57
Vecchio, P.C. (1994) 23
Vingard, E. (1994) 8
Vinokur, A.D., Price, R.H. & Caplan,
 R.D. (1996) 122
von Weiss, R.T., Rapoff, M.A., Varni,
 J.W., Lindsley, C.B., Olson, N.Y.,
 Madson, K.L. *et al.* (2002) 108

Wainapel, S.F., Thomas, A.D. &
 Kahan, B.S. (1998) 25
Waite-Jones, J.M. & Madill, A.
 (2007) 112
Walco, G.A., Varni, J.W. & Ilowite, N.
 (1992) 194
Walker, L.S., Ford, M.B. & Donald,
 W.D. (1987) 98
Wallander, J.L. & Varni, J.W.
 (1989) 93
Wallston, K.A. (1992) 75, 147
Wallston, K.A. (1993) 73
Wallston, K.A., Wallston, B.S. &
 deVellis, B.M. (1978) 74
Wallston, K.A., Wallston, B.S., Smith,
 S. & Dobbins, C.J. (1987) 75
Walsh, J.D., Blanchard, E.B., Kremer,
 J.M. & Blanchard, C.G.
 (1999) 106
Ward, M.M. & Leigh, J.P. (1993) 105
Ware, J.E., Snow, K.K., Kosinski, M. &
 Gandek, B. (1993) 90
Warsi, A., LaValley, M.P., Wang, P.S.,
 Avorn, J. & Solomon, D.H.
 (2003) 198
Wegener, S.T. (1991) 32, 34
Wehmeyer, M.L., Sands, D.J., Doll, B.
 & Palmer, S. (1997) 160
Weinberger, M., Tierney, W.M. &
 Booher, P. (1989) 142
Weinberger, M., Tierney, W.M.,
 Booher, P. & Katz, B.P. (1989) 157

Weiner, C.L. (1975) 44, 51, 52–3
Weinman, J. (1990) 155
Weiss, K.A., Schiaffino, K.M. &
 Ilowite, N. (2001) 112
Wells, K.B., Golding, J.M. & Burnam,
 M.A. (1988) 67
Wells, K.B., Golding, J.M. & Burnam,
 M.A. (1989) 67
Wetherall, M.A., Byrne-Davis, L.,
 Dieppe, P., Donovan, J., Brookes,
 S., Byron, M. *et al.* (2005) 163
White, P.H. & Shear, E.S. (1992) 121
Wilkins, K.E. (2000) 81
Williams, G.H. (1989) 31
Wolfe, F., Anderson, J.J. & Hawley,
 D.J. (1994) 12
Wolfe, F., Hawley, D.J. & Wilson, K.
 (1996) 77
Wolfe, F., Mitchell, D.M., Sibley, J.T.,
 Fries, J.F., Bloch, D.A., Williams,
 C.A. *et al.* (1994) 12
Wolfe, F., Zhao, S. & Lane, N.
 (2000) 10
Wong, A.L., Harker, J.O., Lau, V.P.,
 Shatzel, S. & Port, L.H.
 (2004) 183
Woolhead, G.M., Carr, A., Wilkinson,
 M. *et al.* (1996) 142
Wordsworth, B.P. & Mowat, A.G.
 (1986) 118
Wright, G.E., Parker, J.C., Smarr, K.L.,
 Schoenfeld-Smith, K., Buckelew,
 S.P., Slaughter, J.R. *et al.*
 (1996) 70, 76
Wright, V. & Hopkins, R. (1990) 134

Xin, L. (2006) 122

Yelin, E. (1992) 117
Yelin, E. (1998) 13
Yelin, E., Henke, C. & Epstein, W.
 (1987) 117

Yelin, E., Lubeck, D., Holman, H. &
    Epstein, W. (1987) 101
Yip, Y.B., Sit, J.W., Fung, K.K., Wong,
    D.Y., Chong, S.Y., Chung, L.H.
    et al. (2007) 183
Young, L.D. (1992) 81

Zaadstra, B.M., Seidell, J.C., Van
    Noord, P.A., te Velde, E.R.,
    Habbema, J.D., Vrieswijk, B. *et al.*
    (1993) 9
Zant, J.L., Dekker-Saeys, A.J., Van
    den Burgh, I.C., Kolman, A. &
    Van der Stadt, R.J. (1982) 31
Zautra, A.J., Burleson, M.H., Smith,
    C.A., Blalock, S.J., Wallston, K.A.,
    DeVellis, R.F. *et al.* (1995) 81
Zautra, A.J., Hamilton, N.A. & Burke,
    H.M. (1999) 29, 34–5

Zautra, A.J., Hoffman, J.M., Matt,
    K.S., Yocum, D., Potter, P.T.,
    Castro, W.L. *et al.* (1998) 34
Zautra, A.J., Johnson, L.M. & Davis,
    M.C. (2005) 87
Zautra, A.J. & Smith, B.W. (2001)
    69
Zautra, A.J., Yocum, D.C., Villanueva,
    I., Smith, B., Davis, M.C., Attrep,
    J. *et al.* (2004) 35
Zigmond, A.S. & Snaith, R.P.
    (1983) 95
Zimmerman, M.A. (1990) 160
Zochling, J., March, L., Lapsley, H.,
    Cross, M., Tribe, K. & Brooks, P.
    (2004) 25
Zochling, J., van der Heijde, D.,
    Dougados, M. & Braun, J.
    (2006) 15

General Index

absenteeism
  from school 115
  from work 116
acceptance-resignation 78, 178, 180
accommodation strategies 95
acetaminophen 10
achievement scores (school) 88
action-oriented strategies 81
active remediation 85
active strategy 80, 82, 85
activities
  daily 86, 97, 114
  planning 77
  play, games and sporting 102, 103,
    126, 173
  restrictions on 46–9
  school 97
  see also household; leisure activities;
    valued activities
acupuncture 21, 24, 26
adaptation 82, 115, 124–5, 152, 190,
  194, 214
adherence (as term) 141
adjustment 65, 84, 87, 109, 212, 214
  disorder 89
  lack of 93
adolescent arthritis and rheumatism
  (AAR) 89
adolescents 150
  anxiety in 154

and education 115
isolation of 61
and JIA 58–9, 63, 89, 92, 93, 112–13
and parental involvement 63
and parents with RA 111
and psychological adjustment 90
and psychosocial distress 41
and stress 33–4
adults, young 150, 201–2, 218
advocacy groups 215
aetiology 11, 14, 151
affective disorder 88
affirmational support 196
African Americans 88, 184–5
Africans, Sub-Saharan 11
age
  and AS 14, 31
  and CAM 25
  and OA 8, 9, 10, 111, 144
  and onset of arthritis 101–2, 111,
    113–14, 120, 142, 152, 173
  and popular beliefs about arthritis
    16, 101–2, 113–14, 142, 173
  and RA 31, 119
aggression 90
aids
  in home 111
  to mobility 10
  in workplace 152
AIMS-Depression scale 110

allied health care 136, 137
allied health professionals 146
alternative medicine *see* complementary
   and alternative medicine
altruism 214
ambition 31
American College of
   Rheumatology 7
anaemia 12, 139, 211
analgesia 10, 13, 21, 68, 142, 143,
   221
   and use of CAM 25
anger 65, 114, 168, 213
   and diagnostic delay 212
   and knees 20
   and loss of independence 49
   normalising 52
   in parents 63, 104, 126, 212
   in pre-diagnostic period 37, 38
   problems of 47
   and RA 28
   and restrictions 47
   and stress 163
   suppressed 19, 20, 33, 36, 42, 214
   as term 46
ankylosing spondylitis (AS) 1, 7,
   14–16, 47
   aetiology 14
   and CBT 162
   and emotional disclosure 164
   exercise and 144–5, 148, 170–4
   and fatigue 120
   onset 15
   prevalence 14
   psychosocial aspects 173
   sex ratio 8, 14, 210
   and social support 111
   trigger factors 14–15
   and work disability 118–19, 124
ankylosis 15
anti-depressants 68, 122
antigens 14

anti-tumour necrosis factor (anti-TNF)
   13, 15–16
anxiety 3, 66, 99–100
   and CBT 162
   and coping ability 39
   and depression 40
   failure to assess 91
   following assault 33
   about future 213
   and HRQOL 90
   in inpatients 133
   and JIA 88
   levels 214
   low and high trait 164
   NICE guidelines 215
   and pain 67, 82, 150
   in parents 63, 95, 98, 156
   and personality 29
   and PIL 87
   and self-efficacy 78
   in widows and divorcees 105
   about work 120, 123
appetite loss 17, 68
appraisals 72, 79–80
   primary and secondary 80
aromatherapy 24–5
Arthritis Care 124, 154, 175, 188–9,
   191, 194
Arthritis Foundation (US) 218
Arthritis Helpbook 166, 175, 185
Arthritis Impact Measurement
   Scale 110, 201
Arthritis Parents: Learning,
   Understanding and Sharing,
   A-Plus 196
Arthritis Research Campaign 155
arthritis resource centre, community-
   based 153
Arthritis Self-Efficacy Function 76
Arthritis Self-Efficacy Scales 76, 78
Arthritis Self-Management Program
   (ASMP) 27, 123 (Table 6.1), 163,

169, 175–86, 189, 190, 202, 204,
    206, 207–8, 217
  impact of 218
  programmes based on 181–8, 207
Arthritis Society 134
arthrogram 221
assertive actions 54
Assessment in Ankylosing
    Spondylitis 15
asthma 99, 163, 220
attack on self 20
attentional coping 80
attitudinal barriers 113–14, 120
attrition 195, 204, 205
audiotapes 156
Australia 157, 183, 187, 217
autogenic exercises 195
autonomic nervous system (ANS)
    36
autonomous behaviour 160
avoidance 78, 96, 165
avoidant coping 80, 81, 82, 94, 165

babies 102
back disease 152
back pain 28, 31, 201
Barefoot, Jane 170
behaviour patterns 22
  changing 168, 176, 202–4, 206
  and health education 147
behavioural expectancy 75
behavioural psychology 147
behavioural techniques 194, 207
'being seen' and 'being believed' 129
biofeedback 22–3, 195, 200
biographical disruption 44, 46, 64
biological therapies 13
biomedical factors 106
bitterness 49
black people
  Caribbean 11
  in information-giving study 158

see also African Americans
body
  changes to 50, 65
  negative views of 59
  non-conforming 48
  shape 222
bone density, and OA 9
Bone and Joint Decade (2000–10) 3
booklets 181
booster sessions 183, 208, 218
Bowen technique 27
bracketing 133
breast cancer 33, 74, 167
bronchitis 114
buildings, access to 114, 120
buses 114

camps, summer 155, 194, 195
Canada 89, 117, 121, 134, 157, 183
Canadian Community Health
    Survey 71
cardiovascular disease, and RA 12
caregivers 97–8, 106–7, 112, 126,
    202
cartilage, loss of 9, 12
catastrophising 82–3
causality 69
Centers for Diseases Control and
    Prevention (CDC) 2–3
change
  motivation to 202–4
  stages of 203–4, 203 (Table 8.3)
  see also behaviour patterns,
    changing
Child Behaviour Check List
    (CBCL) 90, 91
childbearing and rearing years 102
childbirth
  lack of sleep following 103
  pain of 45
childcare 101–5, 152, 188
childhood, trauma in 32

children 41
  death of 32
  descriptions of pain 57–8
  and JIA 16–18, 34, 38, 57–64, 88–91,
    100, 126, 130–1, 146, 146–7, 154,
    194–7, 207, 209
  locus of control 195
  and parents 111–13, 126, 149–50
  physical functioning 98–9
  play, games and sporting activi-
    ties 102, 103, 113, 126, 173
  and psychological distress 91
  and public attitudes to
    arthritis 113–14
  social interaction 113
  and social support 108
  and stress 33–4
Children Have Arthritis Too
  (CHAT) 154
chiropractic 24, 26
choice, loss of 49
Chronic Disease Self-Management
  Course (CDSMC) 183–5
cleaning 101
cluster analysis 84, 203
co-morbidity 10, 78, 88, 89, 119, 151,
  199
COAching for eXercise in AS
  (COAX-AS) 172–4
Cochrane Review 198
cognitive appraisals 100
cognitive behavioural techniques/
  interventions (CBT) 22, 54, 77,
    160, 161–2, 185, 194, 198–208, 215
cognitive functioning 77
cognitive restructuring 162, 163, 165
cognitive strategies 81, 82, 84
  for symptom management 177,
    179, 185
communication 55
community health centre 134
community support networks 215

complementary and alternative
    medicine (CAM) 2, 21, 22–7, 142,
    159, 202, 216
  non-prescribed 24
  practitioners 25–6, 27
  usage rates 23–4
compliance (as term) 141
computers 156, 157, 194, 195–6,
  207
concordance (adherence, compli-
    ance) 18, 140–6, 158, 194
  psychosocial factors 142
  as term 141
confrontation 78
constant comparative method 55
consultants 135
consultations
  focus in 134–5
  interactivity in 129–30
  length of 134
'consumer' views 43–4
contemplation, of change 204
contraception, oral 11
contracting (goal-setting) 178, 202
control
  loss of 46, 47, 213
  perceived 73, 75
  personal 74
control cognitions 73
control groups 135, 164, 170–1, 181,
    187, 205
  and children with JIA 92–3
  lack of 195, 217
  leaflet-only 199
  and siblings 93
  waiting-list 165
controlled trials 216–17
convenience, samples of 91
coping ability (of patients) 39, 50, 65,
    108 (Fig. 6.2)
coping modes questionnaire 77–8
coping skills, training in 161–2

coping styles and strategies 52, 72,
79–85, 100, 174, 214
active and passive 165
affective 84
confrontation, avoidance and
acceptance-resignation 78
emotion-focused 165
maladaptive 84, 109
problem-focused 165
repertoire of 85
spiritual and religious 56
variability in 81
copper bracelets 24
corporeality 48
corticosteroids (steroids) 13
cortisone injections 222
cost of disease 2, 13–14
cost-benefit analysis, of ASMP 178–9
cost-effectiveness analysis 217
counselling 121
Coventry University 211
Applied Research Centre in Health
& Lifestyle Intervention,
Self-Management Programme 3
Sports Centre 172–3
COX-2 inhibitors 13
Crohn's disease 14
cross-sectional analysis 107
cystic fibrosis 99

death, premature 12
decision-making 137–8
demographic variables 94
Department of Health, Expert Patient
Programme (EPP) 183
depression/depressed mood 3, 29,
33, 34, 35, 48, 49, 52, 100, 188
and AAR 89
adaptation to 213
in AS 37
and ASMP 179
and CBT 162

clinical and non-clinical 110
and coping strategies 81
and emotional disclosure 164
failure to assess 91
and fatigue 110
and HRQOOL 90
in JIA 41
levels of 214
mild 215–16
in mothers 94–5, 95 (Table 5.1), 98
NICE guidelines 215
and non-responders 205
in parents 94–5, 104
in partners 106
and patient education 198
and PIL 87
prevalence 67
in RA 39–41, 66–72, 86, 143, 199, 215
and self-efficacy 76, 78
and social support 108
symptomatology of 100
and unemployment 122
vulnerability to 101
in widows and divorcees 105
in women 86
and work disability 119, 123
see also anxiety; pain, and depression
diagnosis
delays in 133–4, 212
focus on 134
problems of 37–8
psychiatric 88
receipt of information on 137–8, 216
diet 9, 24, 26, 82, 112, 202, 216
differentness, sense of 114, 210
disability 45, 72, 82
benefits 53, 120
high 106
invisibility of 114, 120, 122
and JIA 91
medical and social models 113,
189, 193

disability (*cont'd*)
  physical 70, 107
'disabled', 'disability', as terms 53, 189
disease activity, intensity of 69
disease burden 45, 89
disease-modifying anti-rheumatic
    drugs (DMARDS) 13
disease severity 77, 91
disintegration of self 55
dispositional coping 80
distraction 54, 225
doctors *see* physicians
driving 47
Drug Information Centre Arthritis
    Project 157
drugs *see* medication
duration, of disease 38–41, 69, 106,
    119, 152–3, 166

economic impact, of RA 12
education
  impact on 60, 115, 120
  post-secondary 118
  and social support 167
education level 31, 151, 188
  and AS 145
  and CAM 25
  and information-seeking 153
  and RA 11, 12, 119
education programmes, group *see*
    group education programmes
effect sizes 181
Egypt, ancient 7
e-Health technologies 215
embarrassments 111
EMG biofeedback relaxation
    training 22–3
emotional awareness 163
emotional disclosure 163–5, 178, 200,
    206, 207, 214, 217–18
  low take-up in studies 164–5
  written 164

emotional support 196
emotion focused strategies 80, 81, 82,
    83, 193
emotions 19–22, 35, 36, 41, 46–9, 67,
    87
  of adolescents 58, 59–60
  and AS 104
  of children 58, 59–60, 112
  contagion of 112
  and JIA 90
  negative 49, 53, 65, 189
employability 49, 126
employment 43, 49
  advisers 193
  barriers to 121, 212
  enhancing potential 190–4, 206
  and fatigue 46
  nature of 119
  see also work; work disability;
    workspace
empowering and disempowering
    processes 167, 199
empowerment, psychological 160,
    178
energy
  lack of 46, 47
  and spirituality 88
energy field healing 27
energy healing 24
environmental barriers 113, 114, 120
ergonomics 124
ESR (erythrocyte sedimentation
    rate) 36, 41
essential oils 25
Ethics Committee 164
ethnic minority groups 202, 210
Europe, treatment in 10
exacerbation 12, 31, 85, 102, 107
exercise 29, 83, 159
  and ASMP 179
  children and 62, 150
  concordance with 140, 142, 143–4

and disease severity 171
group sessions 50, 182
and health education 147, 148
at home 170, 172, 173, 181–2
home-based intervention 171–2
motivation 203
in multi-component self-
  management interventions 206
psychologists and 216
reinterpretation 176–7
to relieve pain 80, 144
and self-efficacy 172
as therapy 10, 13, 15, 18, 24, 31
at workplace 125
see also ankylosing spondylitis
  (AS), and exercise
expectations 72
family 51, 54–5, 126
outcome 161
as parent 102
of partners 105
patients' 138, 142, 146
self-efficacy 170
social 114
externalising symptoms 90
extroversion 29, 32

faith 82
family
breakdown 46
cohesion 93, 95, 111
conflict 105, 135
coping ability 112
expectations of members 51, 54–5,
  102, 126
interaction with 45, 97, 101
JIA and 62–3, 195; *see also* juvenile
  idiopathic arthritis (JIA), parents
  of children with
relationships 43
resources 93, 94, 95
retreats 194

studies 93
support by 49, 112, 118, 149
fantasising 109
fat distribution, and OA 9
fathers 102, 126
depression in 94–5, 95 (Table 5.1)
fatigue in 104
and older children 103
self-efficacy 97
and small children 103–4
see also parents
fatigue 12, 17, 19–20, 22, 37, 45–6, 59,
  65, 68, 71, 85, 159
beliefs about controlling 74
causes 100, 211
in children 33, 58, 89, 97
and depression 110
and education 115
exercise and 216
and home life 46
and JIA 89, 92
in RA 41, 52, 77, 106, 121
relief from 138, 139
self-efficacy and 76, 77
and stress 163
and work disability 116, 120, 124
fear 168
of disclosure 122
of future 188
of joint injections 132
suppressed 33, 212
about work disability 121
Federation of Patient and Consumer
  Organisations 166
feet 20, 101
fibromyalgia 167
fibromyalgia syndrome (FMS) 28,
  87
financial problems 49
fine motor functioning 91, 101
Finland 13, 118, 152
fitness suites 172

flares, disease 34, 112, 115, 122, 151,
    169, 204
fluctuation of disease 114, 120, 122
fluidity, lack of 20
focus-group discussion 56–7, 121,
    140, 192, 193
folk medicine 26
Football Association 221
footballers, and OA 8–9, 83, 220–5
friends 51, 60, 97, 204
frustration 46, 49, 52, 63, 65, 104, 126,
    213
    in children 58
functional disability 2, 16, 58, 70, 73,
    83, 94, 106, 119, 198
    and JIA 89
    and marriage 105
    and PIL 87
functional impairment 12, 43, 47, 49,
    70, 86, 90
furniture, ergonomically adapted 124

gender
    and AS 14, 15
    and CAM use 25
    and children and adolescents 41
    and OA 9
    and RA 11, 12, 13
    and work disability 117
    see also men; women
general practitioners (GPs) 10, 133–4
    patient-initiated visits to 181,
        185–6
genetic predisposition, to RA 11
genetic screening 36–7, 213
Germany 89
goal importance 78, 79
goal-setting 178, 202
gout 1, 211
grandparents 102, 104–5, 111, 112, 126
group education programmes 52,
    146, 186, 207

guilt 20, 49, 102, 120
gyms 172

handbook, for use with carers with
    arthritis 104–5
*Handbook for Parents and
    Grandparents* 212
hands 101
happiness 94
headache, chronic 92
healing modalities 21
health, definition 213
Health Assessment Questionnaire 17,
    180, 182
health behaviours 110
health beliefs 110, 147
health care
    costs 166–7, 181
    patient satisfaction with 137–40
    providers *see* nurses; physicians
    systems 23, 113
    unmet demands 136–7
health communication campaign 3
health locus of control 73–5, 87, 100,
    187
health management, traditional 152
health professionals 208
    as educators 166
    and information distribution 153,
        154–5
    interventions by 199
    as source of feedback 204
health promotion 147
health psychology 147
health-related quality of life
    (HRQOL) 89–90, 124
health-risk behaviour 112
heart disease 88, 114, 158
helplessness 63, 71, 72–3, 100, 117,
    143, 154, 176
herbal treatments 24, 26, 222
heredity 36–7

and AS 102
and JIA 63
and OA 9
and RA 11
hip
  OA in *see* osteoarthritis (OA), hip
  replacement 10, 13, 78, 130, 142,
    154
Hippocrates 7
Hipwell, Alison 210–11
holistic approach 26, 160, 175
home care 136, 137, 140
home exercise *see* exercise, at home
home life 46
homeopathy 21, 24, 26
Hong Kong 183
hope 55
Hospital Anxiety and Depression
  Scale 95 (Table 5.1)
hospitals
  attendance at 112
  and 'caring stigma' 172
  general medical wards 132, 133
  inpatients in 131–3
household, activities in 86, 101, 107
'hurt', as term 57
hydrotherapy 16, 170
hyperactivity 90
hypertension 88
hypnosis 200
hypochondriasis 29
hypothalamic-pituitary-adrenal
  (HPA) axis 36

identity, linked to work 122
illness
  arthritis not considered as 75
  threat 81
  visible signs of 59
illnesses, common 47
immobility 188
immune system 20, 33

functionality 70
and stress 34–5
impatience 104
implementation studies 217, 218
inadequacy, feelings of 49, 102
income 105
inconvenience, arthritis as 46
independence 122, 189–90
  children and 63
  loss of 43, 47, 49
India 25
indigestion 13
inflammation *see* joints,
  inflammation of
inflammatory bowel disease 118
inflexibility 19, 20
information
  acquisition of 150–3
  delivery settings 157–8
  internet-based 156
  and JIA 154, 196
  multi-media 156
  unmet needs for 151–2, 159
information packs 186, 196
information-seeking 81, 82, 109,
    153
inhibition 20
injections, joint 132, 133
injuries *see* trauma
inpatients 131–3
  experience of care 131–2, 215
  expert and novice 132
  satisfaction level in 138–9
insecurity 20
internal disease pathology 58
internal locus of control 160
internalising symptoms 82, 90
internet, programmes delivered
    by 207
internet-based information 156–7,
    159, 215, 216
interpersonal sensitivity 29

interventions 84, 94, 135
  child-centred 154
  at community health centres 134
  educational/self-management 123
    (Table 6.1), 124, 146–7
  employment-related 123–4, 123
    (Table 6.1)
  and exercise adherence 146
  recipients of 149–50
  socially oriented 155
  see also personal development
    interventions; psycho-educational
    interventions; psychological
    interventions
interviews 43, 48–9, 193, 197
INTO Work Personal Development
  Programme (IWPD) 190–3, 191
  (Table 8.1)
intrapersonal factors 100
introversion 32
iritis 17
irritability 17, 104, 126
isolation 114, 115, 155, 213
  social 52, 61, 65, 89, 90

job
  autonomy, low 119
  satisfaction 49
  security 120
  see also employment; work
job-seeking 193, 207
joints
  bony enlargement of 9
  changes in 85
  inflammation of 16, 17, 19, 90,
    162
  injections 132, 133
  loading of 218
  protection 148
  replacement 10, 13, 77
  swollen 12, 17, 39, 41, 45, 73
  tender 73, 200

juvenile idiopathic arthritis (JIA) 1,
    16–18, 57–64
  children with *see* children, and JIA
  and education 115
  information and 154
  interventions in 194–7, 206
  mortality 16
  onset 16
  parents of children with 34, 38, 57,
    61, 111–12, 126, 130, 207
  prevalence 8, 16, 93, 197
  and psychiatric disorders 41
  psychosocial consequences 130
  and social support 111
  subgroups 16–17
  terms used for 16
  and use of CAM 25

karma, non-serving 21
kidney disease 114
knees 20, 71
  instability of joint 45
  OA of *see* osteoarthritis (OA), knee
  replacement 13, 45, 78, 83, 87, 222,
    223
Knowledge Questionnaire (for RA
  patients) 151–2
Korea 156

lay leaders/tutors 182, 185, 206, 208,
    214, 216
  with arthritis 175, 176
leaflets 151–2, 155–6, 197, 198–9, 200
learning disabilities 202
lectures 166
leisure activities 46, 47, 86, 101, 113,
    114
libraries 156
life expectancy 12, 112
lifestyle 39, 216
liver disease 99
liver transplant 98

London Coping with RA
   Questionnaire 81–2
loneliness 166
   see also isolation
longitudinal studies 106, 219
loss, sense of 47
Lund, Sweden 187

Macdonald, Malcolm 220–5
McFarland, Lorraine 173
mail-based programmes 186, 207
manual-based intervention 216
marginalisation 88, 114
marital satisfaction, lower 84
marriage 117
   and RA 34, 105
massage 24
mastery experience 79
mediators 96–9
medical insurance 25
   in US 23
medication 15, 17, 43, 60, 83, 106, 202
   anti-depressant 68
   benefits 143
   complementary and alternative *see*
      complementary and alternative
      medicine
   concordance with 140–5, 147, 194
   decreased need for 219
   dosage and frequency 143
   effects 198
   focus on 134
   NICE guidelines 215
   parents and 112
   side effects 1, 63, 97, 98, 113, 142–3,
      151, 211
   trials 198
   and walking 168
meditation 216
Medline 90
men
   and AS 31, 111

as hard to reach 218
   and work 118, 119
   see also fathers
mental health 77, 90, 197
mental support 152
mentoring 193, 196
meta-analyses
   of psychological intervention
      199–201, 201 (Table 8.2), 208
   of publications 36
metaphysical explanations of
   arthritis 18–22
methodological notes 30–1, 56–7, 68,
   74–5, 92–3, 99, 133, 139–40, 181,
   195, 197, 200
migraine 114
mild disease 92
Minnesota 12
Minnesota Multiphasic Personality
   Inventory 29
mobile phones 113
mobility 10
   limited 58, 101, 104, 119
modelling 176, 178
moderator and mediator 72
monitoring
   of disease progress 146
   remote 215
   of wellbeing 151
mood
   improving 30, 163
   and pain 33
   swings 49
   see also depression, depressed
      mood; positive mood
mortality rate, and RA 12
mothers
   anxiety in 98
   appraisals by 96
   with arthritis 102
   of children with JIA 34, 94–5, 95
      (Table 5.1), 97

mothers (*cont'd*)
  as primary carers 97–8, 126
  psychological distress 99, 195
  stress in 98 (Table 5.2), 103
  see also parents
motivation 171, 202
multi-component interventions 206
  focused on exercise 168–74
  self-management 174–88
Multi-Dimensional Health Locus of
    Control Scale (MHLC) 73–4, 75
multi-disciplinary teams 131
multilinguality, in volunteer staff 153
muscle weakness 71
myths (about arthritis) 16, 101–2,
    113–14, 142, 150, 173

National Ankylosing Spondylitis
    Society 15
*National Arthritis Action Plan: A Public
    Health Strategy* (NAAP) 2
National Arthritis Advisory Board
    (NAAB) 147–8
National Health Service 212
National Institute for Clinical
    Excellence (NICE) 215
National Population Health
    Survey 89
neck 20
negative affect 81, 83, 87, 121, 143
  and PIL 87
negative aspects of arthritis 44
negative thoughts 163
  identification and monitoring 162
Netherlands 12, 41, 117, 124, 136,
    165, 167, 182
neuroendocrine response 35
neuroticism 29, 32, 37
New Zealand 183
non-steroidal anti-inflammatory
    drugs (NSAIDS) 10, 13, 14, 19,
    33, 141, 186, 198

side effects 14
normalising 52–3, 65
normality 64, 65
  sense of 60
North America 7
Norway 137
NSAIDS *see* non-steroidal anti-
    inflammatory drugs (NSAIDS)
nuisance, arthritis as 46
nurse-led and doctor-led care 134–5,
    138–9
nurses 129
  specialist practitioners 131, 134–5,
    138–9, 146, 204
  women as 134
nutrition 202
  see also diet

obesity 9, 144, 150, 218
occupational therapy 1, 3, 146,
    211–12, 218
occupations OA 8–9
older people 188–90, 210
online support groups 167–8, 207
onset (of arthritis)
  personality and 28–32
  stress and 32–7
  see also age, and onset of arthritis
operations 69
ophthalmology clinics 18
oppositional body behaviour 90
optimism 29–30, 31–2, 42, 87, 107, 214
organisational barriers 113–15, 120
orthopaedic care 136, 137
orthopaedic surgery 10, 13
oscillation (between hope and
    despair) 61
Oslo 77
osteoarthritis (OA) 1, 8–10
  age at onset 111
  and ASMP 180–1
  and CBT 162, 168–9

and coping styles 82–3
diet 9
educational interventions for 148,
    186
effects 224
exercise in 142, 145–6
and helplessness 73
hip 20, 101, 130
knee 77, 83, 101, 144, 145, 146, 168,
    183, 220
and obesity 9, 144
occupations and 8–9
and pain management 128–9
and partners 202
patients' needs 152
patients' perceptions 54
personality 28
prevalence 8, 13
risk factors 8–9
self-management behaviour in 202–3
and social support 111
treatment adherence in 141–2, 143,
    145–6
osteopathy 24
osteophytes 9
osteoporosis 15
outcome expectancy 75
outpatients 133–7, 187
    appointments 134
    clinic 50, 186
    satisfaction level in 138–9
over-protectiveness 57, 63, 98

pacing 54
paediatricians 130, 146
pain 9–10, 12, 19, 59, 65, 67, 85
    and AAR 89
    and AS 37
    assessment of 185
    back 28, 31, 201
    biopsychological model of 161
    and CBT 162

children 61, 97, 112
chronic 28–9
coping strategies 30
and depression 42, 70, 72, 73, 82
high and low levels of 79, 82, 84,
    159, 216
intensity of 185
and internalised anger and
    fear 212
and JIA 89, 90, 91, 92
and lack of sleep 103
as major symptom 44–5, 54, 158,
    170, 188
management of 86, 128–9, 139, 169,
    194, 197, 200–1, 202, 211
and negative affect 87
and NSAIDS 198
and parents 94, 104
public perception of 113–14, 120
and RA 41
and relaxation 22–3
relief 138
as risk factor 71
self-efficacy and 76, 79
thresholds 77
tolerance of 77
trigger factors 33
and walking 168
and work disability 116, 119
see also stiffness
pain disability 69, 71, 198
painkillers *see* analgesia
paracetamol 10, 13
parents 101–5, 111–13, 126
    adjustment 96
    'at risk' 95
    avoidance behaviour 96
    behavioural responses 96
    as carers 210
    communication with child 197
    competence of 112
    dysfunctional 93

parents (*cont'd*)
    emotional consequences for 63
    expectations as 102
    helplessness in 154
    importance of role 211–12
    interventions targeting 196–7
    and JIA 34, 38, 57, 61, 130–1, 194, 210
    over-protectiveness 57, 63, 98
    poor adaptation 94
    psychological wellbeing 94
    ratings of children's HRQOL 91
    as recipients of information 149–50,
        154
    see also fathers; mothers
Parent's Arthritis Self-Efficacy Scale
        (PASE) 96
partners
    criticism from 109
    dysfunction in 94
    expectations of 105
    in group programmes 183, 202
    impact of disease on 106
    support from 47, 48–9, 84, 149
partnerships in health care 128–31
passive strategy 80, 81, 84, 85
patient education 134, 146–58, 216
    definitions 147–8
patients
    beliefs of 142, 158
    desire for information 150
    education of *see* patient education
    expectations 138, 142, 146
    as experts 160
    involvement in decision-making
        137–8
    knowledge possessed by 151
    mutual support 133
    non-Caucasian 153
    and providers 128–58
    satisfaction 135, 137–40, 158
    see also inpatients; outpatients
pattern of control beliefs 74
pauciarticular onset 17

peer groups 59–60, 178, 205
peer involvement 60, 61, 64
peer support 94, 113, 204
pension plans 120
perseverance 85
personal development interventions
    188–90, 206
personal independence
        courses 188–90
personality, and onset of arthritis
    28–32
persuasion 79
Perth, Australia 187
pessimism 29–30, 87, 107, 142, 214
phenomenological study 132–3
physical fitness 218
physical functioning 139, 180
    impaired 122
    and social support 108 (Fig. 6.2)
    and work disability 116, 119
physical limitations 85, 90, 114, 119,
    151
physical therapy 3, 10, 112
physicians
    communication with 180
    and patients 129
    women 134
    see also consultations; general
        practitioners
physiotherapy 1, 15, 16, 18, 146, 172–4,
    182
Pima Indians 11
planning, long-term 44
play *see* activities
podiatry 1
polyarthritis, progressive 12
polyarticular JIA 17
population-level data 32
positive affect 81, 86–7, 179
    and PIL 87
positive growth 94
positive mood 56, 73, 74, 87, 114, 155,
    163, 180

positive psychology 100
positive reappraisal 165
postpartum period 102
powerlessness 63
prayer 24
preconceptions, researchers' 133
pre-contemplation, of change 203
pre-diagnostic period 37–8, 42
pregnancy 11, 102, 103
preparation, for change 204
'Preparing for Work' 194
prevalence rates 2
prevention 150, 174, 218
primary care (by GPs) 133–4, 215
Problem-Based Education
    Program 188
problem-focused strategies 80, 81
problem-oriented instrumental
    support 106
problem-solving sessions 178, 202
productivity, loss of 122–3
prognosis 1, 12, 17
proton-pump inhibitors 13
pseudotherapy 22
psoriatic arthritis 1, 14, 211
psychiatric disorders 89
psychiatric morbidity 82
Psychinfo 90
psychodynamic therapy 200
psycho-educational interventions 4,
    54, 79, 146–50, 149 (Table 7.1),
    160–208, 215
  effectiveness 197–205
  group 165
psychological adaptation 91
psychological distress 7, 68–72, 106
  in children 90–2
  and coping strategies 82–3
  in mothers 99, 104
  and pain 79
  risk factors 91
  and social support 126
  and work 119, 122, 123

  see also psychological wellbeing
psychological dysfunction 88
psychological intervention 112, 114, 144
  see also psycho-educational
    intervention
psychological pathology 100, 214
psychological techniques 77
psychological wellbeing 43, 66, 108
    (Fig. 6.2), 201
  and coping strategies 81, 83
  and disease duration 39–41
  and fatigue 46
  in husbands 107
  impact on 122–4
  and information leaflets 155
  and IWPD 191
  and JIA 64, 90, 91, 93, 210
  mediators and moderators 72–86
  positive aspects 86–8
  promotion of 213
  and RA 39, 199
  and self-efficacy 137, 170
  and SMC-AS 171
  in women with RA 105
psychologists 21–2, 218
psychopathology 86, 91, 93
psychosocial adjustment 29–31, 39,
    73, 108
psychosocial care 136, 137
psychosocial rheumatology 3–4, 14,
    43, 66, 75, 92
psychosocial symptomatology 94, 100
psychosocial wellbeing/functioning
  in AS 173
  children's 90–1, 94
  and depression 99
  in JIA 88–9, 90–1, 93, 115, 154, 210
  and play and leisure 113
  in RA 106, 162
  and self-management 174
public health approach 2–3
punishing responses 83
purpose in life (PIL) 87

qualitative and quantitative studies
43, 177–8, 192, 193, 214
quality of life 130, 201, 213
    health-related 89–90, 124

ramps 114
reactive arthritis 14, 89
recall, of ASMP 180
reconstruction of self 55
reflexology 21, 24
Register of Qualified
    Aromatherapists 24
regression analysis 71, 83, 87, 110,
    118, 137
rehabilitation 10
reiki 27
reinterpretation 79, 176–7
Reiter's syndrome 14
relapse prevention 169
relaxation 22, 24, 54, 77, 83, 179, 195,
    200, 216
religion, religious worship 54, 56, 87
remission 11, 12, 17, 44, 52, 85, 92,
    102, 107, 122
remittive agents 33
research wish list 209, 219
resignation 82
respect 178
responders and non-responders
    (in interventions) 204–5
rest 82
    need for 19, 31, 54
restriction, sense of 19
retirement 126, 212
    early 120
retrospective data 30–1
reversal, healing by 21
'rheuma' (as term) 7
rheumatic conditions, classification 7
rheumatoid arthritis (RA) 1, 2, 10–14
    aetiology 11
    age, advancing 119

and CBT 162
educational interventions in 148,
    187
and emotional disclosure 163, 164
and fatigue 121
feet 101
hands 101
and helplessness 73
and information-seeking 153
and joint protection 148
Knowledge Questionnaire 151–2
management of 135
and mental health 101
metaphysical explanations of 20–1
and neuroticism 29
and pain management 128–9
patients' needs 152
personality 21, 38
prevalence 8, 10–11
psychological studies 99
and psychological well-being 66,
    67, 213–14
self-efficacy in 76
self-management behaviour in 203
seronegative 11
and social support 111
treatment adherence in 141
women with *see* women, and RA
and work disability 116, 117, 123,
    124
Rheumatoid Arthritis School 188
rheumatologists, variation in
    practice 136
rheumatology clinics 1–2, 13, 18, 23,
    54, 67, 77, 134, 186
    attendance at 140
    in US 68
rheumatology wards 131–3
rigid thinking 19, 20
risk factors 8–9, 71, 91, 93
    hereditary 102
    for poor adaptation 115

for types of arthritis 150
for work disability 119, 126–7
Rockport Walking Program 169
role-modelling 79, 136, 176, 193
role quality 110

sacroiliitis 15
sadness 168
samples
  recruitment 179, 185, 187, 197, 205
  size 91, 93, 99, 162, 194, 197
satisfaction
  with abilities 85–6, 100
  with life 166, 191, 193
  with social support 179–80
Scandinavia 119, 121
school
  support from 113
  work 60–1
Scleroderma 1, 211
scoring system for disease burden 45
search engines 157, 209
segregation, in education 115
self-advocacy skills 121
self-awareness 54
self-blame 81
self-care 18
  as preventative strategy 174
  as term 174
self-concept, level of 92
self-confidence, loss of 49, 59, 114, 121
self-criticism 19, 20
self-determination 160
self-efficacy 71, 72 (Fig. 5.1), 75–9, 89,
  97, 100, 112, 115, 122, 135–6, 147
  and ASMP 175–6, 179, 182, 183,
    206, 217
  and CBT 162
  in children 196
  and concordance 143, 146
  and empowerment 161
  and exercise 172

expectations 170, 176
  and IWPD 191
  and psychological well-being 137
  in RA 76
  scale to measure change 176
  and Sidewalkers Walking
    Program 168–9, 198
  and SMART programme 185
  and SMC-AS 171
  value of 217
  and Working Horizons 193
self-employment 120, 125
self-esteem 82, 108, 111, 114, 195
  low 47–8, 49, 66, 119, 121, 122, 188
  parents' 96
self-help strategies 168, 215
self-image, negative 88
self-love, lack of 20, 33
self-management 84, 85, 135, 137,
  139, 143, 150
  community-based 175, 185
  in ethnic minority groups 210–11
  health professionals and 218
  lay-led interventions 214
  receipt of information on 137–8
  stages of change in 203–4, 203
    (Table 8.3)
  strategies 53–4, 177, 195, 225
  as term 174
  training 22, 24, 27, 162, 173, 190, 202
Self-Management Arthritis Relief
  Therapy (SMART) 185–6
Self-Management Course for People
  with Ankylosing Spondylitis
  (SMC-AS) 170–2
self-monitoring 170, 194, 204
self-neglect 29
self-regulation 81, 160, 174, 192
self-report questionnaires 71
self-worth
  increased 214
  lack of 19

seronegative spondylarthropathy 14
service provisions, statutory 94
severity, disease 94, 96, 110, 112, 119,
    131, 145, 170, 171, 177, 211
sexual abuse/assault 32–3, 212
shame 20
sharing 55
shattered self 55
shopping 101
shoulders 20
siblings 62, 93, 112, 207
    as carers 112
    rivalry 64
sick leave 116, 119
sickle cell disease 92
Sidewalkers Walking
    Program 168–70
significant others *see* partners
single-site recruitment 91
situational coping 80
Sjogren's syndrome 1, 211
skills mastery 176
sleep 22
    in children 97
    disturbed 37, 47, 66, 71, 92, 103,
        221
    problems 69
smoking 147, 203
    and OA 9
    and RA 11
social cognition models 147
social comparisons 50–1
    downward and upward 178
social exclusion 59, 88, 112, 114
social function 118
social impact (society) 113–15
social interaction 47, 51–2, 109, 113, 188
    negative 166
social network 51–2, 101, 112–13, 205
social support 34, 35–6, 42, 72, 85, 87,
    96, 105–11, 108 (Fig. 6.2), 126,
    150, 160

and exercise adherence 146
interventions 165–8, 206, 207, 218
lack of 20
positive and negative
    effects 108–11
positive and problematic 51–2,
    109–11, 126
satisfaction with 179–80
see also family; friends
social well-being 43, 46, 60
socio-economic status, and RA 11
somatoform disorder 89
South Asians 211
Southwood, T., Young, S. and
    Cheseldine, D. 195
Spanish Arthritis Empowerment
    Programme 183
special needs concept 115
spine 20, 210
spirituality 56, 87–8, 185
splints 10, 13, 17, 61, 140
spondylo-arthropathy 26
spontaneity, lack of 225
sports 47, 61
    therapists 218
spouses *see* partners
state arthritis programmes 3
state health departments 3
stereotypes 31
sthenia 31
stiffness 45, 212
    in AS 37
    beliefs about controlling 74
    in children 58, 59, 60, 90, 97
    and JIA 17, 59, 60, 89
    metaphysical explanations 19, 212
    in OA 9
    and PIL 87
    in RA 12
    and work disability 119
stress 18, 22, 83, 87
    adaptation to 79–80

emotional disclosure and 163
family 93
interpersonal 34–5
life events 94
managing 165, 200, 212, 216
and OA 32
and onset of arthritis 32–7
and RA 11, 12, 28
vulnerability to 101
stress-buffering and direct
 models 107–8, 109, 111, 126
suicide 28
 thoughts of 48
supernormalising 53, 65
support groups 114
surface description 58
Sweden 187, 188
Sydney, Australia 187
symptom identity 82, 151
symptomatology 102, 116, 123
 and impact 44–6
synovial membrane 12
systemic lupus erythematosus 1, 152, 211
systemic onset disease 17
systemic sclerosis 152

teachers 60, 61
technology, support from 113
telephone
 intervention by 157–8
 interviews 169, 181
 support by 186
 see also mobile phones
television 113
tension 163
terminology 92
thoracolumbar activity 15
three blessings exercise 214
toilets, disabled 114
token reinforcement pro-
 grammes 194

transport, access to 114, 120, 121
Transtheoretical Model of
 Change 202–4
trauma 220–1
 childhood psychological 32
 and OA 9
 and RA 11
treatment regimes 113, 119, 122
tricyclics 68

UK 119, 121
ulcerative colitis 14
uncertainty 44, 54, 65, 72, 119, 122, 213
under-researched groups 209–11
understanding, lack of 114, 120, 121
unemployment 69, 117, 122, 123
unmitigated communion 29
unpredictability 119
 of symptoms 85
unprepared action 204
USA
 and ASMP 175, 181, 183–4, 204, 206
 and CDSMC 183–4
 OA in 8
 RA in 11, 12, 117
 websites based in 156–7
 young people with arthritis in 121

valued activities 47, 48, 70, 79, 80, 86, 127, 212, 213
vegan diet 26
victimisation 88
videos 113, 156, 194, 195–6, 207
 children and parents on 130–1
visibility, of disease 59, 97
visual analogue scale (VAS) 201
vitality 90
vocation 60
vocational guidance 121
voluntary organizations 50

volunteer staff 153
vulnerability 120

walking 29, 168–70, 198, 206
wash-out period 198
weather, and OA 9
websites on arthritis 156–7
weight loss 148, 203
weight-management specialists 218
WHO 199
willow bark 26
wishful thinking 81, 109, 165
withdrawal 61
women
    and AS 14, 15, 31
    and CAM 25
    depression in 86
    with high role quality 110
    as 'home-makers' 102
    in information-giving study 158
    and interpersonal stress 34–5
    as members of hospital staff 134
    and OA 9, 29, 83, 87, 209
    older 87
    as patients 134
    as physicians 134
    problems with babies and tod-
        dlers 103
    and RA 11, 28, 29, 31, 48, 55, 70, 81,
        86, 101, 102, 110, 153, 209

and self-efficacy study 79
spiritual experiences of 88
widowed or divorced 105
and work disability 119
see also mothers
work 101, 126
    changes in 49, 123
    dysfunction 77
    flexible hours 124
    and identity 122
    part-time 124–5
    psychologically demanding 118
work disability 12, 115–27, 188, 190,
        207, 212
    definition 116
    masked 118
    prevalence 116–19
    prevention 124–6
    risk factors 119, 126–7
    studies of 117
Working Horizons 193
workspace
    aids in 152
    limitations of 123
World Health Organization 3
written word
    information by 152, 153–6, 208
    release of feelings through 36

yoga 216